the fat switch

the fat switch

Learn what causes obesity and and simple methods to fight it

RICHARD J. JOHNSON, M.D.

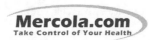

Mercola.com
Take Control of Your Health

The Fat Switch
by Richard J. Johnson, M.D.
Copyright © 2012 by Richard J. Johnson
ISBN 978-0-615-64800-2
Library of Congress Control Number: 2012940330

Disclaimer
Based on discoveries presented in this book, Dr. Johnson and several of his collaborators have
patent applications and patents related to the development of new treatments for obesity and
prediabetes.

Previous books by Dr. Richard J. Johnson:
The Sugar Fix : The High-Fructose Fallout that is Making You Fat and Sick by Richard J.
Johnson with Timothy Gower, 2008, Rodale Press, New York, 304 pp

Printed in the United States of America by Mercola.com   First Edition

Enter these pages to learn why you are getting OBESE and how IT CAN BE REVERSED!

Supporting Obesity Research and Participation
in Clinical Trials

For those individuals who are interested in the research presented in this book or obesity in general, and who would like to learn more about how to support the research programs, please contact the University of Colorado Foundation (www.cufund.org/) and mention either the Colorado Obesity Research Initiative or this specific book. The contact is: Stephanie.Spence@cufund.org

For those individuals who are interested in participating in diet studies or clinical trials involving the new therapies in this book, please contact the Colorado Health and Wellness Center (www.coloradocenter.com). The email contact is info@coloradocenter.com

TABLE OF CONTENTS

CONTENTS

ILLUSTRATIONS

FOREWORD
THE CHALLENGE TO FIND THE CAUSE AND CURE OF OBESITY: THREE VIEWPOINTS

For the General Reader

by Dr. Mercola

mercola.com

It is no mystery that two-thirds of Western cultures suffer from weight control issues and there have been many explanations for this trend. Wouldn't it be nice to have some solid science to explain why this is happening and how you can apply this knowledge to optimize your own health?

It appears the answer to the riddle to the increasing tendency toward weight gain is found in the tension between having enough food for survival and our recent industrial abundance of food. The process of storing fat has not only been a survival strategy for humans for millennia but is something all animals have learned to do to help them survive and prepare for a time when they know food will not be available. This commonly occurs in the winter because they require increased fat stores during periods of food deprivation that is typical during this season.

Survival of the fattest was the key to survival and still is for many animals during certain times of the year. Species that could improve their ability to store fat had the best chance to survive during times of famine. The last century however has brought advances that provide an abundance of food to the bulk of Western cultures. The virtual elimination of starvation and famine threats has caused genes that previously served to extend the survival of the species to actually become detrimental to our health.

By understanding these ancient protective mechanisms and the fact that they are no longer useful for our survival, it is now possible to optimize our biochemistry for weight loss and a far healthier fat composition which can allow us to live longer and healthier lives.

Dr. Johnson provides powerful empirical and anecdotal confirmation of the idea that the recent obesity epidemic is related to the activation of this ancient protective fat switch. He has done many careful experiments in his research lab documenting the switch that is responsible for turning on this protective biochemistry. He has published these findings in some of the most prestigious and well-respected medical and science journals in the world, and he provides an extensive bibliography to these and other studies in *The Fat Switch*. Additionally, his style is easy to read as he seeks to be an impartial and objective observer and not overwhelm you with his view, but merely provide you with the evidence and allow you to be the judge.

History Provides the Clues to Weight Gain

Dr. Johnson has also carefully reviewed the historical literature to provide a solid basis to understand the evolution of obesity over the last few centuries and the historical factors that most likely contributed to it. This provides strong evidence to counter the long standing conventional belief that excess weight was merely related to "over-nutrition" and was simply a matter of rebalancing calories in and calories expended through exercise. This view partially contributed to the vilification of fats as they are twice as dense a source of calories as proteins or carbohydrates.

Most people now realize that the goal in weight management is not to strive for an ideal body weight, but rather an ideal body composition or percentage of body fat. One can weigh far more than ideal, such as a body builder or professional football player, and have a very low body fat and high lean body mass and still be very healthy.

The Fat Switch Responsible for Weight Gain

Dr. Johnson provides a brilliant and detailed explanation of how this ancient fat switch operates and how one can monitor simple blood tests like uric acid to help to effectively control this switch. Interestingly, he found that you could be underweight and have an elevated uric acid level and a remarkable risk for obesity, high blood pressure, and fatty liver and metabolic syndrome.

The major energy currency in your body to fuel most of the reactions in your body is ATP which drives chemical reactions in your cells by donating a high energy phosphate bond. Most of the ATP is produced inside your cells in an organelle called the mitochondria. Interestingly ATP is structurally related to RNA and one of the major breakdown products of nucleic acids is uric acid. When uric acid levels become elevated it has a very potent inhibitory effect on your mitochondria and tends to shut down the production of your body's primary energy source of ATP, and this is one of the reasons why people with increased uric acid levels have noticeably less energy.

So rather than simply being a waste product, uric acid likely has a very powerful biological signaling effect that also tends to influence cellular physiology by increasing insulin and leptin resistance. If you are a starving animal this is actually highly beneficial because it will help you rapidly replace your fat stores. However, if you are overweight, this is not at all useful as it will tend to make you even fatter.

Many of you may realize that humans long ago lost the ability to produce vitamin C which is why it is so important to obtain it from your diet and/or supplements. Interestingly, losing the vitamin C ability also improved our ability to make and store fat. This gave humans a powerful historical survival advantage, but with the advent of pervasive food availability this has actually become a serious contemporary handicap leading to increased levels of obesity and chronic disease.

Along similar lines there is another enzyme that a number of animals lack but humans have and that is called fructokinase. There are genetic disorders in humans in which they actually lack this enzyme and it turns out that these individuals don't become fat. This is powerful confirmation of Dr. Johnson's concept and compelling evidence to support dietary attempts to modify this potent fat causing enzyme.

Read this Fascinating Book to Understand How to Optimize Your Weight

There is solid evidence compiled in this book which documents the powerful influence that gut bacteria has on the fat switch. Additionally, it provides clear details on the destructive influence of sugar and damaging effects it has on intestinal cells that can result in a leaky gut and cause gaps that allow incompletely digested food particles to enter the blood stream and contribute to food allergies and other chronic illness.

Dr. Johnson has carefully analyzed diets and found a number of foods that are potent activators of this switch. If you are very lean or planning on hibernating for a few weeks, then these foods would be useful for you. But the vast majority of the population would be well served by largely avoiding certain foods until they optimized their body composition. *The Fat Switch* provides you with a detailed blueprint to implement this strategy.

This seminal work provides leading edge scientific confirmation that the time honored strategies of eating whole unprocessed foods, exercising and living close to nature, will maximize your genetic potential to live a long and healthy life. It is my belief that the best chance of extending your life beyond the typical 75 years expected life span is to optimize your fat switch and to slow down the aging process.

So if you are interested in optimizing your body composition and are passionate about understanding the solid science that could help you implement an effective strategy to do so then I strongly recommend reading *The Fat Switch*. It is a fascinating book that reads like a detective thriller and will be hard to put down. When you finish this book, you will understand more about the complex mystery of how people become fat.

A Physician's Viewpoint
By Dr. Richard J. Glassock
Emeritus Professor of Medicine
David Geffen School of Medicine at UCLA

Imagery and symbolism play important roles in human communication. In his *magnum opus*, Dr. Richard Johnson, uses these devices to alert the reader to the nature of the process underlying the storage and dissolution of fat. According to Dr. Johnson, the switch from fat storage, and its outward manifestation of obesity, to fat utilization, as a manifestation of starvation, has its origins in evolution, migrations of our early ancestors, climatic changes and mutations of crucial enzymes responsible for uric and ascorbic acid (vitamin C) acid production eons ago. These precursor events, summarized as the origination of the "anti-thrifty genes" that favored survival, by storage of calories as fat in fluctuating periods of feast or famine, have made modern man vulnerable to excesses of contemporary and mostly artificial dietary constituents. These now harmful un-natural "foods," predominantly sucrose (table sugar) and fructose, favor the switch to be more in the ON (fat storage) than the OFF (fat dissolution) position thus encourage the "banking" of calories as fat in fat cells (called adipocytes). Although the fat switch is analogized with the common light switch found on the walls of homes and offices, it is really more like a dimmer (or rheostat) under the ever varying influence of environmental factors and conditions present within the cell (mostly in the vicinity of mitochondria, the energy machines of the cell—symbiotic parasites acquired millions of years ago).

Conventional Wisdom Overturned

This stunning discovery turns the table on the conventional wisdom that fat storage (obesity) is simply an imbalance of energy input and output—too much food, too little exercise. A new paradigm emerges, less ridden with guilt associated with gluttony or sloth and more optimistic for eventual modification of the "epidemic" of obesity and its disastrous complications for society and individuals. Those of us who are obese eat more because of a faulty switch (or dimmer) and exercise less because of a low energy state. The central roles of fructose in the diet (or produced aberrantly by the liver from glucose) and of uric acid in modulating the fat switch (or dimmer) located in the mitochondria (the energy machine of the cell—a parasite obtained millions of years ago) is carefully integrated into the biology of the individual fat cell and the organism as a whole, by a series of inductive reasoning steps. The experimental and observational support for this new paradigm of fat storage and dissolution is enormous, but one should be careful in accepting it as a final truth- the ultimate solution to a long-standing mystery. The 18th century Scottish philosopher, David Hume, cautioned that *truth* cannot ever be reached by recitation of facts derived from observations through inductive reasoning. The 20th century philosopher, Karl Popper, also stated that true science must be falsifiable. Thus, the novel paradigm proposed by Dr. Johnson must withstand experimentation designed to refute the framework underlying the "fat switch hypothesis" before it can be fully accepted as new dogma.

Implications for Control of the Obesity Epidemic

Nevertheless, the concepts elaborated in *The Fat Switch* do generate exciting new vistas for control of the "Black Plague"-like epidemic of obesity that is sweeping the world and causing great concern with diversion of scarce resources into what may well be a controllable disease. Imagine the prospects for universal labeling of processed foods for fructose or sucrose content; contemplate warnings on products containing large amounts of high-fructose corn syrup; envisage new drugs able to safely lower the intra-cellular content of uric acid and/or influence the position of the fat switch; visualize diets embracing natural foodstuffs that promote utilization of energy without fat storage. Pharmaceutical drug development, weight-loss programs, exercise salons, food supplement commerce, clothiers, food addiction psychology and many other fields of endeavor could be dramatically altered. But such elaborate visions mean that the scourge of obesity can be conquered and that Dr. Johnson's book may outline the pathway to success. Perhaps these visions are too grandiose and imaginary, but the arguments posited in *The Fat Switch* are very persuasive and the stakes are too high for them to be ignored. The transforming effect of a world without obesity is almost too enormous to contemplate, but too empowering to be brushed aside.

Insights, Opinion, Guilt Avoidance and Hope—Prospects for the Diligent Reader

The *Fat Switch* is a book worth reading and reading again. For the layperson, the biology may be imposing or even intimidating, but the story is compelling. Darwin would have enjoyed it greatly as an example of his "survival of the fittest" transformed into the "survival of the fattest." Dickens and his Joe the "fat boy" in *The Posthumous Papers of the Pickwick Club* would have obtained greater insight into the condition of "portliness." In sum, *The Fat Switch* will illuminate, alter fixed opinion, abdicate guilt and furnish hope to sufferers of obesity and those who rightly fear it. If followed by explicit action, the prospect for eventual control of the evolution-related scourge of obesity looms large on the horizon.

An Evolutionary Viewpoint
By Dr. Steven Benner
Founder, Foundation of Applied Molecular Evolution

It is now undisputable in biology that we humans are the products of four billion years of Darwinian evolution. It is difficult, however, to find this truism reflected in standard medical practice.

Our Genes Tell Only Part of the Story

On the contrary, the last century of biomedical research has seen the triumph of chemistry over natural history as a source of inspiration in medicine. By the end of that century, researchers had described metabolism at the level of single metabolite molecules, determined the three-dimensional structures of enzyme molecules that catalyze each metabolic step, and built computer simulations of the overall process. The regulation of metabolism, growth and development had been tracked through complex pathways. Many of its defects are now attributed to single changes in specific DNA molecules of individual cells.

As for the DNA, we now almost know it all. At least for a handful of our fellow humans, who have had their genomes sequenced. The sequencing of the human genome was viewed by many to be the "Holy Grail" of genetics, the end of a quest to understand the chemistry at the core of our human biology. For that handful of humans, we can say to high accuracy where every carbon atom, phosphorus atom, oxygen atom, nitrogen atom and hydrogen atom lies in the molecules that they will pass to their children.

And yet, something is missing. First, despite all of the controversy relating to health care in the body politic over the last few years, essentially none of our long-term health is determined by the kind of health insurance that we carry.

Rather, as we approach the three score and ten years biblically allotted to each of us, our individual health is determined largely by how we live. Whether or not we smoke, of course. Whether or not we sensibly exercise, yes. But also, it is now more than clear, how we eat, what we eat, and how much we eat determines how often we will visit our doctor and why we will visit them.

Again, the problem has been dissected at the molecular level. After a battery of tests, we will know from our doctor how much cholesterol, glucose, fats, urea nitrogen, well, you name it, is found in an ounce of our blood. Some of these are good. Some are bad. And not just cholesterol. Without glucose in the blood, we die.

So which is it? Good or bad? And why is it? For all of the deconstruction of human biology to its underlying chemistry, and for all of the efforts by systems' biologists to put it back together within computer models of the "system," chemistry is unable to answer the *"Why?"* questions.

This sentiment lay in part behind the exclamation of Carl Woese, that the "strange claim by some of the world's leading molecular biologists that the human genome is the "Holy Grail" of biology is a stunning example of a biology that has no genuine guiding vision." Curiously, Woese is a chemist. In the 1960s, he deconstructed the chemistry of RNA molecules to recognize that life on earth forms from not one or two, but rather three kingdoms that reflect convergence of life longer than three billion years old. Perhaps it takes a chemist to recognize the deficiencies of chemistry in its description of biology.

The Importance of Natural History in Understanding Medicine Today

And, perhaps, it takes a physician to restore natural history as a key element of medicine. Rick Johnson is a physician who has spent much of his professional life focusing on the kidney. However, that focus has not prevented him from offering a guiding vision for medicine. This book lays out a convincing demonstration that natural history *does* matter in medicine. My medicine. Your medicine.

Forty million years ago, in the Eocene, the earth was tropically warm across most of its landmass. Flowering and fruiting trees with their uplifting branches had replaced the conifers and ferns of the Jurassic. These invited our primate ancestors and the surviving dinosaurs (now called "birds") to dwell above the forest floor, take shelter in their arboreal third dimension, and to feed on their succulent fruits. With no ice at sea level anywhere near, and with winter no more severe than winter in Florida across most continents, the warm earth was (in Dan Prothero's characterization), a Garden of Eden.

But the accidents of continental drift did not let it remain so. Antarctica drifted away from South America. The Drake Passage opened, allowing a new ocean current to flow around the Antarctic continent, isolating it from currents that brought heat from the equator to the South Pole. Antarctica frosted over. While the details are not entirely clear, the white Antarctic continent apparently reflected energy from the sun, leading to further cooling of the earth. The great savannas of grassland opened across swaths of the major continents. The accidents of continental drift also formed Panama a few million years later. That land bridge joined North America and South America, and separated two large oceans on earth, the Pacific and the Atlantic, the first such separation in a billion years.

Although paleoclimatologists do not know enough to model the physics of the earth with any predictive accuracy, it appears that such events set in motion the climate catastrophe known as the Ice Ages. Glaciers advanced as far as New York City and then retreated, again and again, with the global temperature fluctuating wildly. Pity our poor primate ancestors. In an event that was biblical in its import, we were thrown out of the Eocene Eden into a Pleistocene Purgatory. One millennium, we could be enjoying the nectar from a tropical tree. The next could see us swinging for our lives to the south to find trees that survive global cooling. And so we humans learned to run and hunt. But even that was not sufficient for an earth where climate change was the norm. One week, we could be feasting off the fat of a mammoth that our tribe had slain. A month later, we could be near starvation.

The climatic oscillations of the Ice Age occurred too fast for natural Darwinian processes to "keep up." Climate change provides advantage for the right kinds of mutants, of course. But with glaciers coming and going on the millennium timescale, Darwinian evolution never had time to catch up; it could not deliver optimality. At most, a species selects for adaptability. Of course, human culture provides precisely that. Today, we adapt to changing conditions not by bearing mutant children, but rather by creating new

instruments, clothes, and shelters that we pass to our children, not genetically, but by education.

Civilization, Culture and Modern Adaptation to Change

Until lately, cultural adaptation has been a weak tool to adapt to changing
conditions. Therefore, the human genome adapted to manage the privation
that comes with change, storing fat in the good times to be prepared for the
lean times. By building into our instincts certain cravings for specific kinds
of nourishments that we might soon lose access to. By creating cultural
norms that value, among other things, obesity.

Then, as Rick points out, came advanced civilization. Civilization is
superimposed upon our genetic inheritance that prepares us for paucity as
well as gives us our attraction to salt and sweets. Since the Industrial
Revolution, we have had the opportunity to use civilization to indulge our
cravings. But without the famine that goes with them.

In our escape from our natural history, Rick finds the roots of many of the
diseases of the modern world. Obesity, hypertension, and diabetes are
among these. But Rick does not stop there. He makes the connection from
these natural historical insights back to the centuries-old tradition of chemistry in medicine. He identifies some of the molecules (uric acid, fructose,
vitamin C) whose metabolism has changed with the changing environment.
He proposes chemical mechanisms for the signals to allow organisms to
respond and how they lead to the epidemic diseases in the modern world.

A great read.

PREFACE
In Search of the Thrifty Gene

The evolutionary biologist, Jared Diamond, has reviewed the sad story of how diabetes entered the country of Nauru,[1] and it is such a powerful story that it is worth retelling. The remote island of Nauru lies in the Pacific Ocean and is one of the tiniest countries in the world. Separated from other islands by hundreds of miles, it was not colonized until hundreds of years ago when people of Micronesian descent reached the island by boat. A small island of only 7.7 square miles (20 square kilometers), the people survived on fish, breadfruit, coconuts, beach almond, paw paw, and the Noddy bird. The sparse life resulted in the people suffering intermittent starvation. The island was insulated from the world until the early 1800s, when Europeans first visited its shores. Initially the European presence was minor, but a major transition began in 1906 when rich phosphate rock was discovered on the island. By 1922 a large company began mining, providing royalties to the Nauruan landowners. The Nauruans suddenly became wealthy, and would buy the western foods brought in by the ships. One of the favorite foods was sugar, and by 1927 the average intake of sugar was reported to be a pound per day.[1]

For the Nauruans, who had suffered from intermittent famine, obesity had always been viewed as desirable. It was a custom to fatten women to make them more attractive. With the onset of new wealth, however, obesity increased to levels never before observed, and diabetes appeared for the first time. The first case of diabetes was reported in 1925, and the second case in 1934. During World War II the island fell under control of the Japanese, and consumption of sugar fell—many of the native people were sent to the island of Truk where they had limited food supplies and even starved. Following the war, however, the Nauruans returned and by 1968 were collecting royalties amounting to $37,500 dollars per year per person, and with this they resumed their love of sugar and western foods. As they became rich, they hired laborers to work in the mines and they became progressively sedentary.

Cars were brought in so the people could drive for even the shortest distances on the small island. Obesity and diabetes soared. Even today, with the exhaustion of the phosphate mines and a much more shaky economy, the Nauruans maintain the honor of being the most obese people in the world, with over 90 percent of the adult population overweight or obese, and with more than one-third with diabetes.

Unfortunately, the story of Nauru is not new in history. Dramatic increases in obesity and diabetes have been seen with the introduction of western culture time and time again. Examples include the Native American Indians, the Maori of New Zealand, and the Australian Aborigines. It is also not peculiar to indigenous peoples. Today obesity is occurring in all peoples, especially among the young. It does not matter whether you live in Tibet, Mongolia, or the Amazon. Wherever western culture is being introduced, obesity and diabetes are increasing.

In 1961, the anthropologist, James Neel, suggested that the rise in obesity and diabetes observed throughout the world today was due to the presence of "thrifty genes" that we acquired in our past. According to this theory, survival for early humans focused on having sufficient food stores to survive periods of famine. While the storage of food would be helpful, another way would be if the individual could increase their own fat stores. Neel suggested that during these periods of famine, those individuals who carried genes that would favor the greatest accumulation of fat would be more likely to survive, and these genes would then be passed on to subsequent generations. Over time the population would be enriched with these "thrifty genes" that would maximize survival during famine. However, when food would suddenly become plentiful, the beneficial effects of these thrifty genes would have an opposing, negative effect, and that would be to increase the risk for obesity and diabetes.[2-3]

The search for the thrifty genes has remained elusive for more than 50 years, and some have even doubted their existence. Today many authorities view the problem of obesity as simple. We are eating too much and exercising too little. As such, many books on obesity emphasize the controlling of behavior as the key to treating obesity, emphasizing wise food selection, avoidance of excessive television and developing daily exercise routines.

Others concentrate on the psychological issues, such as breaking the dependency on foods, dealing with the guilt of food bingeing, and simply speaking, how to deal with the desire for foods, especially those rich in calories and poor in nutrition. Still other books focus on obesity as a disease associated with a wide host of health problems from fatty liver to high blood pressure and heart disease. Treatment plans abound, ranging from regimented programs with calorie counting, exercise and behavioral modification, to quick solutions involving fad diets, herbal remedies, and even laxatives and enemas. Unfortunately, none of these approaches are satisfactory, as obesity and diabetes continue to be rampant. It seems like something is missing, and we still do not know how to stop this epidemic.

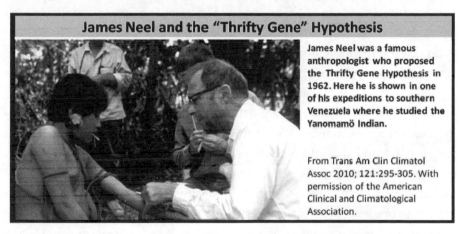

James Neel and the "Thrifty Gene" Hypothesis

James Neel was a famous anthropologist who proposed the Thrifty Gene Hypothesis in 1962. Here he is shown in one of his expeditions to southern Venezuela where he studied the Yanomamö Indian.

From Trans Am Clin Climatol Assoc 2010; 121:295-305. With permission of the American Clinical and Climatological Association.

In this book, we revisit Neel's hypothesis and the world of evolutionary biology. We show that the process of storing fat and becoming insulin resistant is not peculiar to humans, but something all animals have learned to do to help them survive. More importantly, most animals have developed ways to become obese like clockwork, often to prepare them for a period of time when they know food will not be available. Mammals and reptiles become fat prior to hibernation in winter, the lungfish becomes fat before burrowing in the mud to survive the droughts of summer, the whale gets fat prior to leaving the Arctic to mate in Baja, and many birds get fat prior to long distance migration. Even insects get fat prior to becoming a pupa and making a cocoon. Many of these animals not only become fat, but also become insulin resistant. However, the major difference between obesity among these animals and humans is that for animals in the wild, the obesity is temporary and highly regulated, and weight returns to normal once the migration is completed or the winter has subsided. In contrast, humans are getting fatter and fatter, in an apparently unregulated, out of the control way. Why is this happening?

Our approach to solving this paradox was to study how animals turn on and off their fat, and in so doing, we discovered that the animals use a biochemical "switch" to make this happen. This "fat switch" occurs in the energy factories of the cell known as mitochondria, and when this switch is turned on, the animals preferentially shunt energy from food into fat. In turn, the relative reduction in energy produced acts as a stimulus to the brain to encourage the animal to eat more. The relatively lower production of energy also makes a person prefer to be sedentary. In effect, when the switch is turned on, the individual will eat more than they need, exercise less, and store more fat. A corollary of this is that those in which the fat switch is turned on are not eating more because the custom of our culture is to give larger helpings, but rather we are demanding bigger helpings since we have lost control of our appetite. We are not exercising less because the TV shows are so good and the internet irresistible, but rather because we have less energy to exercise. This does not detract from the effects of advertisements and cultural practices to stimulate the obesity movement, but the primary problem appears to be a biological change in us rather than our culture. In other words, western culture is responding to our body needs from activating the switch, and not the reverse.

Storing fat is regulated and is turned on like a switch.

By identifying a fat switch that can convert animals from lean to obese and vice versa, we were able to determine how animals have altered their genes to maximize their ability to become fat. Perhaps more importantly, the discovery of the fat switch allowed us to develop a strong argument for how the switch is being activated in humans and the underlying reasons we are so susceptible to becoming obese. In this book we will show that the primary means for activating this pathway is from the intake of sugar, and to a lesser extent from other foods such as beer. Our susceptibility to becoming obese with these foods is due to both the nature of how the foods activate the switch, as well as specific mutations that we acquired during periods of famine in our past that make us sensitive to the effects of these foods to increase fat. One of the more important mutations resulted in an increase in our blood level of uric acid. While a well known consequence of a high uric acid level is a type of arthritis known as gout, uric acid may also have an important role in causing high blood pressure and amplifies the effects of sugar to stimulate fat accumulation.

> *Many of us have unwittingly activated the "fat switch" to become obese.*

The knowledge of why obesity is occurring provides new insights into the prevention and treatment of obesity and its complications. Animals have already learned how to turn on the switch to become fat, and how to turn off the switch to become lean. Based on new studies, we propose a variety of treatments that should reverse this switch. While it has often been said that obesity can be treated but never cured, our studies strongly suggest this is not true. Indeed, cures are just around the corner. We will discuss these novel therapies, that are only a few years from the clinic, and which carry a high chance for curing obesity and bringing health back once more.

PROLOGUE
THE GREATEST EPIDEMIC IN HISTORY

Most epidemics are due to infections that spread through the population, causing death in days to weeks. The greatest epidemic, however, is not due to infection, kills over decades and is right in our midst. Look in the mirror, as there is a good chance you are already "infected."

Epidemics frighten the public and humble physicians. Consider AIDS, which was unknown until 30 years ago. In April 1981 Sandra Ford, a technician working for the Centers for Disease Control (CDC) in Atlanta, noted an unusual number of requests by physicians for pentamidine. Pentamidine was an "orphan" drug used to treat pneumocystis infection, a rare type of pneumonia that typically affected patients whose immune system was weakened, such as in people who were being treated for cancer or who had received a kidney transplant. However, in the cases for which the pentamidine had been requested, the individuals were young men that had been previously healthy. Ford became concerned and alerted her superiors, leading to an investigation by the CDC that resulted in the recognition of the new disease.

AIDS is due to two different viruses, known as HIV1 and HIV2. Molecular biologists have shown that HIV1 originated from the chimpanzee and that it entered into human population in central Africa, likely in the 1920s. The first confirmed case was identified from historical samples in the Congo in 1959. HIV2 also originated from a primate, the sooty mangabee. It arose in western Africa where it was probably introduced into humans in the 1940s. The first documented case of HIV2 infection occurred in Guinea-Bissau in 1966. Early on HIV1 spread to Haiti, largely because many Haitians worked in Central Africa. HIV1 also spread to most of the larger cities in the world, and also to central and sub-Saharan Africa. Today 33 million individuals are infected with HIV, with 20 percent of infected adults living in sub-Saharan Africa.

Initially AIDS was fatal, with most dying 7 to 10 years after being infected with the virus. With newer anti-viral therapies, survival has increased to 20 years or more, although treatment is life-long and expensive (amounting to > $600,000 dollars per lifetime). Unfortunately, only a minority of people who need antiviral therapy are receiving it. Today over 25 million people have died from the infection, and the epidemic is not over.

The Spanish Flu Epidemic of 1918

While the AIDS epidemic wins awards for being one of the worst epidemics of all time, there was another epidemic earlier in the twentieth century that was also devastating. While it is commonly referred to as the Spanish Flu Pandemic of 1918, its roots likely began in a rural community in southwestern Kansas.[4] Haskell county, with a population of less than 2000 people for its 578 square mile area, was a farming community known for raising cattle, hogs, chickens and grain. Very little excitement occurred in this quiet county—that is, until January 1918 when a local physician, Dr. Loring Miner, began to see patients with a particularly severe form of influenza. Symptoms included high fever, chills, headache, and cough, often with severe fatigue. A curious blue-lavender color (termed cyanosis) of the lips and extremities would develop, with violent coughing of frothy pink material, and several patients died. Dr. Miner recognized that he was dealing with an outbreak, and he alerted national public health experts.

Soldiers stationed in local Fort Riley became infected and were likely responsible for taking the infection to France as part of the American deployment effort of World War I. Infection spread rapidly in Europe and then throughout the world, including Asia, Africa, and even the Arctic. Most deaths occurred between September and December of 1918. By the end of the pandemic, between 3 and 6 percent of the world population had died, amounting to 40 to 50 million individuals. Compare this with the total number of soldiers and civilians who died in World War I, which amounted to 16 million.

The Black Plague

While both AIDS and the Spanish Flu Pandemic of 1918 were major epidemics of the last 100 years, few epidemics were more terrorizing or more fatal than the Black Plague. The Black Plague is caused by the bacteria *Yersina pestis*, which is carried by fleas. Originally, this infection was limited to certain regions of central Asia, such as around Lake Issyk-kul near the Tien Shan mountain range which separates China from the great Russian steppes. Here it was endemic in the local bobak marmot.

Sometime during the early 14th century the infection spread to humans. Lake Issyk-kul was a favorite stopping place on the Silk Road, a major trading route that connected Europe with China. While the marmot was not a regular food, during periods of famine the marmot became an important food source. Infected fleas from the marmots may have directly infected humans, and then also spread to the black rat (*Rattus rattus*), that would travel with the caravans.

Individuals infected with the plague developed painful swelling of the lymph nodes in the groin, armpit, and neck that could rapidly increase in size, sometimes to the size of a chicken egg before rupturing. High fevers accompanied the swellings, and the subject would lie in bed, devoid of energy, often with the spontaneous development of bluish bruises over the body. Death usually occurred within one week, although rare persons survived.

Large numbers of deaths from the plague were first noted in the Lake Issyk-kul region in 1336. By 1347, the first cases in Constantinople (now Istanbul) were reported. Rapidly the infection spread, sweeping Europe between 1347 and 1349, where it killed more than one third of the population. Some cities, such as Venice and Paris, lost more than half of their inhabitants. The plague also spread across China and India. By 1350, the pandemic had subsided, leaving 45 million people dead, with 20 million from Europe and 25 million from China and India.

The Greatest Epidemic of All

The Black Plague could be considered the worst pandemic of all time when one factors the rapidity of the illness and the percentage of the population that died. Similar to AIDS and the Spanish Flu, each epidemic led to between 20 and 45 million deaths, which could occur in days (Black Plague), days to weeks (Spanish Flu) or years to decades (HIV). The impact of these pandemics has been immense.

In *The Fat Switch* we discuss another pandemic, one that has progressed more slowly, but with a higher toll, causing the death of more than 100 million individuals. While not caused by an infectious agent, it nevertheless is spreading uncontrollably throughout the world.

Great Pandemics of History			
	Black Death	**1918 Flu**	**AIDS**	**Obesity**
Origin	Asia	USA	Africa	England
Duration	Days	Weeks	Years	Decades
Source	Bacteria	Virus	Virus	Diet
Cause of Death	Sepsis	Pneumonia	Infection	Heart Disease
Deaths (millions)	45	40	25	>100

The epidemic of obesity is largely considered to have been active for only 30 or 40 years. However, we will show that its roots lie earlier, beginning sometime in 17th century England and Holland. Before this period obesity was rare, present in less than 5 percent of the adult population. Today over 1 billion people in the world are overweight, of which 300 million people are obese.[5] Two-thirds of the United States population are overweight or obese.[6-7] The highest frequencies of obesity are from countries in the Pacific islands and Persian Gulf, but the United States is not far behind. In the Pacific Island of Nauru, 94 percent of the population are overweight or obese.

> *Obesity has taken more lives than all previous epidemics. Unlike epidemics that kill in days (Black Death), weeks (influenza), or years (AIDs), obesity kills over decades.*

While some view obesity not as a disease but as a condition, it nevertheless carries an increased risk for mortality which has been known since the early 1900s from data provided by life insurance companies.[8] Obesity increases the risk for mortality in 50-year-old people by two- to threefold.[9] Obesity also increases the risk for other diseases, such as type 2 diabetes, high blood pressure, fatty liver disease, stroke, and heart disease. Obesity is also associated with increased risk for cancers, including breast, colon, prostate, endometrial, kidney and gall bladder cancer.

Prevalence of Overweight and Obesity in the World	
Persian Gulf (Kuwait, Qatar, Dubai, Saudi Arabia)	61-74%
USA	66-70%
Mexico	68%
Europe (UK, Germany)	60-64%
South America (Argentina, Chile, Venezuela, Peru)	60-69%
South Africa	50%
North Africa	30-50%
India	30-35%
China	20-25%
Central Africa	10-20%

While deaths directly attributable to obesity are about 300,000 per year, when one considers the role of obesity in these other diseases, the mortality escalates. Today there are 220 million people with diabetes worldwide, and in 2005 alone over 1 million of these people died from complications related to this disease. Hypertension is largely driven by obesity and is the primary cause of congestive heart failure and stroke. High blood pressure and diabetes also make up the two most common causes of chronic kidney disease.

Obesity is costly. In the United States approximately 100 billion dollars is spent per year on obesity.[10-11] When one considers the role of obesity in other conditions, and calculates both the direct health care costs and the costs from loss of productivity, then the costs escalate. In the United States alone the total direct and indirect costs for heart disease is 170 billion, for hypertension is 312 billion, for type 2 diabetes is 132 billion, for stroke is 36 billion, and for chronic kidney disease over 16 billion.[12]

The obesity epidemic is killing millions of people. Ironically its current furor is countered by a prior time in history in which obesity was associated with a greater chance for survival. As discussed in the Preface, the anthropologist James Neel proposed there were "thrifty genes" that humans acquired to help them survive famine in the past but which now predispose to diabetes today.[3] Neel, however, did not know what genes these were or how they acted to cause this epidemic. In this book we present an explanation of how genes and environment have sadly interfaced to cause the rampant rise of the great killers of today: diabetes and heart disease.

Section 1
Why Obesity was Once Good

chapter 1

Survival of the Fattest

This principle of preservation, or survival of the fittest, I have called Natural Selection.[1]
—Charles Darwin, *Origin of the Species,* 1859

What does the word "survival" make you think about? How you have "survived" a boring lecture, a terrible traffic jam, or another day at work? Or perhaps "survival" makes you think of young, healthy and good looking individuals romping on the beach in swim suits playing games of elimination for the television masses? At least for most of us, we are not thinking day to day of our personal survival. Yet, this is not true for most species living in this world, where life follows the principles laid out by Charles Darwin more than one hundred years ago. For most animals, every day provides major challenges as they try to find enough food to survive and at the same time to evade predators that would feast on them.

There are incredible examples of survival. Primitive bacteria-like organisms called *Archaea* can live in thermal vents in the ocean floor or in steaming hot geysers. The *Pompeii worm*, which got its name from the famous Italian town buried by the volcano, can live at temperatures close to boiling (176 degrees Fahrenheit). In contrast, ice crawlers (*Grylloblattidae*)

1

are wingless insects that live in Siberia where they scavenge organic material off glaciers. The simple wood frog (*Rana sylvatica*) is one of the most interesting animals. Every year when winter comes, it freezes like a rock in the ice, only to reemerge in the spring. Animals that survive extreme conditions are called extremophiles. Extremophiles are interesting, for there is something about surviving extreme conditions that is attractive.

While it is fun to think about how animals survive in extreme environments, an overarching fundamental principle in survival is to develop ways to protect against famine. To do so, all species have developed means for storing energy to protect themselves during periods of food shortage or starvation. For animals, the principal form of energy stored is fat, which is converted to energy if there is not enough food provided in the diet. All animals have learned how to store fat, whether it is a hibernating bear, a whale, a migrating bird, or even an insect preparing for metamorphosis into a pupa. Being able to increase fat stores is critical for survival. Indeed, the more fat you can store, the longer you can survive during famine. Fat rats, for example, live much longer than lean rats when they are starved. Thus, while Darwin emphasized the principle of the survival of the fittest, there is an equally important concept of *survival of the fattest*.

Obesity and the Emperor Penguin

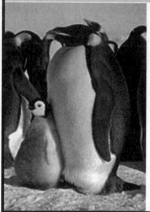

The male Emperor Penguin doubles its body fat during the Antarctic summer by eating squid and fish. It then marches inland where it will incubate the egg laid by its mate until it hatches. During this time the penguin may survive without food for as long as 4 months. Shown here is a an Emperor Penguin and its chick, both getting fat in preparation for the winter.
Photo by Guillaume Dargaud with copyright permission

One of the most interesting aspects is that the process of storing fat to protect oneself from subsequent famines is often scheduled. The 13-lined ground squirrel routinely doubles its fat content in late summer in preparation for hibernation during winter. The Emperor penguin also doubles its weight in fat prior to protecting and warming its eggs during the fierce Antarctic winter. The bar-tailed godwit markedly increases its fat in its liver and blood prior to migrating thousands of miles to its winter home. The grey whale increases its fat in the Arctic, and then fasts during its long distance migration to Baja California. For all of these animals, the periods of weight gain (fat accumulation) and weight loss (fat burning) occurs regularly and predictably.

An extremely important aspect is that the increase in fat that many animals undergo is *not only scheduled, but also tightly regulated*. This has been shown by several investigators, most notably by Richard Keesey.[2-3] Specifically, Keesey and his colleagues have shown that animals maintain their weight within a half percent, with little deviation. Indeed, if you force-feed a rat to induce it to gain weight, the increase in weight will not be sustained. Rather, after the force feeding is stopped, the rat will rapidly lose its weight and go back to its regular weight. Similarly, if a rat is starved for a period of time, it will also regain its weight after it is provided food. Interestingly, in both cases the rat doesn't go back to the original weight, but rather to the weight it would have been had it not been force fed or fasted. In other words, the rat is able to go to its trajected weight for its age and the time of year!

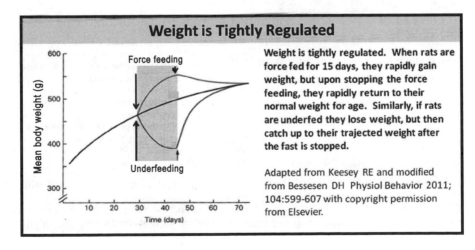

Weight is Tightly Regulated

Weight is tightly regulated. When rats are force fed for 15 days, they rapidly gain weight, but upon stopping the force feeding, they rapidly return to their normal weight for age. Similarly, if rats are underfed they lose weight, but then catch up to their trajected weight after the fast is stopped.

Adapted from Keesey RE and modified from Bessesen DH Physiol Behavior 2011; 104:599-607 with copyright permission from Elsevier.

The same has been shown for hibernating animals or birds preparing for long distance migration. For example the garden warbler, which migrates each winter, will normally become fat during the summer and late fall in preparation for its long flight. If it has fasted during the period normally associated with fat storage, the bird will lose weight. However, as soon as the fast is lifted, the bird will rapidly gain fat back to its projected weight in preparation for its long flight.[4] This same phenomenon has also been shown for hibernating mammals, including hibernating ground squirrels and woodchucks.[5]

> *Obesity by Design. Most wild animals have learned to become obese by design; they store fat in their fat tissues, liver and blood in preparation for periods of fat storage. This process is programmed and tightly regulated.*

Perhaps more interestingly, animals that have shifted into a fasting mode often reject food even if it is available.[5] For example, the red junglefowl is a type of hen that becomes fat prior to nesting, and then sits on its nest for 20 days during which time it leaves the nest no more than 20 minutes per day, taking in a minimal amount of food. During the nesting period the bird will lose 10 to 20 percent of its weight. However, if food is placed next to the nest so that it can both nest and eat at the same time, it will not significantly increase its food intake.[5] In other words, the hen is following a set internal program that involves specific periods of weight gain and loss.

This loss of appetite even when food is available can also be observed in hibernating mammals. When animals hibernate, they quit eating and go into a deep sleep (torpor) in which their body temperature falls and their overall metabolism slows down. During this time, these animals break down fat into energy which is then used to help run the normal body functions. By slowing their metabolism, they can minimize the energy required to maintain key body functions, such as the energy required for breathing and maintaining circulation. This way the animal can survive for a long time without food.

The interesting aspect of hibernation is that these animals often will quit eating and start to drop their metabolic rate BEFORE they actually go to sleep and drop their body temperature.[5-8] This means that something in the body is "triggered" to alert the animal that it is time to switch from fat accumulation to fat utilization, and the process can literally occur overnight.

> *The Reverse is also True. Animals will switch from a fat accumulating phase to a fat burning phase on demand. This process is also tightly regulated.*

So it is as if all animals have "set points" for their weight, and they can adjust these set points depending on changes in food availability. Under most circumstances the animals know ahead of time when they need to store fat, such as in preparation for winter, for nesting, or for migrating long distances. For insects, the larvae accumulate fat in their "fat bodies" prior to turning into a pupa where they live in cocoons without any food or liquid. Under some circumstances, however, the triggering for fat accumulation may not be based on scheduled times. For example, a sudden change in climate can alert insects such as mosquitoes to go into "diapause" in which they suddenly accumulate fat in preparation for some adverse change in weather or conditions.[9] These survival mechanisms are inherent to all species. Indeed, even plants have developed means for storing nutrients to survive long winters.

If weight is so tightly regulated, then what happened to us? Why has obesity skyrocketed throughout the world? Why are our pets also getting fat? And if the storage of fat is good, then why are we seeing obese people dying early with such severe conditions as fatty liver, diabetes, high blood pressure and kidney disease?

> *If weight is so tightly regulated, then what has happened to us? Why are over two thirds of our population overweight or obese?*

CHAPTER 2

THE BENEFITS OF BEING FAT

Becoming fat is a key survival strategy that all animals have learned to help them live through periods of food shortage. Depending on the species, different strategies are used.

When I was a boy my mother read to me the story of the Grasshopper and the Ant from Aesop's Fables. All summer long the grasshopper would sing, dance and play, while the ants would be scurrying around to bring food to their nest. The grasshopper would laugh at the ants while they worked, jesting at them for not having fun and enjoying the summer. But when the first frost came and the ants retreated to their home with plenty of food stored for the winter, the grasshopper was left on his own with nothing to eat, and though much bigger and stronger, succumbed with the onset of winter.

Being prepared can be a very good thing, especially when it comes to having food to eat. Animals (even the grasshopper) know this, and will purposely get fat, often in a scheduled and highly regulated way. As we will show in the next few chapters, gaining weight is NOT simply eating more, and losing weight is not simply about eating less. If it were that simple, then it would be easy to cure someone with obesity. Rather, animals activate a "switch" in their metabolism that allows them to gain weight, and then they turn off this switch when they want to lose weight. Obese humans, however, have turned on the fat switch and if it's stuck in the "on" position it will lead to development of diabetes.

In order to understand how this switch works, and why many humans have been caught with the lights stuck on, I think it is important to review a few aspects about obesity in animals.

Where do Animals Put on Fat?

Where you store fat can be important. Most animals store fat similar to humans, collecting it in specific fat cells (adipocytes) that are present in the subcutaneous regions of the skin and in the abdomen. Animals, especially birds, also store much fat in their liver. The hummingbird drinks so much nectar throughout the day that its liver will become creamy white from fat by evening.[10] Many animals also store fat in their blood in the form of triglycerides. The serum from the Minke whale, for example, will be cloudy from fat during the feeding season.[11] This pattern of visceral fat, fatty liver and elevated triglycerides is similar to what is seen in obese humans.

Other animals have unusual places they store fat that may have special benefits. Take the water holding desert frog (*Cyclorana platycephalus*), for example, which lives in the Great Sandy Desert of Western Australia. It is well known for its ability to retain large amounts of water which it uses for survival during droughts. However, it also stores fat in the pads in its feet, and these pads can become fat-laden and large during periods where food such as insects are plentiful; indeed, the overall fat pads can become so large that they amount up to one-fifth of the total weight of the frog. It is a perfect place to store fat, as storing the fat here might actually help insulate the frog from the hot sands whereas putting it in the subcutaneous areas might interfere with breathing (as the frog breathes in part through its skin). When a drought occurs, the frog burrows into the sand and uses its water and fat stores to survive. In addition, it drops its heart rate and respirations, resulting in a decrease in its energy needs. When a frog does this, it may survive for *years* without food. However, this depends on the overall fat stores. For example, only 10 percent of frogs can survive a five-year drought, and this only occurs with the fattest, the ones that stored 20 percent of their weight in their fat pads. The other 90 percent would die over this period of time.[12] For this frog, having fat feet is critical for survival.

Lizards store fat in their tails. It is a convenient site, for they can drag their fat around without having to carry it, and they can also use it to help their balance if they sit up on their hindlegs, cantilevering them which helps to defend or frighten predators. The importance of balance may also help explain why the kangaroo preferentially stores fat in its tail.[13] Other animals such as horses store fat in their neck ("cresty neck"), possibly because too much in the abdomen might interfere with its ability to run. The whale puts some of its fat in its subcutaneous blubber to help insulate it from the cold Arctic sea. Fat also helps whales communicate, as a fat pad between the mandible and middle ear is used to amplify sound waves, as they lack an external ear. The male gorilla, while storing fat much like humans, also puts a little of his fat in a "cap" on the top of his head, the latter which may act to attract a mate.[13]

As with most animals, humans preferentially store fat in specialized fat cells (adipocytes) in their subcutaneous and abdominal areas. However, humans also can develop fatty liver and elevated serum triglycerides just like most other animals. There are some significant differences in fat distribution in men and women. For example, women store relatively more fat in their upper legs and buttocks. In some ethnic groups, such as the San (Bushmen) and Khoikhoi (Hottenot) people in southern Africa, accumulation of fat in the buttocks can be marked, resulting in a condition called steatopygy. There is some evidence that steatopygy represented a sign of beauty for these groups, as well as a source of fat stores for periods of food shortage.[13-14] Finally, for those who like trivia, one difference between men and women is that the latter have fat around their Achilles heels.[13] However, it is usually not necessary to use this information to help determine the sex of an individual!

How Much Fat is Important: Bigger is better!

The amount of fat that you can store can make a big difference. Salmon, for example, quit eating when they migrate from the ocean to the fresh water streams to spawn. During the migration, they survive on their fat, and may lose up to 60-80 percent of their fat en route to their spawning site.[15] The more fat they have, the longer they can migrate, with some sockeye salmon traveling as much as 1300 km up the Fraser River in British Columbia.[16] If the fat stores become depleted, the fish will die.

Some animals can store an enormous amount of fat based on their weight. Small mammals such as the desert gerbil (*Psammomys obesus*) and the tenrec (the Madagascar hedgehog) can become incredibly fat; the western jumping mouse, for example, can gain so much fat that it accounts for 80 percent of its dry weight.[17]

Nevertheless, an important principle that has been known for a long time is that the larger an animal is, the more fat it can store relative to its energy needs.[18] This is because energy needs relate more to the body surface area whereas energy stores relate more to body volume, and as we increase in size, the body volume increases more than the surface area. It was for this reason that German scientist Christian Bergmann proposed in 1847 that species become larger as latitude increases.[19] This is because as the climate gets cooler with longer winters, the need for increased fat stores becomes evident.[20] This rule is thought to be the reason that the largest penguins, such as the Emperor Penguin which can achieve a weight of 75 pounds, lives in the Antarctic whereas the Galapagos penguin which lives at the equator is much smaller (weight of 4 to 5 pounds). It also explains why fasting elephant seals that weigh 3000 pounds can fast 60 days, whereas harbor seals that weigh 220 pounds only last 19 days.[21] Whales are the largest mammals in the world and have enormous fat stores. The Gray Whale ingests as much a one ton of shell-less, shrimp-like crustaceans a day (called amphipods) during the long summer days in the Bering Sea in northern Canada and become extremely fat. In October the whales depart for a 5000 to 7000 mile (8000 to 11,000 kilometer) migration to shallow bays in Baja Mexico, where they breed and calve. During the 6-month journey to Baja and back the whale fasts. Whales can lose as much as 30 percent of their weight, especially for the females that are lactating.[5,22] Importantly, the shorter the feeding season, the larger the whale, likely because it needs to survive a longer fast.[22]

The fact that larger size is associated with the ability to survive famine longer could be relevant to humans. Indeed, there has been a progressive increase in size during the evolution of primates that led to humans, from early apes (proconsul) to *Australeopithecus, Homo erectus*, and eventually humans consistent with evolutionary pressures to store more fat to safeguard against times of food scarcity. So if you want to have a lot of fat, it is good to be tall, for you can carry more. But I think all of you already knew this—for a big man can hide 10 pounds of fat much better than a petite woman.

More than Fat: The Importance of Reducing Energy Needs

Being fat is great if you want to survive famine, but it is also important to reduce your activity. Being a slug is good if you want to live longer when food is not available, as you will use less energy. Recall that food is converted into energy in the body, and that we use this to do our daily work. Some of this work oversees basic processes such as providing the energy to pump our heart, breathe and excrete wastes, and other energy is used for activities that can be controlled, such as how physically active we are. The "metabolic rate" of an organism can dramatically affect how much food is needed on a daily basis.

> *Reducing your activity and metabolism is a key way to maximally maintain your fat stores.*

The need for energy, either from food or from the fat we store, is dependent on this overall metabolic rate. For example, cold blooded reptiles, such as the Green Sea Turtle (*Chelonya midas*), require little energy to survive. This magnificent creature can reach five feet in length, weigh 500 to 600 pounds, and live up to 80 years. Every year, Green Turtles feast on sea grass to increase their fat stores prior to leaving Brazil for an incredible 1400 mile (2200 kilometer) journey across the Atlantic to Ascension Island, a volcanic and barren island in the mid South Atlantic. Swimming at a steady rate of 1.6 miles (2.6 kilometers) per hour, they reach Ascension in 37 days, all the time fasting. Here they mate and then the female lays up to three clutches of eggs, of approximately 120 eggs each. After staying at Ascension for approximately two months, the turtles return to Brazil. During the entire 140–145 day trip, the turtles eat minimally.[21] They survive during this time on their fat stores. Because they are cold blooded, they have lower metabolic rates than mammals or birds, and as such they on average lose only 19 percent of their weight, which is much less compared to similar sized mammals such as seals.[21] Indeed, compared to a warm blooded mammal, a cold blooded reptile uses twelve times less energy.[23] Some reptiles are even more effective at conserving energy. For example, a desert tortoise expends the same amount of energy in one year as a similar size mammal does in 3.5 days.[24]

In contrast, the highest metabolic energy is expended by birds and insects. Birds spend 20 times more energy than the same sized reptile, and insects utilize even more.[23] An excellent example, and also somewhat of an unusual story, is the work of Dr. Weis-Fogh who studied the desert locust in the early 1950s.[25] Dr. Weis-Fogh imported desert locusts into his laboratory in Denmark, and then carefully studied them over many months. Among other things, he would trim off the bottom of their legs and dip the tips in wax so they would not jump and hurt their wings, and he also set up a round-about where he could clock their speeds. Based on his work, he was able to calculate that each locust must eat 1.5 to 3 times its weight in vegetation in preparation for a long flight. He even calculated that a large swarm of African desert locusts, amounting to a weight of 15,000 tons, would eat the same amount in one day as 1.5 million men.

Most swarms of locusts leave two to three hours after sunrise and typically fly for 6 to 8 hours. During flight, they utilize fat for more than 85 percent of their energy needs.[25] While most swarms fly for only 8 hours, there have been examples where swarms have traveled for more than 24 hours, including one swarm that flew an impressive 600 miles (966 kilometers) from southern Morocco to Portugal. According to Weis-Fogh's calculation, the degree of fat stores would be critical in this situation, with those having 10 percent fat only lasting about 12 hours whereas those with 15 percent body fat content lasting 20 hours or more. As such, in such a journey many locusts would not have survived the crossing and would likely have drowned in the Mediterranean Sea.[25]

The marked difference in metabolism between cold-blooded reptiles and birds may be relevant to the extinction of the dinosaurs that occurred approximately 65.5 million years ago following the impact of the Chicxulub meteor north of the Yucatan in Mexico.[26] It is thought that the dinosaurs may have died from starvation associated with marked cooling of the planet due to the dust and ash that entered the atmosphere and that blocked the sun. The discovery that dinosaurs were warm blooded[27] suggests that they likely had a relatively high metabolic rate, which likely countered the benefits of being large in size. This could provide one explanation why these animals did not survive compared to cold blooded reptiles and the smaller, warm-blooded mammals.

Hibernation

One of the more powerful ways to conserve energy is to hibernate. This is a process in which an animal will go into a deep sleep associated with a decrease in body temperature and energy metabolism (torpor). For example, when the Arctic ground squirrel (*Spermophilus parryii*) hibernates, it will decrease its heart rate to an average of 6 beats per minute, its breathing to approximately 5 respirations per minute, and its body temperature to ambient levels.[28] All things slow down in the hibernating animal, and the metabolism drops to 1 to 5 percent of normal levels. This results in the tissues in the animal needing less calories to function. Once hibernating, these animals may remain asleep for 6 or more months.

Hibernation does not require the presence of winter. In some places in the world, it may occur when temperatures become extremely hot (summer hibernation, also known as estivation). For example, the Malagasy fat-tailed dwarf lemur hibernates in a small hollows in trees for up to 6 months of the year.[29] An even better example is the African Lungfish. This is a very primitive fish that can breathe by lungs as well as by gills. It lives in freshwater lakes and marshes in Africa, and unfortunately, many of these lakes dry up during the summer, leaving mudflats with little water. To survive, the fish increases its fat stores, and then burrows into the mud, creating a cone-like hole through which it breathes. To conserve water, it will coat itself with slime, and it will minimize energy consumption by reducing its metabolic rate by as much as 50-fold. It stays in a light sleep (a type of torpor) and lives off its fat. In this process, it can survive until the next season, and possibly even longer provided it has sufficient fat stores.

Some animals drop their metabolic rate "on demand." For example, the hummingbird drinks a lot of nectar (which is sugar) all day which is converted into fat in the liver and elsewhere. However, it has an extremely high metabolic rate (the highest of all birds), with a heart rate of 1200 beats per minute, so it burns much of the fat at night while it sleeps. Occasionally it will burn off most of its fat before the morning arrives. When this happens, it will spontaneously drop its metabolic rate to as low as 3 to 10 percent of baseline until the morning when they can start feeding again.[30]

By now you are thinking it might be good to be physically inactive, and to have abdominal obesity, fatty liver, and elevated triglycerides. This is not what I am saying. Rather, there has been strong evolutionary pressure for all animals to learn how to get fat. Or perhaps you are reacting to my comments by thinking that the comparison of obesity in wild animals and insects with humans is not fair, as humans are not simply becoming fat, they are also developing diabetes and other diseases. If the comparisons are valid, should not wild animals also develop prediabetes or even frank diabetes?

CHAPTER 3

IF FAT IS GOOD, WHY ARE WE BECOMING DIABETIC?

Animals prepare for famine by not only storing fat, but by becoming insulin resistant or prediabetic. Insulin resistance is another way animals protect themselves from famine.

After all, it isn't just about *FAT*. Yes, humans are becoming fatter, and yes, this is not a good thing. But it is not the fat that doctors are worrying about. Fat is often accompanied by diabetes, by high blood pressure, and by liver, kidney and heart disease. People with obesity are commonly prediabetic, meaning that they are showing signs of being resistant to the hormone, insulin. Insulin is a key hormone that is released from the pancreas by eating and helps drive glucose that is in the blood into tissues where it is used to generate energy. Many tissues use insulin, including fat cells (also called adipocytes), muscle and liver. In obese people the tissues often become resistant to insulin, and blood glucose stays elevated for a longer time following a meal. The response of the pancreas to the increased blood glucose levels is to secrete more insulin. Initially, this helps overcome this effect, and glucose levels return to normal, but at the expense of higher serum insulin levels. Unfortunately, as insulin resistance gets progressively worse, the pancreatic islet cells that secrete insulin slowly give out, and the elevation in blood glucose becomes persistent, even when food is not present. Now the person is diabetic, and it is called type 2 diabetes as it results from the progressive resistance of tissues to insulin. This separates this type of diabetes from type 1 diabetes in which the primary problem is a destruction of the beta cells in the pancreatic islets that produce insulin.

In the days before obesity was common, the clinical diagnosis of type 1 or type 2 diabetes was relatively simple, as individuals presenting with type 1 diabetes were classically lean and type 2 diabetic individuals were usually overweight or obese. In fact, the use of this approach to diagnosing these two types of diabetes dates back to the studies by the French physician Étienne Lancereaux (1829-1910), who separated "lean diabetes" (*diabetes maigre*) from fat diabetes (*diabetes gras*) in the late 1800s.[31] Unfortunately, today so many people are overweight, that this distinction no longer holds.

Identification of a prediabetic state among obese individuals was not known until the twentieth century. Prediabetes, however, does not simply mean insulin resistance. Rather, people with prediabetes often show a constellations of signs, including obesity that favors the abdominal regions, the presence of fatty liver, elevated fats in the blood (primarily triglycerides), a reduction in the "good" cholesterol (HDL cholesterol), and elevations in blood pressure. The frequent clustering of these findings led to the recognition that it is a clinical syndrome.[32] Features of this "metabolic syndrome" were first described by the Swedish physician Eskil Kylin in the 1920s,[33] and later by Haller,[34] Singer,[35] and Phillips[36] in the 1970s, but the syndrome became widely known following a paper by Gerald Reaven in the late 1980s.[37] Today over 25 percent of U.S. adults fit the criteria for having metabolic syndrome.[38]

Insulin Resistance is a Component of Fat Storage

You might think that insulin resistance is an abnormal condition, but it is not. Insulin resistance turns out to be a key survival strategy for animals,

15

similar to the importance of storing fat. Animals preparing for a period of food shortage not only become fat, but also become insulin resistant. Marmots and squirrels, for example, become fat and insulin resistant in preparation for hibernation.[6,39] The European Garden Warbler (*Phylloscopus collybita*) is another example. This bird doubles its weight by increasing its fat stores in its visceral fat, liver and blood in preparation for its epic journey across the Sahara so it can winter in subtropical Africa.[4] It also becomes insulin resistant.[4] The desert gerbil (*Psammomys obesus*) or fat sand rat, has learned to become obese to help it survive the Egyptian deserts; when it is given a regular laboratory diet, it rapidly develops diabetes suggesting that it was in a prediabetic state in nature.[40]

Metabolic Syndrome

1) Abdominal Obesity determined by waist circumference (Men > 40 inches (102 cm); Women > 35 inches (88 cm)
2) Triglycerides ≥ 150 mg/dL
3) Low HDL cholesterol levels (Men < 40 mg/dl, Women < 50 mg/dL)
4) Blood pressure ≥ 130/≥ 85 mmHg
5) Fasting glucose ≥ 110 mg/dL

The Metabolic syndrome is defined as the presence of at least 3 of the 5 listed risk factors. Definition of the Adult Treatment Panel III of the National Cholesterol Education Program (NCEP-ATPIII).

Some animals actually become diabetic during the period of fat storage. The hummingbird, for example, lives on nectar from flowering plants, which consists of about 40 percent sucrose (table sugar). In a period of just 12 hours these birds may ingest up to 4 times their weight in nectar. While hummingbirds weigh only 2 to 8 grams and at baseline have about 21 percent fat content, their fat content can increase to 40 percent of their body weight after feeding. During the day, the liver can double its weight in fat, making it one of the fattest livers observed in birds, and resulting in a creamy white color.[10] Blood sugars are high in hummingbirds, being close to three times that observed in humans at baseline (300 mg/dl) and rising to as high as 700 mg/dl after meals.[30] Raising their blood sugar and storing fat is critical in these animals, especially in preparation for migration. Indeed, some hummingbirds will fly across the Gulf of Mexico to winter, a distance of over 600 miles (966 kilometers). During flight the birds rapidly use the glucose and fats that they store, as they have an exceptionally high metabolic rate, with a heart rate of over 1200 beats per minute, a respiratory rate of 250 breaths per minute, and even a higher body temperature (39 degrees centigrade). Since the glucose and fat are so rapidly utilized, the hummingbird never develops evidence for diabetic complications.

The most magnificent example is the wood frog (*Rana sylvatica*) that lives in Canada and the northern United States. This frog never learned how to burrow well, and had to develop a way to survive the cold winters. In preparation for winter, it stores huge amounts of glucose in the liver in the form of polymers of glucose called glycogen (which is similar to starch in plants). As winter ensues, it releases a massive amount of glucose into its blood and then actually freezes. Despite having 65 to 70 percent of its tissues frozen, it remains alive with a heart rate of only a few beats a minute. The blood does not completely freeze as the huge concentrations of glucose (which can amount to over 3000 mg/dl, or 30 times that observed in man) acts like antifreeze. Since the high glucose levels also act as a nutrient, this is one of the few animals that does not depend on fat stores. Indeed, since its metabolic rate is so low, it can survive simply from the glucose in its blood.[41]

> *The metabolic syndrome should actually be renamed the fat storage syndrome. It is not an abnormal process; animals purposefully develop metabolic syndrome to help them survive periods of food shortage.*

Insulin Resistance is a Survival Factor

Since insulin is critical for driving glucose into the cell, then how does glucose in the blood help an animal to survive if it is insulin resistant? The answer is that not all organs are resistant to insulin. In particular, the brain does not require insulin for the uptake of glucose. So in insulin resistant states, it can still utilize glucose as its energy source. This is particularly important as brain cells cannot utilize fat. In contrast, tissues such as skeletal muscle can use fat as their energy source. When these tissues become insulin resistant, they will use fat as their primary energy source. This allows preservation of blood glucose for the brain.

Insulin resistance is a great way to assure glucose delivery to the brain. However, when an animal fasts for a long time, other ways take over to provide energy to the brain. Before we discuss this other mechanism, however, let us address a question you may never have considered, which is why can't humans hibernate?

CHAPTER 4

FAT, HIBERNATION, AND BEAUTY

> *Having fat is important in pregnancy, for food shortage can result in the loss of the baby. Early humans likely desired having their young women fat to ensure a successful pregnancy.*

No discussion about obesity in animals is complete without reviewing the relationship of obesity and pregnancy. Just as animals have to look after themselves, they must also look after their young; this includes making sure they survive gestation and the nursing period.

Different strategies are used between small and large animals. As discussed earlier, larger animals can store more fat than small animals relative to their needs. This gives them a greater chance to survive a long period of famine. However, being larger turns out to have some disadvantages when it comes to pregnancy. This is because the length of pregnancy depends substantially on the size of the animal. For example, the gestation period of the mouse is 18-19 days, for the hamster it is 15-18 days, and for the squirrel and chipmunk it is 30 to 40 days. Contrast this with seals and sea lions (350 days), the rhinoceros (450 days), the elephant (616 days) and the sperm whale (480 to 590 days). For humans the length of pregnancy is about 266 days (8 days shy of 9 months), and this is similar to the great apes, such as the chimpanzees (237 days), gorilla (257 days) and orangutan (260 days). As such, larger animals may carry more fat, but they also have to be able to maintain a pregnancy during seasons in which food sources may become scarce. In contrast, smaller animals can wait until the winter subsides to mate and reproduce. With such a short gestation, smaller animals can give birth to their young when it is still summer and there is plenty of food. This allows the young to be maximally prepared when the winter comes the following fall.

The fact that small mammals do not have to carry a pregnancy during the winter months provides an additional advantage, and that is the ability to undergo hibernation. As discussed earlier, true hibernation is associated with profound reductions in metabolism (rates to 1 to 5 percent of their basal metabolism) that cannot sustain pregnancy in which a fetus is actively growing. As a consequence, only small mammals (17 pounds or lower) that can wait to become pregnant in spring can be true hibernators.[18] This is why humans cannot hibernate, for if they did, they would not be able to maintain a successful pregnancy. But what about bears? Bears, however, are not true hibernators, in the strict sense of dropping their body temperatures to near freezing and slowing their heart rate to imperceptible levels. Rather, hibernating bears go into light torpor and remain easily arousable, dropping their body temperatures to only 30 to 36 degrees centigrade. During this time they drop their metabolic rate only 20 to 50 percent but do not urinate, defecate or eat for 3 to 6 months.[42] Since they do not drop their metabolic rates to drastically low levels, they can remain pregnant throughout the winter.[42]

Most large animals would prefer not to give birth during the period of food shortage. This can be a problem if an animal with a long gestation period becomes pregnant in the spring, for as a consequence delivery may not occur until the winter when food is scarce. One way some animals have dealt with this is to find a way to delay pregnancy. The roe deer has developed such a clever means. These deer mate in July but the fertilized egg remains unattached in the uterus for several months, simply living off the fat in the egg. In December or January, the egg will attach to the uterine wall where it will trigger the normal processes that lead to the development of a placenta that allows the growth of the fetus. By delaying implantation of the egg, the deer can avert having the young from being born during the winter. This process of delayed implantation is also true of a number of other animals, including bears, the kangaroo, the badger and the grey seal.

Many animals also maintain fat stores so they can help feed their young without leaving them vulnerable to predators. Having sufficient fat stores is especially critical for the female, as lactation can rapidly deplete fat stores as breast milk is rich in fat. For example, female fur seals fast ashore for the week following giving birth while they nurse their pups.[43] Some birds, such as pigeons and the Emperor penguin, vomit up a milky-like substance consisting of fat-rich tissues sloughed from the esophagus (crop milk) that they use to feed their young so they do not have to leave the nest to get more food.

Other animals have developed unusual ways to protect their eggs or young that also involves fasting. The African Cichlid, a beautiful fish often kept in tropical fish aquariums, quits eating so it can incubate its eggs in its mouth for 3 to 5 weeks until they hatch,[5] and the same is true for the Arowana (Dragon Fish) from southeast Asia. Once hatched, the fish can still retreat safely into the mouth of their mother if frightened or threatened. Similarly, the Nile crocodile will fast while nesting, and then will carry their young in their mouth for up to 3 months.[5]

A particularly interesting animal was the gastric brooding frog (also known as platypus frog) of Queensland. These frogs lived in the rain forests and protected their eggs by swallowing them into their stomach. The eggs secreted a compound (prostaglandin E) that blocks acid production by the stomach, and also a substance that allows the eggs to attach to the wall of the stomach. Once hatched, the frog would regurgitate the tadpoles and then once again be able to eat. Unfortunately, the last gastric brooding frog was seen in the early 1980s, and it is now thought to be extinct.

Humans, Fat, and Reproduction

The importance of having sufficient fat stores is critical for human reproduction, and especially for the female.[13] For example, the onset of menarche

21

is dependent on fat stores; and once initiated, as little as a 10 to 15 percent decrease in weight can cause menstruation to stop.[13,44-45] According to Frisch and McArthur, an 18-year-old girl needs about 35 pounds of fat to maintain normal menstruation.[46] This is the reason anorexia nervosa is associated with irregular or absent menstruation. It also explains why female marathon runners and ballerinas frequently have irregular menses.[47] Some authors believe that the reason men are the hunters in most hunter-gatherer societies is to allow the women to maintain their fat stores so the pregnancies can be successful.

Maintaining fat stores during pregnancy is critical in order to provide sufficient nutrients to the fetus. The high energy demands in pregnant or nursing mothers make them susceptible to losing their fat stores quickly and vulnerable during periods of famine.[48-49] Pregnant women may need even better nutrition than most animals, as humans are one of the only species in which the baby is born with relatively high amounts of fat.[50] The relatively high percentage of fat is maintained throughout early child-hood.[51-52]

Early humans likely knew about the benefits of having sufficient fat stores in order to have a successful pregnancy, and this may have translated into viewing obesity as something desirable since it could be viewed as important for successful reproduction. The earliest evidence comes from the Venus figurines, hundreds of which have been found throughout Europe. These figurines date to 20,000 to 35,000 years ago, at the same time when early humans were creating their first art in the caves of southern France. Venus figurines, such as the Venus of Gagarino, were small carvings typically 2 to 8 inch in length and made from stone, ivory or bone. Most depict the torso and head of extremely obese women, with dramatic abdominal fat and large hanging breasts. Similar figurines can be found much later in the Neolithic period throughout Crete, Greece, and Turkey, and are referred to as "Mother Goddess" figures.[53-54] Art objects depicting fat women have also been found in predynastic sites in Egypt, in which the women sometimes show massively enlarged hips, buttocks and thighs.[14]

The Venus of Gagarino

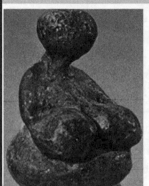

In the late 1920s an old house pit was excavated in Gagarino, Ukraine on the bank of the Don River. The site included bones of the rhinoceros and mammoth, hundreds of flint tools and blades, bone artifacts, and several figurines including the 5.8 centimeter Venus carved out of rock.

Photograph from the Pictorial Encyclopedia of The Evolution of Man by J. Jelinek (London: Hamlyn Publishing Group, 1975) with permission of Aventinum Publishing

The Venus of Gagarino
Ukraine, 22,000 B.C.

The symbolic meaning of the Venus and Mother Goddess figurines is not known. Some have proposed they represent fertility figures, and that the figurines depict pregnant (and obese) women. Others have suggested they may represent symbols of health, prosperity, and happiness. I tend to believe both concepts are correct. To be fat would be both a symbol of health and success and also highly desirable as it would increase chances to carry pregnancy during a period of famine or starvation.

The observation that our ancestors linked fertility with obesity may explain why certain cultures viewed it desirable for the women to be fat. William Wadd wrote in his book on obesity in 1816 that in Tunisia the young ladies were kept in rooms and fattened in preparation for their weddings.[55] John Speke, the explorer who discovered that the White Nile originated from Lake Victoria, talked about how King Rŭmanika of Karague (the kingdom on the west side of Lake Victoria) had a very fat wife "whose flesh hung down like large, loose-stuffed puddings" and who had a sister-in-law who "was another of those wonders of obesity, unable to stand excepting on all fours."[56] Obesity was something so desired that members of the royal family were forced to be obese. Speke noted a 16-year-old girl who was forced to drink pot after pot of milk. As he wrote, "the daughter, a lass of sixteen, sat stark-naked before us, sucking at a milk-

23

pot, on which the father kept her at work by holding a rod in his hand; for, as fattening is the first duty of fashionable female life, it must be duly enforced by the rod if necessary. . . . Her features were lovely, but her body was as round as a ball."[56]

> *"Being fat is beautiful"* as it ensures a successful pregnancy for those who cannot predict if there will always be food on the table.

A specialized type of obesity is the remarkable large buttocks (steatopygy) observed in the Khoikhoi (Hottentot) and San (Bushmen) women that live in the arid regions of southwest Africa. These have been described by Peschel as "fatty cushions of the buttocks which project above like inverted steps and then gradually merge into the thighs."[57] Milder forms of steatopygy were also reported in the 1800s among the pygmies living in the Congo and in the Nilotic Bongo people of Central Africa.[14]

Shattock wrote how the British explorer, Sir Harry Johnston, noted that the protruding buttocks were viewed as a sign of beauty by the men whereas women viewed it as effeminate if it was present to any extent on the men.[14] Darwin also quotes the explorer Richard Burton as saying that Somali men chose their wives by lining them up and then determining whose buttocks extended behind the most.[58]

Johnston wrote that steatopygy was an important source of fat for the women, and that it would decrease during periods of food shortage.[14] Others also commented how the buttocks was used to store fat and how it would decrease markedly in size during severe droughts and famine.[57] It seems likely that the development of enlarged buttocks was an evolutionary adaptation that allowed additional storage of fat that would confer a sign of fertility and hence attractiveness. One might consider that the attractiveness of "curvy" figures today as a carryover of our desire to have young women have sufficient fat stores to maintain pregnancy.

Steatopygy and Beauty

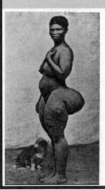

A photograph from the 1800s of a San woman with steatopygy. Steatopygy allowed the storage of fat that was important to assure successful pregnancy, and also was a sign of beauty.

Original in the Museum of the Royal College of Surgeons. Published by SG Shattock in the Proc Royal Soc Med 1909; 2:207-70

One of the most famous painters in history was Peter Paul Rubens (1577-1640), a Flemish painter who is famous for drawing beautiful women who were overweight or "full-figured." Rubens travelled to Spain in 1603 during his early years just after a major famine had spread through that country (1599-1601). During the following decades, Holland would be seeing the first emergence of obesity (see later chapters). While totally speculative, I wonder if his early visit to Spain and the subsequent contrast with the flourishing culture in Holland may have influenced his concept on health and beauty.

To summarize, an overriding principle of evolution is to develop ways to survive periods when food is not available. One of the best ways to do this is to become fat and insulin resistant and also reduce energy needs. Having fat stores is especially important for the mother to assure a healthy baby. This led to early humans viewing obesity as both desirable and representative of fertility.

A striking finding about obesity in animals is that it is highly regulated and frequently (but not always) scheduled. This seems incongruent with the complete lack of regulation of weight we observe in humans today. Yet is this the case? In the next section, we will look at human obesity and see if there is evidence that it is regulated as well. Then, we will go back to our animal studies to figure out how this regulation occurs, and to see if we can identify whether a "fat switch" has been inadvertently turned on in our population that is causing us to become fat and diabetic.

CHAPTER 5

IS HUMAN OBESITY REGULATED?

> *Obesity results not because we choose to eat larger portions or to exercise less. Rather we have activated a "program" to become fat. This causes increased appetite, resulting in more food intake, and decreased energy output, resulting in exercising less.*
>
> *The equation is the same. Too much food intake plus too little exercise equals Fat. However, the interpretation is different. Obesity is not from gluttony and idleness, but rather because we have activated the same program all animals use to increase fat stores.*

If the increase of wealth and refinement of modern times have tended to banish plague and pestilence from our cities, they have probably . . . increased the frequency of corpulency.

—William Wadd, 1816

William Wadd, the author of *Cursory Remarks on Corpulency or Obesity Considered as a Disease* wrote in his textbook of 1816 that he was concerned that increased inactivity, somnolence, and overeating were driving the marked increase in obesity of his day. He noted that life was easier for the working Englishman, and he related this, of all things, to the sudden increase in chimneys for ordinary homes that occurred in the mid-16th century that allowed cooking and eating without one having to leave the home. "Hollingshed, who lived in Queen Elizabeth's reign, speaking of the increase in luxury of his days, noticed, 'the multitude of chimnies lately erected; whereas in the sound remembrance of some old men, there were not more than two or three, if so many, in the most uplandish towns of the realm.' How far corpulency has kept pace with the number of chimnies, I pretend not to determine; certain it is that Hollingshed and his contemporaries, furnish no account of the front of the house, or the windows, being taken away to let out, to an untimely grave, some unfortunate victim, too ponderous to be brought down the staircase."[55, 59]

Just as Dr. Wadd complained that obesity increased when life became easier with houses equipped with chimneys, today we can also argue that obesity is the result, at least in part, of overeating coupled with lack of exercise. However, as we will discuss below, associations do not prove causality, and in this case it is not quite this simple.

Obesity: Eating too much, exercising too little

Simply put, energy balance is often explained by the first law of thermodynamics. In essence, the energy ingested equals the energy expended. In many cases, the individual who eats more will have greater energy to expend, and will

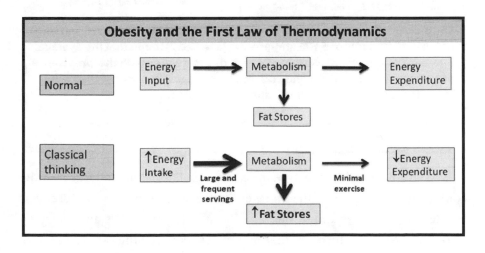

27

remain in balance. However, if one expends less energy than one consumes, the excess energy ends up being stored as fat, resulting in weight gain.

According to this law of physics, the cause of obesity is straightforward—the problem is that we are eating too much food and exercising too little. There are cultural, economic and behavioral factors that support these concepts. We are eating too much because of the availability of fast food restaurants that allow one to ingest massive amounts of calories in only a few minutes; all you can eat buffets; the increasing size and supersize of soft drinks and their automatic refills at local restaurants. It is compounded by the food industry that tries to encourage bad food habits. For example, one study reported that the average child is exposed to 40,000 food advertisements a year of which 72 percent are for fast food, candy and cereals.[60]

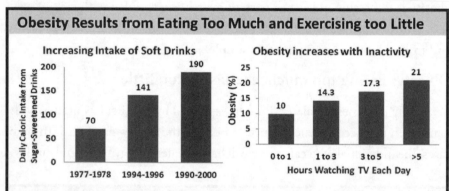

Obesity Results from Eating Too Much and Exercising too Little

Increasing Intake of Soft Drinks
(Daily Caloric Intake from Sugar-Sweetened Drinks)
- 1977-1978: 70
- 1994-1996: 141
- 1990-2000: 190

Obesity increases with Inactivity
(Obesity (%) vs Hours Watching TV Each Day)
- 0 to 1: 10
- 1 to 3: 14.3
- 3 to 5: 17.3
- >5: 21

The daily intake of soft drinks in Americans increased between 1970 and 2000 (left panel). A study of 6,671 adolescents (age 12-17) found that the average number of hours spent watching TV each day correlated with the prevalence of obesity (right panel). Studies such as these suggest obesity results from ingesting too many calories and insufficient exercise.

Left figure with permission from the New Engl J Med 2009; 360:1805. Right figure shows data from Pediatrics 1985; 75:807.

We are also exercising too little, due to television and the remote control; increasing use of the internet; the general reduction in exercise as the days seem busier and busier; and because technology is always trying to reduce physical effort, whether it is the escalator or the car. The less we exercise, the less energy we burn and the more energy that will be converted to fat. In one study of adolescents, for example, the number of hours the child sat in front of the TV correlated closely with his or her risk for being obese.[61]

This is not simply the case for humans. Pets such as dogs and cats can also become obese, likely related to the same process of being provided excessive amounts of food coupled with a reduction in exercise. Evidence such as this suggests there is a strong role for cultural and behavioral mechanisms in driving obesity. Furthermore, environmental, genetic, and congenital factors are also likely to modify these behaviors.

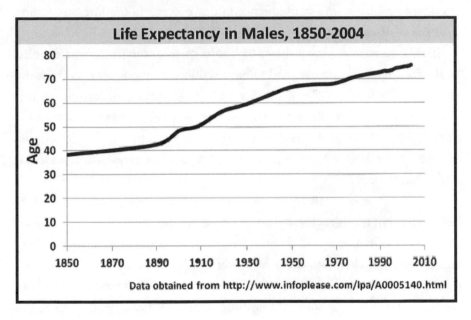

Obesity: the natural consequence of better health?

The concept that obesity may reflect increased food availability and technological advances that reduce our needs to perform physical work may lead to the idea that obesity may be the undesired consequence of advances in our civilization. Some experts have even suggested obesity is the consequence of better health.[62] In the 1800s life was frequently short due to deaths from infections. Tuberculosis, pneumonia, typhoid fever and cholera were common causes of death in the 1800s, and others succumbed to rheumatic valve disease that developed as a consequence of a strepto-coccal infection. However, with the advent of improved hygiene and antibiotics, people are living longer. The average lifespan in the United States for white men has increased from 47 years in 1900 to 78 years in 2004, and to 81 years old in white women.

With fewer deaths from infection, humans live longer and can enjoy the pleasures of life. With better food availability and technical advances that require less exercise, we should be expected to become obese. Like the future generations as depicted in the Disney-Pixar movie Wall-E, obesity and its attendant problems are a consequence of our success, not failure, in battling the evils of disease.

In this scenario obesity is the *passive consequence* of living longer, enabled by the fact that older people tend to have reduced metabolic rate and a more sedentary life with unaltered or increased food intake. According to this hypothesis, obesity results from an "epidemiological transition" from a life censored by infectious diseases to a longer life but at the cost of developing diseases associated with aging, such as type 2 diabetes, cardiovascular disease and obesity.

The hypothesis that obesity is a success story about human health, however, is not tenable. Obesity is not a passive consequence of living longer due to better hygiene and fewer infections, for obesity is also affecting adolescents and children. There were plenty of young children who did not have tuberculosis or typhoid fever in the 1500s, but obesity was not commonly observed in them at that time. Obesity is not a healthy response; obesity actively increases the risk for death and is associated with remarkable increases in type 2 diabetes and coronary artery disease.[63] While the risk for becoming obese might increase with longer life spans from better public hygiene and a reduction in infectious diseases, one can certainly live a long life without becoming obese.

Are there other Factors besides Overnutrition and Inactivity that may be driving the Obesity Pandemic?

A classical viewpoint of obesity suggests that our culture and behavior are to blame; and obesity is a consequence of our choice to eat as much as we desire and to minimize our daily exercise. I remember traveling to Europe in the mid-1980s and hearing from some European friends about the stereotypic "fat American tourists" who fill their stomachs with fast food and exercise so little. The problem was a lousy lifestyle, and no desire to change. It was all a problem of the behavior, economics and lack of fortitude of the American people.

The concept that obesity is a consequence of voluntary behavior has also been argued based on the finding that obese people tend to form social networks in which their behavior patterns can be reinforced.[64] The government apparently agrees, as there are 21 states that have "personal responsibility" laws that protect fast food companies and restaurants from obesity related tort claims.[65] In essence, it is our responsibility, not that of the public domain, that we eat too much. If you don't want to overeat, just don't overeat!

While I agree there should be some personal responsibility to food selection and exercise patterns, over the last decade there has been increasing evidence that obese individuals may engage a process that makes us want to overeat and to exercise less. In other words, the process of overeating and exercising may be a regulated response in those destined to become obese and diabetic.

Obesity Requires an Abnormal Appetite with Reduced Satiety Response

A breakthrough in our understanding of the cause of obesity was made when Dr. Jeff Friedman and his laboratory discovered a central mechanism for controlling appetite. Specifically, when an animal eats, there is a signal to the brain that tells it when it is full ('satiety signal'). When this signal occurs, the animal will quit eating. Therefore, there are specific mechanisms in place that help the animal to maintain a normal weight.

Friedman showed that the key player in this satiety response is a hormone called leptin. Leptin is a protein released into the blood from fat tissues following eating and acts as a satiety signal to the brain. When Friedman used special techniques to inactivate the leptin gene in the mouse, it became massively fat due to uncontrolled food intake.[66]

Since Friedman's seminal work, other hormonal mechanisms have also been identified that help regulate our food intake, including insulin (released from the pancreas) and ghrelin (released from the stomach). Ghrelin has some functions which act oppositely to leptin, for when it turns on, it signals to eat; hence it is sometimes referred to as the hunger hormone. Together, ghrelin, leptin and insulin help control our appetite. It is actually difficult to make an animal fat if these hormonal systems are operating normally, although they can be overruled if the animal decides to do so.

These hormonal systems are not operating normally in obese individuals. Just as obesity is associated with "insulin resistance," obese persons often become resistant to the effects of leptin. Since leptin does not effectively signal satiety in response to food, leptin levels rise to compensate, just like insulin levels rise in response to insulin resistance.

This has led to the recognition that obesity is not simply the consequence of cultural and behavioral factors, but there is also a defect in the inability of the obese person to sense when their intake fulfills their needs to maintain their energy balance. As such, they may continue to eat beyond their needs, and start to accrue fat. Obesity might therefore be considered to be a consequence not only of our western culture, but also of some underlying mechanism that alters the regulation of satiety. Thus, obesity could be viewed as a "dysregulation" in which there is an interference of metabolic processes aimed at keeping us at a normal weight.

While the development of leptin resistance is one reason we are eating too much, many obese individuals also develop an addiction for food, and especially for sweets ("foodaholics").[67] Food addiction also has a major role in driving food intake and obesity. We will discuss how food addiction happens, its consequences, as well as how to prevent or reverse this later in the book.

Obesity as a Consequence of a Reduced Ability to Burn Fat

There is also increasing evidence that the reason obese people may not exercise enough is not due to their preference to watch TV or work on the computer, but rather because they lack the energy to exercise. A study was performed in 192 school children in which half reduced their television and video watching from 23 hours per week to about 13 hours per week for a 6 month period. The hypothesis was that reducing time in front of the TV would result in an increase in physical activity and a reduction in weight. However, physical activity did not increase with reducing TV, and in fact tended to decrease. The group that reduced their time watching TV showed slightly less weight gain than the control group, but the effects were modest (only a difference of 1 to 2 pounds).[68]

Why would physical activity not increase spontaneously if one quit watching TV? One possibility is that an individual may not have the energy to exercise. The body generates energy by making ATP (adenosine triphosphate), primarily from carbohydrates and fats. All living things use ATP as their way of running the chemical reactions that are necessary for metabolism and growth. ATP can be viewed like currency or money that the cell uses to perform their day to day functions. As such, much of the food we eat is used to create ATP.

The oxidation or "burning" of fatty acids from fat is very effective at generating ATP. This process occurs in the mitochondria, which are small structures that exist inside the normal cell. Mitochondria also generate ATP from products of glucose metabolism, although this is not as efficient in producing ATP as from fat. ATP then drives metabolism by its ability to donate phosphate groups, and thus can keep the cell healthy and active.

Obese people have a defect in their ability to burn fat.[69-71] This defect is also found in individuals predisposed to obesity.[72] The defect is associated with a reduction in mitochondria in skeletal muscle as well as the peripheral white blood cells.[73-75] ATP levels are also low in the liver.[76]

A relative inability to burn fat could have several consequences. For example, it may result in inefficient removal of fat, and thereby increase fat accumulation. The inability to make sufficient ATP would also result in a low energy state, causing fatigue and reducing the desire for physical activity and exercise. Fat people fatigue more easily and have less exercise tolerance.[77-79] Obese children also have increased fatigue and tiredness.[80] Not surprisingly, obese people who tire easily have lower ATP levels in their muscle.[81] Finally, low ATP levels in the liver stimulate appetite.[82-84] This likely represents a compensatory response as eating more will generate more ATP to correct the low energy state, but will have the consequence of further increasing weight.

Even more worrisome, the impairment in the burning of fat persists in individuals who lose weight by dieting.[85] This has also been shown in laboratory animals.[86] This explains why most obese people cannot maintain weight loss, and regain most of their weight after a few months.

Obesity is Regulated

Obesity is therefore triggered by an alteration in metabolism, in which leptin resistance results in increased food intake, and a block in energy production leads to preferential conversion of the energy into fat. Therefore, the major reasons we are eating too much is not because we are given larger plates of food, but rather because we are now more hungry and want larger plates of food. The reason we are sitting in front of a TV all day is not simply because the TV is so good, but rather because we do not have the energy we used to have. This does not deny the emotional and behavioral factors driven by the fast food industry, or the advertising and technological advancements that encourage us to eat more and exercise less. The major problem, however, is that we have activated a "program" to become fat.

The major reasons we eat too much is not because we are given larger plates of food, but rather because we are now more hungry and want larger plates of food. The reason we sit in front of a TV all day is not because the TV is so good, but rather because we do not have the same energy we used to have.

The law of thermodynamics remains the same; the only thing we have done is to change what is driving what. In Chapter 1 we talked about how weight is tightly regulated in animals, and how force feeding will only transiently increase the weight of an animal, as it will want to return to its normal baseline weight. In other words, the animal knows its "set point" for body weight. To change this set point, so that one can be larger and fatter, all one needs to do is to activate a program that causes insulin and leptin resistance resulting in more food intake, and at the same time reduce the burning of fat to block energy production.

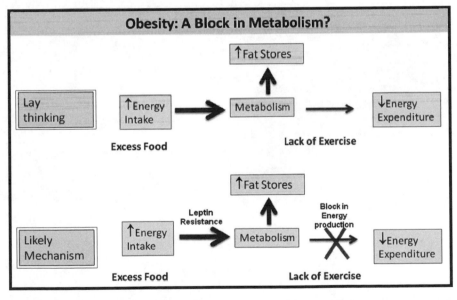

Activating this "fat switch" would remove the normal mechanisms that maintain body weight, and weight gain would occur. Importantly, it would not only persist, but continue to increase weight over time if it remains activated. In the next chapter, we are going to learn that this is a uniform way animals become fat. In other words, to become fat one must activate a process that causes leptin resistance and blocks energy expenditures. Obesity is not dysregulated at all; it is a highly regulated response that is used by all animals to get fat. So what is activating the process that is making us fat and tired?

SECTION 2

IDENTIFICATION OF THE SWITCH THAT CAUSES OBESITY

CHAPTER 6

A DETECTIVE'S APPROACH TO FINDING THE "FAT SWITCH"

One way to understand how animals become fat is to determine what animals do to try to regain weight when they are starved. This approach led to an exciting insight.

It is apparent that those of us who are becoming fat and insulin resistant have activated a program similar to the mammal readying for winter, or the bird preparing for a long distance migration, or the desert frog preparing for a drought. We are all storing fat, but why? What is triggering our body to do this?

One approach we used to answer this will likely catch you by surprise, for it is to study not how animals get fat, but rather what happens when they starve. Fasting is a normal process that all animals prepare for and undergo at different times. If starvation becomes prolonged or unexpected and ends up depleting all of the fat stores, however, then what happens to the animal? We reasoned that if this occurs, then the animal would have to engage whatever mechanisms it could to regain weight, and to do this as rapidly as it could. In so doing, if there exists a switch that turns on the gaining of fat, it would occur at that time.

Much of our knowledge about starvation comes from the seminal work of George F. Cahill, a Professor from Harvard who published many research studies on starvation over the last 50 years.[1] To briefly review, carbohydrates, fats, and protein make up the three major food groups. The first two are the primary foods used for energy storage, whereas protein is reserved for building of muscle. When one undergoes starvation, one first burns off excess carbohydrate stores, then the fat stores, and finally the animal starts to degrade the protein stores in the muscle. This stepwise utilization of carbohydrate, fat, and then protein falls roughly into three stages or phases.

Stage 1 of Starvation: The Carbohydrate Phase

The two major carbohydrates present in the diet are starch and sugar. Starch consists of many molecules of glucose bonded together. Sugar, as I use this word in this book, refers to table sugar, or sucrose, which consists of a glucose molecule and a fructose molecule bound together. Starch, therefore, consists of 100 percent glucose, whereas sucrose or sugar consists of 50 percent glucose and 50 percent fructose.

The principle storage form of carbohydrate in the body is in the form of glucose, which is maintained at a concentration of nearly 100 mg per 100 ml of blood and is also stored in the liver as glycogen, which is the animal equivalent of starch from plants and which also consists of multiple glucose molecules bound together. Glucose, which is sometimes referred to as "blood sugar," is an important energy source for all tissues, but especially the brain. As discussed in Chapter 3, the brain cannot use fat as an energy source, and so it relies heavily on the delivery of glucose.

When food is removed from an animal, the immediate response is to maintain the blood glucose level to assure sufficient nutrition for the brain. As blood glucose levels start to fall, the body responds by reducing its level of insulin, and the glycogen in the liver starts to break down rapidly, releasing glucose into the circulation that can provide the needed energy to the brain and other tissues. Weight loss is significant this first day, as glycogen is bulky and laden with water. Energy production, however, is not that efficient, and for each gram of glycogen burned, only 2 to 4 calories of energy is produced.[2] As long as glycogen is present in the liver, there is minimal burning of fat.

The breakdown of glycogen is the "rapid response" to food shortage.[3-5] In insects and birds, glycogen stores are used up within hours.[6] In mammals such as rats and dogs, liver glycogen stores takes about 12 to 24 hours to be depleted. In humans it can happen within hours if a person is exercising, and in about 12 hours if one is not.[3-5] It is also common to deplete glycogen with an overnight fast.[3-5] Likewise, glycogen can be quickly restored following intake of carbohydrates, such as sugar and starch.[7] Furthermore, liver glycogen levels tend to be higher in obese people.[8]

> *The release of glucose from the liver is the "rapid response" to starvation.*

We will discuss the importance of this phase when it comes to strategies for losing weight in later chapters. The important point to remember is that it is hard to burn fat when one has glycogen stores in the liver. This is one reason why low carbohydrate ("low carb") diets tend to be effective, at least initially, as low carb diets help keep the glycogen levels low in the liver so that fat is preferentially burned.[5]

Stage 2 of Starvation: The Fat Phase

Phase 1 is activated daily, as it is the principal mechanism for providing energy between meals. In contrast, phase 2 is designed to provide energy for prolonged periods of time when food is unavailable. Hence, this is the "professional" phase of starvation, for this is exactly what the animal has planned.

The phase usually begins around 24 hours and is characterized by the burning of fat. Fat is a very efficient fuel, generating 9 calories per gram of fat. With such an efficient energy source, weight loss occurs more slowly, and falls at a constant rate over time.

This phase is well tolerated. Most animals reduce their physical activity, show little agitation, and even appear relaxed. This phase is also associated with reduced energy needs, with a fall in the basal (resting) metabolic rate, including a slight fall in body temperature.[9-10] As we discussed in earlier chapters, some animals will actually drop their metabolic rates even more, such as hibernating mammals and reptiles.

The burning of fat is the "professional response" to starvation.

Since the burning of fat does not generate glucose, the supply of glucose to the brain must come from another source. Initially this is from muscle breakdown, which releases amino acids from the muscle protein that can be used to make glucose through a chemical process (called gluconeogenesis). However, after a few weeks the brain switches its metabolism from using glucose as its fuel to ketoacids which are generated from the burning of fat. This allows the preservation of the muscle mass.

Humans have been studied under starvation conditions. For example, in the early 1900s it was discovered that individuals with uncontrollable seizures (known as epilepsy) could improve during periods of voluntary starvation. When it was discovered that the benefit was associated with the presence of ketoacids (also called ketosis) that occurs during the fat-burning phase, low carb diets were introduced as an alternative treatment since they also result in the production of ketoacids (hence why low carb diets are sometimes called ketotic diets). Starvation has also been used to treat obesity, especially in the 1960s. Others have studied anorexia nervosa, a psychiatric condition in which individuals develop abnormal views of their body image and preferentially reduce or stop eating to decrease their body weight. In all of these conditions the phase characterized by the burning of fat is well tolerated. Furthermore, during this period, humans also decrease their metabolic rate, which reduces the energy needs and allows the fat stores to last as long as possible.[10]

Stage 3 of Starvation: The Protein Breakdown Phase

No animal wants to enter phase 3, for this is when the fat stores have been depleted. In rats this occurs when fat content is down to 2.5 percent of body weight.[11] This was never meant to happen, and when it occurs, it sets off an alarm signal for the animal. In order to survive, the animal has to start breaking down its own tissues to generate energy, resulting in it becoming weaker and weaker as more and more tissue is broken down. With the loss of fat stores, it now becomes insulin resistant again, to help maintain glucose levels in the blood as a fuel for the brain.[12] Time is of essence, and if the animal was hibernating it will suddenly awaken and become agitated. Its metabolic rate will now increase, even to levels higher than that observed in nonfasting animals. It will actively look for food even if it puts itself at risk for being hunted by predators. This "foraging response," as it is called, will last until the animal becomes too weak to continue. At this point, it will go into a coma and die.

> *Once carbohydrate and fat stores are depleted, the animal degrades its protein (muscle) for survival. The animal is now desperate, and must activate processes to maximally help the animal obtain food and regain weight. This is called "the foraging response."*

Only rarely has phase 3 starvation been studied in humans. In one study, five unconscious severely malnourished individuals with a history of anorexia nervosa and/or depression were evaluated following admission to an intensive care unit in a hospital in Paris. The patients weighed between 50 and 60 pounds and had an average body mass index (BMI, see insert) between 9 and 10 (normal is 20-25). These individuals had no body fat, with less than 1 percent compared to healthy controls when it was measured using a fancy test called bioelectrical impedance analysis. Despite being unconscious, they were found to have elevated resting metabolic rates. There were no fatty acids in the blood, but signs of protein breakdown were evident as reflected by elevated nitrogen levels in the urine. Placement of stomach tubes with feeding was attempted, but in spite of these efforts one of the five persons died.[10]

A Measurement of Obesity

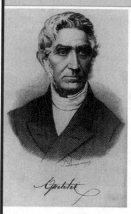

The classical measure for obesity was developed by the Belgian astronomer and statistician, Adolphe Quételet (1796–1874), who introduced a measure based on the height and weight of an individual.

The body mass index (BMI) = (weight in kg)/(height in meters squared)

A value of 20-25 is considered normal weight, 25-30 is overweight, and ≥30 is obese. For some populations, such as Asians, the cutoff values for overweight and obesity are lower (for example, >24 for overweight and >27.5 for obesity).

The portrait is by Joseph-Arnold Demannez and was published in the *Annuaire de l'Académie royale de Belgique*, 1875, vol. 41, p. 108.

Uric acid, Cortisol, and the Foraging Response

If an animal would ever desire to activate a metabolic process to gain weight, it would be during the foraging response. In this regard, one of the most characteristic findings that occurs during this phase is a sudden rise in serum cortisol. Cortisol is a steroid that is produced by the adrenal gland under conditions of stress and has multiple effects on the body. One of them is to break down protein in muscle, and in so doing this helps to release amino acids that can be metabolized for energy. Cortisol is critical in animals during phase 3 starvation for if the adrenal glands are removed, then the breakdown of protein is blocked, and the subsequent generation of energy needed for survival is reduced.[13] The steroids also have a role in awakening the animal and increasing its activity so that it can find food.

The other major characteristic of the foraging response is a rise in serum uric acid. As starvation progresses, muscle cells break down their proteins into amino acids that are released to provide energy. Two important amino acids that are released are glutamine and glutamate, both which have important roles in the synthesis of uric acid. Muscle breakdown also is associated with some release of DNA and RNA from the cells. DNA and RNA are nucleic acids and they become degraded. One of the major products of this degradation process is uric acid. The consequence of these events is that there is a marked rise in uric acid in the blood.[11,14]

An example of this foraging response can be seen with the Emperor Penguin. In the Antarctic summer the Emperor penguins becomes extremely fat from eating fish, squid and krill, and during this time they double their weight. The penguins then leave their feeding grounds and march inland for up to 60 miles (96 kilometers) to their breeding sites on the cold sea ice.[15] During their inland march, which can last a month, they are fasting the entire time. Once they arrive, the female lays the single egg. The male penguin then incubates the eggs by holding it between the top of its feet and its body while the female returns to the sea to obtain more food. For the next two months the male penguin sits quietly on the egg, fasting the entire time. During this time he is comfortable as he is living by burning his fat. Ketones are high in his blood, his activity is minimal, and he is just fine. However, once the fat stores get low, serum cortisol increases, protein degradation occurs, and the serum uric acid increases as much as 10-fold.[16] The penguin awakens, and starts making loud display songs to signal to its mate that she must return to help. For several days they may make these calls, and usually the female will arrive in time to take over incubating the egg, or to help feed the baby if it has just been born (which it does by regurgitating food or producing a milk-like material from the lining of the esophagus (crop milk). However, if the female does not arrive, the male penguin will abandon the egg to look for food.[16]

Another example is what happens to long-distance migrating birds. One of the most remarkable migrating birds is the bar-tailed godwit. The godwit holds the world record for long distance flight, with one documented to have flown 6,800 miles (11,000 kilometers) nonstop from Alaska to New Zealand! During flight these birds burn their fat stores for survival, and they also try to minimize their energy as best as they can by using tail winds and wind currents.[17] Many godwits breed in the Taymyr peninsula on the Arctic Ocean in northern Russia during the summer, and then they migrate 5,600 miles (9,000 kilometers) to Western Africa where they live in the mudflats of Mauritania during the winter. During this migration, they will stop over on Texel Island in the Wadden Sea in Germany, which is the approximate half-way point. Typically they will take 2.5 days to fly the 2,800 mile (4,500 kilometer) distance, and when the birds arrive they are exhausted and will stay for a month to refuel. When they arrive, some godwits still have some fat stores and ketones in their blood. Those birds that have depleted their fat stores are quite weak and have extremely high serum uric acid levels.[18]

In a related study, ten species of migrating birds (warblers, turtle dove, and flycatchers) were caught in the spring after flying at least 310 miles (500 kilometers) from their wintering sites in the Sahara to Ventotene Island off the coast of Italy. Again a relationship was shown between fat stores and serum uric acid. If fat stores were greater than 5 percent, then serum uric acid levels were low. In contrast, if fat stores were less than 5 percent, then there was evidence for protein degradation and serum uric acid and cortisol levels were high.[19]

A final example relates to the need of zoos to stimulate reproduction of their animals. As we discussed earlier, many animals time mating after they emerge from hibernation, as it is very difficult to maintain pregnancy when an animal drops its body temperature and metabolism during torpor. In zoos this has been a particular problem with snakes, as these animals may not hibernate at all when food is available year round. To help solve this problem, some zoo keepers have forced the snakes to go into hibernation by placing the reptiles in cold rooms for 12 to 16 weeks. This often leads to mating after they emerge from hibernation. However, studies have shown that some of these animals may be forced into hibernation without sufficient fat stores. While one would think that they should awaken once fat stores are depleted, some will not fully awaken until the room is rewarmed. Occasionally this can result in snakes that are near death with sky high levels of uric acid. In a few cases the uric acid has been so high that it has formed crystals in the internal organs (which is termed "visceral" gout). Snakes that get visceral gout are extremely sick and death is common.[20]

Are Cortisol and Uric Acid Clues for How Animals Get Fat?

A rise in serum cortisol and uric acid appear to be the two striking changes that occur when fat stores become depleted, and both correlate with the awakening of the animal and its immediate search for food ("foraging response"). Could these substances activate alarm signals to help the organism to survive, including stimulating the reaccumulation of fat and glycogen?

For cortisol, this is well established. Cortisol is a steroid released from the adrenal glands in periods of stress. It has numerous effects that suggest it is an alarm signal. It suppresses sleep, raises blood pressure and causes retention of salt and water, all features that help an animal survive when food, water and salt supplies are low. When steroids are given for a long time, or when there is a pituitary tumor in the body that stimulates excessive secretion of cortisol from the adrenal gland (a disease known as Cushing's syndrome), then fat accumulates, typified by abdominal obesity and the classic "buffalo hump" of fat between the shoulders, and in some individuals by the accumulation of fat in the liver.[21] Some individuals also develop high triglycerides in their blood, insulin resistance, hypertension and diabetes. Cushing's syndrome also causes glycogen accumulation in the liver of some animals such as cats and dogs,[22] although whether this also occurs in humans is less certain.

While cortisol would be considered a great candidate for driving the obesity epidemic, serum cortisol levels are not high in the average obese person. But what about uric acid? When most people hear the word uric acid, they think of the disease gout. Gout is a painful arthritis that commonly occurs in the big toe, but also can occur in other joints such as the knee and wrist. It is caused by uric acid crystals that deposit in the joint space and cause inflammation, resulting in red hot joints that are painful to touch, and is typically seen in people with high serum uric acid levels.

However, most people with gout are obese, insulin resistant and hypertensive. Furthermore, an elevated uric acid is also common in individuals with obesity and insulin resistance, and this was known since the original study by Kylin in 1923.[23] An elevated serum uric acid is so universal in these people that many authorities suggested an elevated serum uric acid should be considered a criteria for this syndrome. Even more striking, even if you are skinny and completely healthy, if you have an increased serum uric acid you have a remarkable risk for developing obesity, high blood pressure, fatty liver, and metabolic syndrome.[24-28] In other words, an elevated uric acid is not only common in obesity, but it also precedes and predicts its development.

Could uric acid activate the metabolic switch to make one fat?

CHAPTER 7

URIC ACID, AN "ENERGY CRISIS" SIGNAL THAT STIMULATES FAT ACCUMULATION

> *Uric acid was long considered important only as a cause of gout and kidney stones. Recent studies are challenging this concept, and suggest it may have a role in the stimulation of fat stores and insulin resistance.*

One can mourn the fatal love affair of Romeo and Juliet, but few stories compare with that of the midnight dance of the marine clam worm, *Platynereis dumerlii*. For six or seven months this worm lives its day to day life, eating algae and other vegetation in the shallow waters of the southern Pacific. When it is time to reproduce, it must perform a memorable but fatal act. Triggered by a change in a hormone from its brain, it quits eating, followed 3 or 4 days later by a complete disintegration of the gut. Unable to eat food, its fat stores become depleted and its uric acid levels rise. Its eyes enlarge, and it changes from its usual dull gray color to a beautiful lustrous yellow shade for the female and handsome crimson red for the male,[29] and then both leave their tubes on one enchanted evening, one week after the new moon, to meet at midnight just 6 inches under the ocean surface. Here swarms of males and females congregate, and when a male finds a female, he releases a pheromone that excites her, causing her to dance by swimming

47

rapidly in tight circles as the males swarm around her. At a climactic moment the female discharges her egg along with uric acid. In turn, the uric acid acts as an aphrodisiac (pheromone) for the male, causing an immediate release of sperm, thereby allowing the eggs to be fertilized. Shortly thereafter both the adult male and female die.[30]

This story is more than a love story—for it shows that uric acid is not simply a marker of the starvation state, but has biologic functions involved in survival and reproduction. Indeed, the concentration of uric acid that stimulates the release of sperm is 1/500th that of the mean concentration of uric acid in human blood.[30] Let us take a closer look at this molecule.

Uric acid and the RNA World

While carbohydrates, fats and proteins are important components of the cells that make up our body, the "brain" of the cell is made of nucleic acids. DNA is the nucleic acid that carries our genes, and RNA is the nucleic acid that directs the production of proteins. While DNA is the driver of most life today, those interested in the origins of life know that the earliest life forms existed solely as RNA, a time known as the RNA World.[31] RNA, or ribonucleic acid, consists of a helical structure containing specific nitrogen-rich compounds (called purine and pyrimidine bases) bound to the sugar ribose and phosphates. One of the unique aspects of this structure is that it can replicate itself, although imperfectly. By making occasional mistakes, it had the ability to evolve, and over hundreds of millions of years it was able to acquire additional features such as DNA, proteins, fats and carbohydrates that constitutes life as we know today.

The RNA World is long past, but some products of RNA-related molecules have carried over to life today. One of the most important is ATP, which is structurally related to RNA. ATP is the energy currency that the cell uses to perform its functions. It is so fundamental that it is used by all living organisms as their energy source. While some ATP is produced in the cytoplasm of the cell, today most of the energy is produced in specialized units in the cell called mitochondria. These mitochondria are energy factories that make ATP. In turn, the ATP drives chemical reactions in the cell by donating phosphate groups, which converts the ATP to ADP (adenosine diphosphate) and AMP (adenosine monophosphate).

The scientist Steven Benner has noted that simpler compounds exist by which an organism could donate phosphate to stimulate these chemical reactions.[32] However, the fact that all life uses ATP indicates that it had such a fundamental function in ancient times that it is still used by life today. In other words, it has been continuously used as the cell's source of energy for generations after generations, all the way back to the RNA World.

Life in the RNA World would also need tactics to survive when under attack. If an early RNA life form was injured, resulting in loss of some of its structure, what would be a better danger signal to the organism than one of its own degradation products? The major degradation product of nucleic acids is uric acid. As we shall see, recent studies suggest uric acid functions as a major alarm signal of the organism, telling it that the nucleic acids that drive all cell functions are under attack. Like ATP, uric acid likely represents a carryover from the RNA world and may have a survival role that is used by all living organisms.

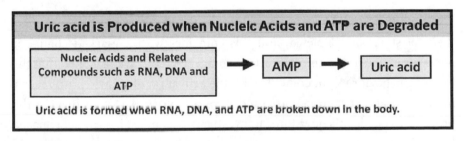

Uric acid is Produced when Nucleic Acids and ATP are Degraded

Nucleic Acids and Related Compounds such as RNA, DNA and ATP ➡ AMP ➡ Uric acid

Uric acid is formed when RNA, DNA, and ATP are broken down in the body.

Uric acid as a Waste Product that Causes Gout

Of course, most physicians do not know about the love affair of *Platynereis*, nor do they think about the RNA World. Rather, since uric acid is produced during the breakdown of nucleotides, many physicians have considered uric acid to be a waste product with little biologic function.[33-34] This belief was bolstered from the observation that some animals, like birds and reptiles, use uric acid as their principal way to rid themselves of nitrogen-containing wastes. Because uric acid has 4 nitrogen atoms per molecule, it is a more efficient way to rid nitrogen compared to urea (which has two nitrogens) and ammonia (which has one nitrogen). This explains why most freshwater fish excrete nitrogen as ammonia as they have plenty of water and can dilute their urine so that ammonia never reaches levels that are irritating to the tissues. In contrast, mammals including humans excrete most of their nitrogen as urea. Reptiles and birds, however, have to conserve water the most, and so they excrete their nitrogen as a chalky uric acid-rich precipitate in the form of bird droppings or guano.[33]

Since uric acid has been commonly viewed as a waste product,[34] few physicians measure it in patients, and the primary concern is that high blood levels can cause gout and kidney stones. As we mentioned in the last chapter, an elevated serum uric acid is extremely common in people who are obese, especially if they have fatty liver or are insulin resistant. A sentiment among many scientists, however, has been that this the elevation in uric acid is a consequence of obesity and insulin resistance, and is not playing a role in causing the obese state.[35] As we shall see, this viewpoint is likely to change.

Uric Acid: A Regulator of Fat Accumulation

Recall that there is a rise of uric acid in the blood of most animals once their fat stores are depleted, and this coincides with a marked change in behavior in which the animal starts to forage for food. We reasoned that this foraging behavior might coincide with the activation of a "switch" to reaccumulate fat, and that uric acid could have a biological role in driving this process. To tackle this question, an investigative team led by Miguel Lanaspa, Laura Gabriela (Gaby) Sánchez-Lozada, and Yuri Sautin performed a series of experiments that resulted in some startling findings.[36]

While the nucleic acids are the brains of the cell, it is the mitochondria that churn out the energy that runs the cell. Like a factory, mitochondria produce ATP, which runs the chemical reactions in the cell, generating heat (like the steam coming out of the power plant) and producing the energy that allows us to run, to eat, and even to think. Without ATP, the cell would shut down and eventually die.

The startling finding was that uric acid was found to affect these energy-producing factories.[36] Specifically, when Miguel and Gaby raised the uric acid levels inside cells, they could detect oxidative stress in the mitochondria. Oxidative stress is a process in which substances that contain oxygen are altered so they are highly chemically reactive with tissues, thereby damaging them or altering their ability to function. Smoking, for example, generates oxidative stress that damages the lung; the ultraviolet rays of the sun generate oxidants that damage skin and cause sunburn. In this case, uric acid causes oxidative stress in the mitochondria, injuring specific enzymes involved in energy production, and at high concentrations actually reducing the total number of mitochondria in the cell.

The way uric acid worked was clever. The oxidative stress induced by the uric acid specifically inhibited an enzyme that led to citrate accumulation, which is a substance that stimulates fat production. Uric acid also inhibited an enzyme required for the burning of fatty acids, leading to less ATP being produced. The net effect was to stimulate fat synthesis, reduce the burning of fat, and reduce energy (ATP) output! In other words, uric acid had altered the mitochondrial energy factories to preferentially convert the energy from food into fat as opposed to producing ATP. This would be an ideal way to replenish one's fat stores!

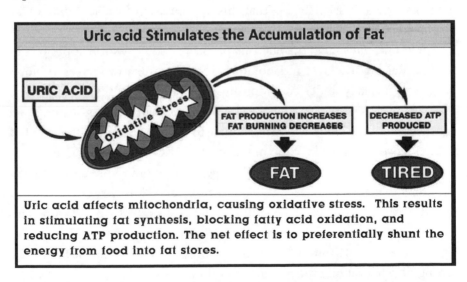

Uric acid Stimulates the Accumulation of Fat

URIC ACID

Oxidative Stress

FAT PRODUCTION INCREASES
FAT BURNING DECREASES

DECREASED ATP
PRODUCED

FAT

TIRED

Uric acid affects mitochondria, causing oxidative stress. This results in stimulating fat synthesis, blocking fatty acid oxidation, and reducing ATP production. The net effect is to preferentially shunt the energy from food into fat stores.

In a starving animal a rise in uric acid would help to maximize the reaccumulation of fat. Energy (ATP) is still being produced from food in the setting of high uric acid levels, but more of the energy from food is being put back into fat stores. While there is a relative reduction in the production of ATP in the setting of a high uric acid, this is good as it helps to keep the animal hungry, as a reduction in ATP in the liver signals the brain to encourage more food intake.[37-38] Food intake would increase, generating more ATP and at the same time increasing fat stores.

Uric Acid as a Survival Factor

In the last decade additional studies have uncovered other biological roles for uric acid that could have beneficial effects during the late stages of starvation. For example, uric acid may have a role in causing insulin resistance. Lowering uric acid improves insulin resistance in laboratory animals, and contrariwise, raising uric acid can increase insulin levels in models associated with insulin resistance.[39-42] Pilot studies in humans also suggest insulin resistance can be improved by lowering serum uric acid levels.[43] Recently, oxidative stress to the mitochondria has been identified as having a critical role in causing insulin resistance.[44-45] Since uric acid causes mitochondrial oxidative stress, it seems likely that this is the reason uric acid may cause insulin resistance.

An animal must also maintain its blood pressure to survive periods of famine. Raising uric acid in laboratory animals results in increased blood pressure, especially under conditions in which dietary salt is limited.[46] The rise in blood pressure was shown to be due to oxidative stress, leading to a constriction of the blood vessels.[47] Similar to insulin resistance, the target of the oxidative stress is likely the mitochondria.[48] Over time the rise in uric acid causes low grade injury to the kidney, resulting in the retention of salt (sodium) that further raises the blood pressure.[49] Thus a rise in uric acid would have great survival benefits by both raising blood pressure and increasing the blood pressure response to salt intake. These effects would protect the animal from a fall in blood pressure that could occur in the setting of dehydration or inadequate salt intake.[49]

A weakened animal must also heighten its immune and inflammatory systems to protect itself against predators or infections. Not surprisingly, uric acid stimulates the release of inflammatory proteins from cells, including the well-known marker, C-reactive protein.[50-51] Animals with high uric acid levels develop low-grade inflammation.[39,52] The immune system can also be activated by uric acid. For example, Ken Rock's group at the University of Massachusetts Medical School showed that when cells die, they release uric acid from the breakdown of nucleic acids that drives local inflammation as part of the immediate defense.[53-55] Uric acid also enhances the action of white blood cells that are important in fighting infection.[56-57] For example, uric acid stimulates the production of antibodies by B lymphocytes and activate other specialized white cells (T lymphocytes) that help clear infections.[58-60] In acute malaria, the release of uric acid from dying cells has a role in stimulating the inflammatory response to the malarial organisms.[61]

The rise in uric acid inside the cell is therefore a "call to arms" to stimulate local inflammation and the immune response to fight infection. However, the animal also needs to protect itself against the oxidative stress generated from toxins or the infectious organisms themselves. In this regard, uric acid, while being an oxidant inside the cells, acts as an antioxidant outside the cell.[62] The ability for uric acid to neutralize external oxidative stress while at the same time activating the immune system allows for a doubly effective way to combat infection.

Finally, an important aspect of survival is the "fight-and-flight response," in which, the animal heightens its response to danger. In this regard, uric acid may act as a neurostimulant, similar to the structurally similar compound, caffeine.[63] Acutely raising uric acid in rats results in increased physical activity and raises adrenaline (norepinephrine) levels in certain regions of the brain, both which are desired features that occur when an animal is endangered.[64-65] As we shall see later, the potential benefits of uric acid on brain function is definitely short lived. Nevertheless, for an animal trying to survive, a rapid increase in uric acid has many potential benefits.

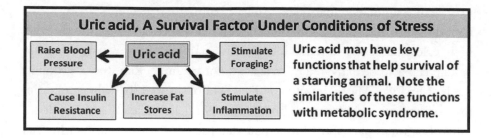

Uric acid, A Survival Factor Under Conditions of Stress

Raise Blood Pressure ← Uric acid → Stimulate Foraging?

Cause Insulin Resistance   Increase Fat Stores   Stimulate Inflammation

Uric acid may have key functions that help survival of a starving animal. Note the similarities of these functions with metabolic syndrome.

Specific Examples of Uric acid as a Survival Factor

The evidence that uric acid is simply a waste product of metabolism no longer seems tenable. Many studies in other animals show that uric acid drives important biological reactions. Recall the female clam worm, *Platynereis,* that secretes uric acid as a way to signal sperm release from its mate so the egg can be fertilized even as the female worm is dying. Uric acid is also important for crayfish and mollusks, where it binds blood cells (hemocyanin) and alters how easily they release oxygen. When oxygen content is low, such as in stagnant water, uric acid levels rise and increase oxygen release from the blood of the crayfish, thereby helping increase oxygen delivery to the tissues so the crayfish can survive.[66-67] In certain bacteria, uric acid can also regulate the expression of genes involved in survival.[68-70]

Uric acid may also be involved in the stress response in insects. While humans release adrenaline, insects release a related substance called octopamine.[71] Both octopamine and uric acid increase in insects during stress and may be interrelated. A great example is the firefly. Fireflies use octopamine to spark their light (bioluminescence) while they use uric acid crystals to reflect the light.[72] The light of the firefly was likely used initially to scare off predators, but over time has evolved as a means for courting and mating. Certainly the relationship between octopamine and uric acid needs to be better defined. However, it is interesting that the enzyme that generates uric acid may also have a role in helping convert dopamine to octopamine (as well as norepinephrine) in the brain.[73]

Summary

To conclude, uric acid should be viewed as a "mayday" signal by the animal under conditions of starvation or stress.[74] Uric acid functions by acting on the mitochondria energy factories where it causes oxidative stress and disrupts energy metabolism. The result is an increase in fat accumulation, insulin resistance, a rise in blood pressure, the stimulation of inflammation and activation of the immune system. These findings are similar to what animals undergo when they activate the switch to maximize fat storage. These findings may also remind you of the metabolic syndrome that affects over one fourth of the American population today.

So this raises important questions. If uric acid is involved in fat accumulation, is there evidence that uric acid levels cycle in animals in which obesity is tightly regulated? Could uric acid be involved in the metabolic switch that animals use to become fat or lean?

CHAPTER 8

TURNING THE OBESITY SWITCH
ON AND OFF

Hibernating squirrels show evidence for a fat switch, in which they convert from a fat accumulating period during summer to a fat burning period during winter. Can we figure out how this switch works?

If a fat switch exists, it would probably be easiest to find in an animal that hibernates. Many hibernating mammals have been studied, including prairie dogs, marmots, the arctic ground squirrel, the Oriental hedgehog, and Syrian hamsters. However, the one we studied is the 13-line ground squirrel (*Ictidomys tridecemlineatus*), which is also known as the striped gopher and happens to be the namesake for the University of Minnesota Gophers, my medical school alma mater.

All of these mammals are true hibernators and show similar patterns. During the summer and fall they gain significant amounts of weight, with up to a 50 percent increase over their spring weight by the time they are ready to hibernate. Most of the increase in weight is due to the accumulation of fat. Basal metabolic rate also decreases in late summer which results in a relatively greater gain in weight and fat for the amount they eat.[75] Animals also become insulin resistant and leptin resistant during this time.

Sometime in the late fall, the animals initiate hibernation by dropping their metabolic rate further and by quitting eating, and over a period of hours they drop their body temperature and go into a deep sleep.[76] The body temperature approaches freezing temperatures (approximately 4 degrees centigrade), and heart rate and respirations become almost imperceptible. The animal may appear dead, but it is alive and survives by slowly burning its fat stores.

Hibernating mammals do not stay in torpor for the entire winter, but rather undergo intermittent arousals in which their body warms up for 10 to 12 hours. The reason for these "interbout arousals" is not known, but it may be to aid the animal in excreting its metabolic wastes as during deep torpor the kidney function ceases.

Uric acid, Hibernation, and the Fat Switch

The sudden switching from a fat accumulating, leptin and insulin resistant obese animal to one that is burning fat is driven by a change in metabolism. The triggering event remains a mystery; while it was originally thought to be due to falling outside temperatures and decreased food availability, studies have shown this is not required.[77] We also know that the decrease in metabolism is the initiating event, and the fall in body temperature follows.[76] Whatever, the process, it does look like a switch has been triggered.

The question, of course, was what could be causing this switch. We knew, as we had discussed in the last chapter, that uric acid could be involved, for we had found that it can cause both fat accumulation and insulin resistance in experimental studies in laboratory animals. There was also suggestive evidence that uric acid might be important in hibernation in the literature, as some studies had reported that uric acid levels tend to be higher in late summer and then fall as animals enter hibernation, only to rise again when they emerge from hibernation in the spring.[78-81]

However, it is not the *serum* uric acid that causes fat accumulation, but rather the uric acid levels *inside* the cell, for we had found that the way uric acid causes fat accumulation is by causing oxidative stress to the mitochondria, and the latter are located inside the cell. Since one of the main sites where fat is both made and burned is the liver, our attention focused on this organ. To our delight, there were already studies that reported that both the 13-line ground squirrel and the arctic squirrel had a dramatic decrease in liver uric acid levels during the time they were hibernating.[80,82] A fall in liver uric acid could theoretically explain a switch in a hibernating animal from a period in which one is accumulating fat to one in which one is burning fat!

In the previous chapter we discussed how uric acid is produced from the breakdown of nucleic acids such as RNA and DNA, or related compounds such as ATP. One of the early breakdown products is AMP. AMP, however, is quite a versatile molecule, and can be further broken down to uric acid, or can be reutilized by other enzymes. If AMP is metabolized by the enzyme, AMP deaminase, which we will call AMPD, the AMP is degraded, eventually producing uric acid. According to our data, the uric acid would then stimulate fat accumulation by both stimulating fat synthesis and blocking the degradation of fat. However, if AMP is metabolized by the enzyme AMP kinase, or AMPK, an opposite effect occurs. Specifically, the activation of AMPK stimulates the utilization of fat by blocking fat synthesis and stimulating fatty acid oxidation. We therefore realized that AMP could sit at the fulcrum where it could be used to stimulate fat accumulation (via AMPD) or fat burning (via AMPK).

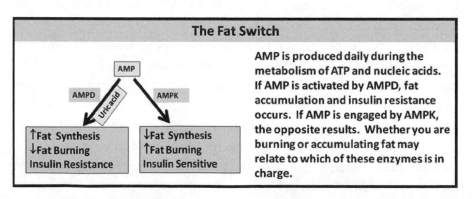

The Fat Switch

AMP is produced daily during the metabolism of ATP and nucleic acids. If AMP is activated by AMPD, fat accumulation and insulin resistance occurs. If AMP is engaged by AMPK, the opposite results. Whether you are burning or accumulating fat may relate to which of these enzymes is in charge.

To test the importance of this fat switch, Miguel Lanaspa from our group took cultured human liver cells and genetically modified them so that they either had very high or very low levels of AMPD. When AMPD was high, uric acid increased inside the cells and fat accumulated due to a block in fat oxidation. AMPK was also inhibited. In contrast, when AMPD was reduced in the liver cells, AMPK became dominant and fat levels fell.[83]

We then collaborated with Dr. Sandy Martin and her colleague, Elaine Epperson. Sandy is a world expert on hibernating mammals and particularly the 13-line ground squirrel. Sandy provided us with liver samples that had been collected from these squirrels at different times of the year. During the summer the livers of the squirrels were actively producing fat. Fat synthesis was stimulated, fat oxidation was low, and the livers showed high AMPD activity and uric acid levels and low levels of active AMPK. However, when the animals hibernated, the exact opposite was observed; AMPK activity was high, AMPD activity and uric acid levels were low, and fat oxidation was high.[84]

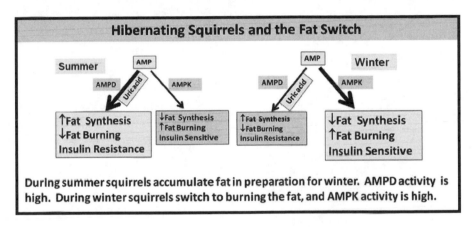

During summer squirrels accumulate fat in preparation for winter. AMPD activity is high. During winter squirrels switch to burning the fat, and AMPK activity is high.

We should state right now that we do not know for certain whether the fat accumulation in squirrels is truly driven by the changes in these two enzymes, although the data is suggestive. We also do not know if this is a universal fat switch. It is interesting, however, that some parallels may be observed in other species, including insects. For example, it is known that serum uric acid levels are high in insects during the larval phase when they are actively increasing their fat content.[85] Once the larva is mature, it will quit eating and look for a place to make a cocoon (wandering phase), and during this time the uric acid production stops and uric acid levels fall in the blood and accumulate in specialized cells in the fat body.[86] Once the pupa is formed, the insect lives off its fats stores, and uric acid remains undetectable in the blood. However, just like the squirrel in which uric acid rises at the end of hibernation, so does uric acid also increase in the blood towards the end of the pupa phase just before the adult insect emerges from the cocoon.[87]

If we have discovered the fat switch that can convert someone from fat accumulating to fat burning, then this raises two key questions. Could humans have activated this switch, and if so, how? That humans may have activated this switch is suggestive, for it is well known that people with obesity and diabetes have low AMPK activity. In fact, the number one drug used to treat diabetes is metformin, which works by inhibiting AMPD and stimulating AMPK.[88] But if we have activated this switch, how could this have happened?

CHAPTER 9

FRUCTOSE, A MASTER DRIVER OF THE FAT SWITCH

> *Fructose, a sugar present in fruits, honey, and table sugar, is the master of all foods in its ability to cause fat accumulation and insulin resistance.*

Every spring tropical rains fall heavily on the Amazon basin, causing the Amazon River to rise and swell. The floods are predictable, and peak in early summer. During this time, the Amazon rises from 20 to 60 feet and floods as much as 27,000 to 116,000 square miles (70,000 to 300,000 square kilometers) of the rainforest.[89-90] As the forest floods, as many as 200 types of fruit-eating fish migrate into the inundated forest searching for food. Here, the trees have timed their fruiting to drop their ripe, succulent fruit into the water, creating a water orchard for the fish. One of the fruit-eating fish is the Pacu, which looks like a piranha but is larger and toothless. The Pacu ingests as much fruit as it can, which benefits the fruit trees as the fish excrete the seeds and thereby help disperse the seeds throughout the forest. In turn, the Pacu convert the sweet fruits into fat which it stores as oils in its liver and tissues. In one study the average fat content of the Pacu reached 28 percent of its weight during the flood.[90] As the waters recede, the Pacu returns to the low water, where food is scarce. During this time the Pacu may not eat for as long as six months, and it survives by living off its fat. By the end of the dry season the fat content of the Pacu may drop to 10 percent or less of its overall weight. With the next coming of the floods, the cycle recurs again, providing a delicate ecological balance that helps both the fish and the trees.

The Pacu fish uses sweet fruits as a means for increasing their fat content. This may challenge your thinking, for we have all been taught that fruits are healthy and good to eat. After all, they contain many wonderful nutrients, including antioxidants such as vitamin C, flavenols, potassium, and fiber. Fruit diets have even been proposed as a way to lose weight. However, not all fruit is the same. The types of fruits humans prefer is often the tart, slightly sweet fruit that has not fully ripened, and is high in vitamin C content and only modestly sweet. As fruit ripens, the sugar content increases while the levels of vitamin C fall.[91] Most animals prefer mature, ripened fruit over immature fruit, as this is the best way to put on fat.

The Pacu fish is not alone in preferring fruit as a means for increasing fat stores. To prepare for hibernation, bears increase their body fat in the fall. One of their favorite sources of food is fruit, especially mature fruit rich in sugar content.[92] The Japanese black bear eats fruits in the autumn, often consisting of huge amounts at one time. American black bears rely on fruits as the main staple in their diet in late autumn and fall, where it can make up 38 to 91 percent of their total diet.[93] In these bears, fruit ingestion can be massive. One bear scat, for example, contained over 60,000 Oregon grape seeds, consistent with the bear eating approximately 10,000 individual fruits within a 24 hour period.[93] While this latter fruit is relatively sour, its sugar content increases dramatically after a frost. Bears that live in warm climates also eat fruit to help to survive during the dry season. The Sloth bear of India likes honey and fruit, the latter of which makes up the majority of its diet during the dry season. Sun bears from Borneo love to eat fruit and honey-rich bee hives. These bears will remain with a fruited tree until all of the fruits have been eaten.[94] Captive bears also prefer ripened fruit. Many carnivores including bears, martens, raccoons, and foxes also eat fruits when they are available, primarily in autumn and early winter.[95] In addition to helping increase fat stores, the ingestion of fruits by carnivores such as bear and martens help with seed dispersal, similar to that observed with birds and the Pacu fish.

Birds also love fruit as a means for increasing their fat content. The migrating European Garden warbler will switch from an insect-based diet in the early spring to fruits in the autumn, which helps stimulate the accumulation of fat and development of insulin resistance prior to their migrations.[96] When they switch to fruit, the warblers reduce their basal metabolic rate by as much as 30 percent and also eat more food than they would otherwise normally do.[96]

Orangutans also crave fruit and will travel long distances to find it. When they do, they will go on a feeding binge, eating as many ripe fruit as they can and as rapidly as they can. Anthropologist Cheryl Knott showed that this was a major way these animals increase their body fat, and this helps them survive during subsequent months when food is less plentiful.[97]

Fructose as an Activator of the Fat Switch

All of these studies suggest that there is something special about ripe fruits that can increase fat content. Our studies suggest that it is fructose. Fructose is the primary sugar present in fruit, and is also present in honey, where it makes up 40 percent of the weight. Another source of fructose is sucrose, or table sugar. Sucrose is made up of fructose and glucose bound together. While sucrose is present in sugarcane and sugar beets, it is also present in the nectar of flowers that insects and hummingbirds drink, in saps of the palm and maple tree, as well as certain grasses such as the sweet sorghum (Guinea corn). One other source of fructose for humans is high fructose corn syrup, in which corn is chemically treated to generate a sweetener that contains both fructose and glucose.

To most observers, fructose and glucose might be considered similar. Both are "simple sugars" of approximately the same molecular weight, and both can be metabolized to produce glycogen and triglycerides. One distinct difference is that glucose is the primary sugar in the circulation and is regulated by insulin. However, as a food source they are commonly viewed as equivalent, as each sugar produces approximately 4 calories per gram. Nevertheless, numerous studies, especially in laboratory animals, have shown that fructose is much more effective at stimulating fat accumulation in the blood, liver, and fat tissues, as well causing insulin resistance when compared to glucose or starch (which consists of multiple glucose molecules).[98-100] This is true even when laboratory animals are fed the exact same number of calories.[40,101] In this case, the fructose-fed rats always develop worse features of metabolic syndrome.

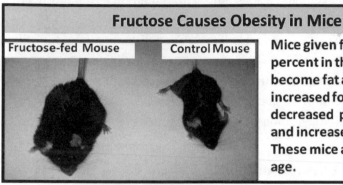

Fructose Causes Obesity in Mice

Fructose-fed Mouse   **Control Mouse**

Mice given fructose (30 percent in the water) become fat and have increased food intake, decreased physical activity and increased fat mass. These mice are the same age.

Why would glucose and fructose be different in how they stimulate fat synthesis? When glucose is metabolized, the cell remains healthy and ATP levels increase. However, a unique feature of fructose is that there is a transient period of time during its metabolism when ATP levels plummet inside the cell. This paradoxical effect in which energy levels fall inside the cell with feeding of a nutrient is distinctly unusual. However, it occurs because the first enzyme in fructose metabolism, fructokinase, consumes ATP while it metabolizes fructose, and it does this as rapidly and uncontrollably as a runaway train. This process not only generates AMP but also activates AMPD, and intracellular uric acid accumulates.[102]

We have done a number of studies to show that this is the major mechanism by which fructose causes fat accumulation. Similar to what we had seen earlier, the activation of AMPD was found to increase fat by a process involving uric acid generation and the development of oxidative stress. Furthermore, Miguel Lanaspa from our group was able to show that he could largely block fat accumulation in response to fructose by specifically blocking different parts of this pathway.[83,84] In other words, if he blocked the activation of AMPD or the accumulation of intracellular uric acid the increase in fat was largely prevented, despite the fact that the fructose was still being metabolized. This provided strong evidence that it is not the calories from fructose that is causing the fat accumulation, but rather the activation of the AMPD fat switch.

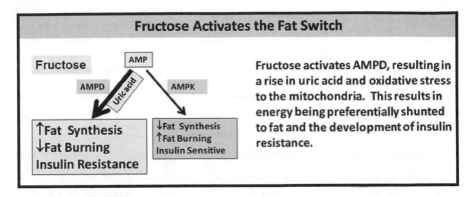

Fructose Activates the Fat Switch

Fructose activates AMPD, resulting in a rise in uric acid and oxidative stress to the mitochondria. This results in energy being preferentially shunted to fat and the development of insulin resistance.

Fructose Induces All Features of the Metabolic Syndrome

We and others have found that fructose induces every feature of metabolic syndrome in rats, including visceral obesity, elevated serum triglycerides, low HDL cholesterol, elevated blood pressure, and insulin resistance.

Fructose also stimulates increased food intake. One mechanism may be due to its sweetness, as fructose stimulates the release of dopamine in the brain where it induces a pleasure response. Repeated administration of sugar to rats can result in symptoms suggestive of addiction, and there is some evidence that it may lead to generalized food addiction.[103] We will discuss this more in a later chapter. The other mechanism by which fructose stimulates food intake relates to leptin. Recall that leptin is the hormone released from fat cells that tells the brain to quit eating. Unfortunately, studies by Peter Havel's group has shown that drinks rich in fructose do not stimulate the release of leptin as effectively as glucose based drinks, and this can translate into a lesser sensation of satiety and the intake of more food.[104] In addition to not stimulating leptin release in response to food, our group also found that rats fed fructose become leptin resistant.[105] This means that even if leptin is released, it will not effectively tell the brain to quit eating, and as a result one will eat more calories than one needs.

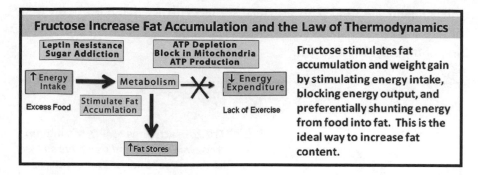

Fructose Increase Fat Accumulation and the Law of Thermodynamics

Fructose stimulates fat accumulation and weight gain by stimulating energy intake, blocking energy output, and preferentially shunting energy from food into fat. This is the ideal way to increase fat content.

Summary

Fructose is distinct from other foods in that it activates the fat switch that preferentially shunts the food we eat into fat. By activating the switch, obesity results from both an increase in food intake and a decrease in physical activity. The law of thermodynamics holds. However, unlike classical thinking, obesity occurring in response to fructose is not due to the animal choosing to eat too much or deciding to exercise too little. Rather, the switch is signaling the animal to eat too much and to exercise too little.

For animals, the ability to increase one's fat content is critical for survival. The king of fructose is the hummingbird which lives off nectar as its primary food. As mentioned earlier, these birds will ingest so much sugar that they increase their fat content to 40 percent of their total body weight and develop the fattest liver of all birds.[106-107] They also develop high serum triglycerides and elevated blood sugar. When they get this fat, it allows them to migrate the 600-mile journey across the Gulf of Mexico without stopping. However, it is also very easy for these birds to deplete their fat stores due to their remarkably high metabolic rate.

This latter point raises an interesting question. What defense measures can animals do when ripe fruits and other foods are not available? One way may be by finding ways to amplify the switch. In the next chapter, we will learn about two major mutations that occurred in our past that helped us amplify the switch during periods of food shortage. Unfortunately, these very mutations may explain why we are so susceptible to obesity and diabetes today.

CHAPTER 10

GENETIC REASONS WHY HUMANS ARE PRONE TO OBESITY

> *Humans are double knockouts, meaning they lost two genes. One gene controlled uric acid metabolism and the other controlled vitamin C synthesis. We believe the loss of these two genes may explain why humans are susceptible to becoming obese and diabetic.*

One might not think that the cause of obesity today may have its origins million of years ago. Yet I believe that the story of obesity may be traced back to the early Miocene. It was at that time, approximately 20 to 23 million years ago, when the earliest apes are found. These apes represented a milestone in evolution, for unlike the monkeys that preceded them, they had larger skulls, weighed over 20 pounds, and lacked tails. They also had broad chests, mobile hips and strong grasping feet. While their brains were still small, approximating one-eighth the size of a human brain, apes such as *Proconsul* still represented an advance over earlier primates.[108-109]

The earliest apes lived in East Africa where they lived in trees and dined on ripe fruits. It was an ideal time for these apes, and in the course of 4 to 5 million years at least 14 new species appeared. Then a change began, subtle at first, but with an impact that carries to this day. The climate began to cool, possibly due to increased volcanic activity in the Rift Valley. The polar ice caps expanded and sea levels fell, and a land bridge formed that allowed animals to escape out of Africa. Around 16 to 17 million years ago many animals made the crossing, including ancient giraffes, rhinos, and elephants, as well as pigs, antelopes, and even aardvarks.[109]

Among the newcomers to Eurasia were the apes. Initially they were able to continue to eat their diet of ripe fruits all year long. But as global cooling continued, the tropical rainforests began to disappear. The apes living in Europe retreated, forming isolated colonies where they tried to survive the changing environment. As temperatures became cooler and more seasonal, there became a relative lack of fruit during the colder months. The anthropologist, Mark Skinner, found evidence that apes (*Dryopithecus*) that lived in an isolated colony in Valles Penedes, Spain were undergoing periods of intermittent starvation as noted by the presence of telltale signs on the teeth.[110] Kelley and colleagues showed similar evidence of seasonal stress in dental specimens from *Kenyapithecus*, a different ape found in Turkey during this time.[111]

With a reduction in fruit availability, the primates expanded their diet to include "fallback" foods such as roots and tubers, and this required both stronger teeth (thicker enamel) and the ability to leave the trees, stimulating early "knuckle walking." Being able to travel longer distances and to improve foraging skills became critical for survival. Certain apes, such as *Dryopithecus*, developed changes in its spinal column that allowed them to stand upright.[112] True walking (bipedalism), however, did not occur until later in history. Despite these adaptations, conditions worsened, and by 8 million years ago there were no more apes in Europe.[113]

Evidence for Starvation Among Miocene Apes

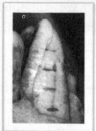 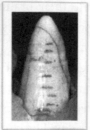

Evidence for episodic starvation can be determined by examining canine teeth from apes during the period that the tooth is growing. The presence of repetitive striations reflects periods of starvation in which the enamel could not adequately develop. Skinner used this method to show that the *Dryopithecus* apes from Valles Penedes, Spain, that lived in the mid-Miocence were undergoing periodic starvation.

Canines from Modern Orangutan With Repetitive Linear Enamel Hypoplasia

Photographs from Am J Phys Anthro 2004;123: 216-235, with permission of John Wiley and Sons

The Back to Africa Hypothesis

The extinction of apes in Europe may appear like the end of another chapter in the evolution of species, another dead end in biology. But this is no longer considered to be true, for there is evidence that some of these apes made it back to Africa before the great extinctions, and these apes may be the ancestors of not only the chimpanzee and gorilla, but also of man.[114] Peter Andrews, an anthropologist from the Museum of Natural History in London, found evidence that one such ape, *Kenyapithecus*, returned to Africa by 14 million years ago.[115] David Begun, another well-known anthropologist from the University of Toronto, argued based on skeletal features that *Dryopithecus* must have travelled back to Africa, perhaps 9 or 10 million years ago, to become the common ancestor of humans and great apes.[116]

A "Thrifty Gene" is Acquired by Starving Apes in Europe

In the first chapter we mentioned the Thrifty Gene Hypothesis, which was proposed by the anthropologist James Neel in the early 1960s. Neel suggested that during periods of famine, our ancestors may have acquired genes that would favor the accumulation of fat. Neel stated that while this would have been a survival factor at that time, it might increase our susceptibility to obesity and diabetes in the setting where food is plentiful.[117]   While this hypothesis received a lot of initial attention, the inability to identify thrifty genes has led to skepticism over whether this hypothesis is true.[118]

This changed when anthropologist Peter Andrews and I proposed that such a thrifty gene may have had a role in the survival of apes in Europe during the mid-Miocene.[119] Indeed, it was around 15 million years ago when a mutation occurred in ancestral humans that affects the way we metabolize uric acid. In most mammals, uric acid levels are low due to an enzyme, uricase, which degrades uric acid, eventually generating allantoin. However, humans and all great apes lost uricase due to a mutation, and as such humans and great apes have higher uric acid levels.

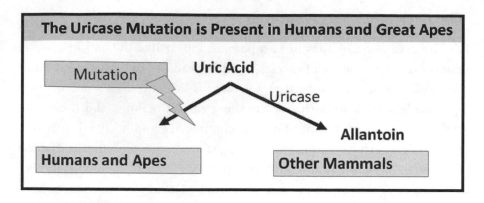

The Uricase Mutation is Present in Humans and Great Apes

One of the consequences of not having uricase is that the uric acid response to fructose is markedly enhanced.[120] Since uric acid has such an important role in how fructose causes fat accumulation, the uricase mutation should amplify the ability of fructose to induce obesity and fat accumulation. Consistent with this hypothesis, Gaby Sánchez-Lozada from our group showed that blocking uricase in rats could enhance the ability of fructose to increase serum triglycerides, insulin resistance, blood pressure, and fatty liver.

A more elegant way to determine the effect of having early apes lose their uricase is to resurrect the extinct uricase and directly test how it affects fructose metabolism. While this may sound impossible, one can use computer modeling to resurrect extinct genes.[121] Recently Eric Gaucher, a leader in such techniques, generated several of these extinct ape uricases for us. Miguel Lanaspa then compared the effects of fructose on human cells that either lacked uricase or that expressed the ancestral ape uricase. As expected, the human cells that lacked uricase showed a greater uric acid response with more triglyceride accumulation in response to fructose. In some respects this provided direct evidence in support of the thrifty gene hypothesis. However, in this case the "thrifty gene" is not the acquisition of a new gene, but rather the loss of an old gene.

Peter Andrews and I proposed that the uricase mutation likely occurred in Europe, for it was here that such a mutation would have provided a survival advantage since European apes were faced with seasonal food shortage. In Africa the effects of global cooling were to cause a retraction of the rainforests but not their elimination, and so primate populations likely fell but fruit remained available all year long. However, once the apes returned to Africa, they may have had advantages that help the European apes to gradually replace their African cousins. Not only had they learned additional skills such as knuckle walking, but the ability to enhance their fat stores could have provided advantages during intermittent famines.

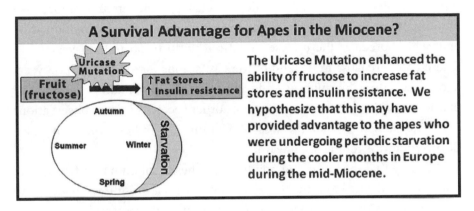

A Survival Advantage for Apes in the Miocene?

The Uricase Mutation enhanced the ability of fructose to increase fat stores and insulin resistance. We hypothesize that this may have provided advantage to the apes who were undergoing periodic starvation during the cooler months in Europe during the mid-Miocene.

The uricase mutation is not specific to great apes and humans, as the lesser apes (gibbons and siamangs) also lost uricase outside of Africa during the same time period, somewhere on their journey to eastern Asia. It is likely that the mutation provided similar survival advantages for these apes. Reptiles and birds also have high uric acid levels due the loss of uricase in a common ancestor approximately 200 million years ago, around the time of the Triassic-Jurassic extinction in which nearly 50 percent of all land species died.[122] It seems likely that birds and reptiles also used the uricase mutation to help maintain fat stores similar to what we observed in mammals. In addition, the uricase mutation may help these species conserve water, as they excrete their nitrogen wastes in the form of precipitates of uric acid.[33,123]

The Loss of Vitamin C: Another Thrifty Gene?

Just as the loss of uricase may have been a way to improve fat stores, another important substance is vitamin C. Vitamin C is an antioxidant and is made by most animals and plants. Some studies suggest that vitamin C synthesis began during the Permian where it helped to block the effects of high oxygen levels that occurred in the atmosphere at that time.[124-125] However, the ability to synthesize vitamin C was subsequently lost in a wide variety of species, including salmon, the fruit-eating bat, the Red-vented Bulbul bird, and a variety of songbirds (a subset of passerine birds).[126]

Most primates, with the exception of lemurs, also lost the ability to make vitamin C. Because the tarsier, which is related to the lemur, cannot make vitamin C, one can date the mutation to approximately 58 to 63 million years ago, which predates the uricase mutation by 40 to 50 million years.[127-128] These dates are close to the end of the Cretaceous Period (65 million years ago), when the Chicxulub asteroid crashed into the Atlantic, causing the extinction of the dinosaurs and multiple other species.[129] These observations raise the possibility that the loss of vitamin C synthesis may have also occurred during a time of upheaval.[130]

I believe that the loss of our ability to synthesize vitamin C enhanced the fat switch and acted as a thrifty gene. There is a lot of indirect evidence to support opposing roles of fructose and vitamin C. For example, vitamin C can partially block the effects of fructose to induce metabolic syndrome in animals.[131] Vitamin C also lowers serum uric acid levels and blocks mitochondrial oxidative stress.[132-133] Vitamin C levels are also low in individuals with obesity and diabetes, and some studies suggest the administration of vitamin C can lower blood pressure and improve the oxidation (burning) of fat. Furthermore, as fruits ripen, fructose content increases whereas vitamin C levels decrease. In animals that make vitamin C, fructose inhibits vitamin C synthesis.[134] Vitamin C is also high in the hibernating mammal during the winter when fat is being oxidized, but falls as the animal emerges from hibernation in association with rises in uric acid.[81,135]

Other Thrifty Genes

Additional thrifty genes are being identified. One may have occurred as late 10,000 years ago when agriculture was being introduced. For sure, the ability to grow vegetables and to domesticate animals improved the chances to avoid periods of famine, and represented a major advance in civilization.

However, one problem was that this forced humans to eat new types of food. One of these was starch, which is the principal carbohydrate stored in many plants. Starch consists of many polymers of glucose and requires an enzyme (amylase) to degrade it so that it can be absorbed.

Recently it was discovered that many humans living in farming populations carry a more active form of amylase compared to populations that subsist by hunting and gathering.[136] The higher activity of this enzyme is due to the duplication of the amylase gene and results in more rapid and efficient digestion of starch. This change is specific for humans and is not seen in chimpanzees and other apes that have continued to live the same way as they did millions of years ago. Unlike the mutations associated with uricase and vitamin C, however, not all humans share the same genetic changes, but rather the alterations in amylase represent a recent change which is still taking over the population.

Summary

Thus, all humans are double knockouts, meaning they lack two important genes. We lack uricase so we have higher uric acid levels. We lack the ability to make vitamin C so we tend to have lower levels of vitamin C than most animals. These mutations enhanced our ability to survive famine, and enhanced our ability to increase fat in response to our original major food source, fruit. However, as we moved from being a fruit-eating species to one that was a hunter-gatherer, and then to an agricultural society, we had a major surprise coming. A sweet surprise, one could say. For the discovery of sugarcane placed us in the perfect storm to become fat and diabetic.

SECTION 3

THE RISE OF SUGAR AND THE FATTENING OF MAN

CHAPTER 11

SUGAR FOR THE RICH

The earliest sources of fructose were from fruit and honey. Later, sugarcane was introduced in India and spread throughout the world. In these early days only the rich could afford sugar, and only the rich developed obesity, diabetes, and gout.

During the age of the monkeys (Eocene and Oligocene) and the age of the apes (Miocene), genetic mutations occurred in vitamin C and uric acid metabolism, respectively, that enabled us to generate and store increased amounts of fat from the fructose present in ripe fruits. As evolution progressed, modern humans arose in Africa, approximately 200,000 years ago, and with this came changes in diet, beginning with a hunter-gatherer society which changed over time to one that was agriculturally based. With these changes came new sources of fructose. One of the oldest and richest sources was honey.

The Discovery of Honey

Wild honey is sweet, delicious, and an excellent source of fructose, containing nearly 40 percent fructose by weight. Honey has been a venerated food source for thousands of years. Cave paintings from all over the world, including from Europe, India, South Africa and Australia have documented the honey hunters in their quest for the golden sweet treasure. Some of the oldest paintings date back to the Stone Age, 10,000 to 15,000 years ago. One famous painting, which is nearly 9000 years old, was found in a cave near Valencia, Spain and shows a person collecting honey from a hive located on a cliff. Similar honey hunting continues today in Nepal, where men obtain honey from hives in the steep cliffs, using fires lit below to smoke out the largest honey bees in the world so the hunters can obtain the honey safely.

Modern Day Honey Hunters

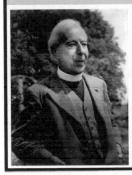

The Reverend Tickner Edwardes (1865-1944), "the bee-man of Burpham" of West Sussex, England, described ways for finding wild honey beehives. One way was to place a small saucer with honey in the woods until numerous honey bees started to feed. A wire mesh would be placed rapidly over the plate to catch the bees. One bee would then be let out. The bee would always fly upward to establish its bearings, and then fly towards the hive. The bee hunter would go to the spot where the bee was last seen, and repeat the procedure, letting another bee out. Eventually he would find the nest, usually in the hollow of a tree.
Photo generously provided by family.

For early humans honey must have been a special treat, for finding wild honey is not so easy and the amount a single hive produces is not so great. It is also not known with any certainty if early humans recognized that honey had survival properties by enhancing fat stores. However, there is some indirect evidence that would support this speculation. As mentioned in Chapter 4, some of the earliest art sculptures from Europe depict obese women, often with large breasts and vulva, so called "Venus" figurines. These figurines have been proposed to represent fertility or prosperity, and would be consistent with the importance of having sufficient fat stores for survival, especially in pregnancy. However, as we discussed earlier, becoming fat is not so simple, as it appears that one has to activate a metabolic switch to become fat. For hunter-gatherer societies this switch could be activated by eating ripe fruits, but of all natural foods, honey is the richest source of fructose, and if sufficient amounts were available, would have been the best way to help increase fat stores.

Some authorities have suggested that the Venus figurines of the Stone Age, and the "Mother Goddess" figurines of the later Bronze Age, are linked with the honey bee. Some sculptures and paintings found during these periods, such as the Neolithic settlement at Çatalhöyük in Turkey (6500 B.C.), refer to bees or honey. Other Venus figurines, such as the Venus of Willendorf (24,000-22,000 B.C., Austria) and the Venus of Kostenky (23,000-21,000 B.C., Russia) have hair that resembles beehives or, in the case of a particular Mother Goddess found in Hacilar, Turkey (7900 B.C.), actually wear a beehive as a tiara (www.thebeegoddess.com). This raises an admittedly wild speculation that science cannot answer—is it possible that early humans might have identified several young females in each tribe for whom they would provide the rare wild honey and ripe fruits as a means to fatten them to ensure that these individuals would be able to have successful pregnancies during unexpected periods of famine, thus allowing the survival of the clan? Recall that the Tunisians of the 1700s would fatten their fiancés prior to marriage[1] and how the explorer John Speke noted that King Rŭmanika would force fatten his wives.[2] Being fat assures sufficient fat stores during pregnancy, and providing wild honey to the young woman would be one of the best ways to ensure this would happen.

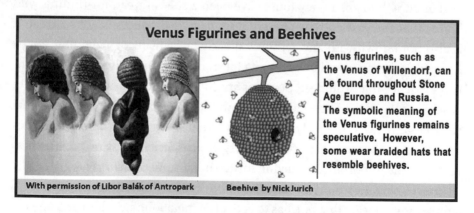

Venus Figurines and Beehives

Venus figurines, such as the Venus of Willendorf, can be found throughout Stone Age Europe and Russia. The symbolic meaning of the Venus figurines remains speculative. However, some wear braided hats that resemble beehives.

With permission of Libor Balák of Antropark   Beehive by Nick Jurich

While searching for wild beehives provides some honey, a breakthrough was the introduction of apiaries during the Bronze Age. The earliest documented apiaries are from ancient Egypt and date to the first dynasty, circa 2400 B.C.[3] Apiaries existed in Turkey as early as 1500 B.C. The Hittites, who lived in Anatolia (Turkey) during that period, viewed honey as a major valuable, and stealing of hives was associated with severe punishment.

Honey was also produced in Canaan where it was so famous that it is referred to in the bible as the "land of milk and honey." One of the earliest sites where apiaries have been found is Tel Rehov, a settlement in northern Israel (860-950 B.C.). Here 180 hives were found, with an estimated capability to produce 300 to 500 kilograms of honey per year.[4] Despite the fact that the number of beehives suggest that they supported more than one million bees, the hives were located in a densely populated area of the city. The archeologists speculated that because honey was so valuable that the hives were kept at this location.[4]

Ancient Egypt and Beekeeping

Honey was also produced in the Nile delta in Lower Egypt. The symbol of Lower Egypt was the bee, and the early Pharaohs were often referred to as the "bee kings." The honey was used not only to make honey cakes and a honey-based beer, but also as medicinals, as salves for wounds, and possibly in mummification. Honey was valuable enough that it was used as offerings for deities, given as royal gifts, or placed in tombs as offerings for the *ka*, or spirit that would arise from an individual after death. Pharaoh Ramesses III gave 15 tons of honey as offerings to the Nile God Hapi, in the 12th Century B.C.[5] Honey was also considered a spoil of war. Thutmose III, a Pharaoh from the 18th dynasty whose numerous victories in the Middle East and elsewhere are well recorded, collected 470 jars of honey as part of the spoils for taking Djahi in the Canaan.[6]

During this period honey was a food only for the nobility and wealthy. As is well known, sugar is strongly associated with the development of dental caries, and studies suggest it is the fructose component that is responsible.[7-8] It is therefore interesting that dental caries, which had been near absent in the Egyptian Predynastic Period, became prevalent among the wealthy and royalty of the Old Kingdom, and this accelerated in the New Kingdom.[9] In contrast, caries were rare or absent among the poor.[9]

Not surprisingly, obesity began to be observed in ancient Egyptians during the New Kingdom (1570-1069 B.C) where it also affected the wealthy and nobility. Several pharaohs, including Hatshepsut (1473-1458 B.C.), Amenhotep III (reigned 1386-1349 B.C., Dynasty XVIII) and Ramesses III (reigned 1182-1151, dynasty XX) were all obese as determined by the presence of excessive skin folds found on their mummies. Hatshepsut may have also had diabetes (see insert).

Queen Hatshepsut, Obese and Diabetic

When her husband, King Thutmose II, died prematurely, the throne passed to Thutmose III, son of King Thutmose II. Because he was a child, Queen Hatshepsut became the co-regent to oversee the Kingdom. However, after two years Hatshepsut proclaimed herself Pharaoh, stating it was her rightful claim as she was the daughter of the god, Amun-Re. For 13 years she ruled, dressed as a man including the wearing of a false beard.

Her mummy was discovered in 2007 by Zahi Hawass of the Egyptian Museum who matched a molar tooth found in a wooden box with Hatshepsut's name with a specific mummy. A CT scan of the mummy provided several surprises: despite statues showing her lean and vibrant, she was obese, with bad teeth, and likely had both diabetes and liver disease. Shown is a statue of Hatshepsut with her name in hieroglyphics flanked by "the sedge and the bee" which acclaims her as the Pharaoh of both Upper (Sedge) and Lower (Bee) Egypt.

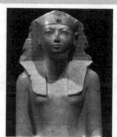

Metropolitan Museum of Art, NYC

Other Sources of Fructose: Grape Syrups and Sweetened Wines

Various sweeteners and drinks were also made from honey and fruit. For fruits that were only available during certain parts of the year, this practice allowed its preservation and year round use. For example, grape juice could be reduced and thickened to make fruit juices and syrups, and this practice was described in the Old Testament. The Romans were particularly fond of grape syrups. They would take freshly squeezed grape juice and heat them in large lead kettles, eventually reducing the volume to a sweet liquid that they would add to their foods. If the juice was reduced to half of its original volume, it was called *defrutum*, and if it was reduced to one-third its volume, it was called *sapa*. In addition to being a rich source of fructose, the lead acetate that would leach from the kettles also gave a sweet flavor (the flavor of lead sugar). Of interest, low levels of lead poisoning also increase uric acid levels, thereby activating the same pathways as fructose in causing obesity and diabetes. As such, this drink may have not only led to lead poisoning in ancient Rome[10] but may also have had a role in the obesity that occurred during this period. Indeed, while Hippocrates of Greece makes no mention of diabetes, the first reports from Europe were made by Aulus Cornelius Celsus (30 B.C.–50 A.D.) and by Aretaeus of Cappadocia (30-90 A.D.) in Rome during the time of Nero.[11] Gout also became prominent during this period and was also linked with the drinking of the lead-laden *sapa*.

Mead was another drink that was developed by fermenting honey with yeast. Mead was developed nearly 8000 years ago, possibly in Crete. Over time it became most popular in northern Europe where grapes were less available for producing wine. Indeed, mead was a popular drink among the Vikings and was considered the drink of the Norse gods. While the fermentation of honey would have likely eliminated much of the fructose, the mead was often supplemented with additional honey or fruit.

The Discovery of Sugar

Sugarcane is a tall grass that likely originated in India and New Guinea. There are six species of sugarcane, four of which are cultivated and two which are wild. The sweetest of the sugar canes, *Saccharum officinarum*, or "noble" cane, probably originated in New Guinea. However, India also had several indigenous sugar cane species and it is in India where the cultivation of sugarcane first began.

Sugarcane was probably harvested during the first millennium B.C. Soldiers in the military campaign led by Emperor Darius in 521 B.C. found that the local Indians were enjoying "reeds that provide honey without bees" that may represent some of the earliest reports of sugarcane. When Alexander the Great led his army into the Indus River valley in 326 B.C, his senior officer, Nearchus, also wrote that the local people were using extracts of the sugarcane as a sweetener.

Exactly how much sugar the local Indian people were eating is not known. They were also not initially making true sugar crystals from the cane, but were rather either chewing the cane or obtaining a sugar-rich liquid from boiled extracts. However, it is interesting that the earliest reports of obesity (*medoroga*), diabetes (*madhumeha or honey-urine*), and angina (*hrit-shoola*) were written by the Indian physician Sushruta. Sushruta lived in Banares (also known as Kashi) on the banks of the Ganges River in north-western India, perhaps around 300 to 500 A.D.[12] The region where he lived, known as the Uttar Pradesh, is currently one of the major regions in India producing the sugarcane. Other Indian physicians, such as Charaka (300 B.C), also wrote about diabetes. Both Sushruta and Charaka linked the development of diabetes with the ingestion of sweets. For example, Charaka attributed diabetes to being lazy, sleeping too much, and eating molasses, whereas Sushruta stated diabetes develops in the individual who follows "sedentary pursuits or is in the habit of taking sweet liquids or fat–making food."[13] According to Chunder Bose, Sushruta viewed madhumeha (or diabetes) as a condition " the rich principally suffer from, and is brought on by their overindulgence in rice, flour, and sugar. The patient feels weak and emaciated, and complains of frequent urination, thirst, and prostration. Ants flock around his urine" (due to the passage of glucose which makes it sweet).[14]

> **Obesity, diabetes and angina were first described in India and it was in India where sugar was introduced.**

The *Sushruta Samshita* contains the writings of Sushruta and has numerous references to sugarcane. The earliest version of this text dates to 300 to 400 A.D. so it is possible that much of the reference to sugar relates to this period. In this book sugar is referred to both as a food and as a medi-cine. The juice of the sugarcane was mixed with a wide variety of foods, including with honey, milk and rice to treat a variety of ailments. Sugar wine (Shakara Sidhu) is described as a drink "sweet in its taste, increases one's relish for food, is appetizing and diuretic. It subdues the deranged Váya and is exhilarating, sweet in digestion, and rouses up the sense organs." Treacle, which is the left over sucrose-rich syrup following the crystalliza-tion of sugar, is described as "sweet in taste . . . and increases fat . . . and corpulency . . ."[15]

The Spread of Sugar into China, Egypt and Europe

Sugar spread to China around 100 B.C., and by 200 A.D. diabetes is first being reported there by the famous Chinese physician, Tchang Tchong-king.[11] While knowledge of the sugarcane reached Greece as noted by Aristotle's pupil, Theophrastus (371 B.C.–287 B.C.), likely from the writings of Nearchus, there is very little evidence that sugar (sucrose) was available to early Greeks or Romans. The physician Galen (129-217 A.D.) mentions the existence of sugar which he stated came from India and Arabia Felix (the southern part of Arabia similar to present day Yemen).[16-17] During his career diabetes was still very rare, as he only saw two cases.[18]

Several hundred years later the sugarcane was introduced into Persia (500 to 700 A.D.). Obesity and diabetes were described a few hundred years later by two famous Persian physicians, Rhazes (also known as Muhammed ibn Zakaria Al-Razi , 865-925 A.D.) and Avicenna (980-1037 A.D.).[11,19] While both Rhazes and Avicenna wrote about sugar as a potential medicinal, such as to stimulate the bowels,[16] neither specifically linked sugar intake with diabetes. However, Rhazes linked obesity with an arthritis which was possibly gout, and suggested that treatments of obesity should include the reduction of sweets and fatty foods.[20]

Sugarcane was grown in Egypt by approximately 600 A.D. Over the subsequent centuries sugarcane was introduced to Cyprus, Crete, and by the Moors to northern Africa and southern Spain. However, sugar was largely unavailable to most of Europe. Indeed, while obesity was known to some physicians in Italy during the Middle Ages, including Oribasius (325-400 A.D) and Alexander Trallianus (6th century A.D.),[21] obesity was distinctly rare and when present was confined to royalty and the wealthy.

The earliest sugar imported into Europe was likely brought from Egypt and Syria through the port of Venice, perhaps as early as 990 A.D.[16] Knowledge of sugar became even more widespread with the return of the Crusaders from the Middle East. The Crusader Albertus Agnensis wrote in 1108 about the "sweet honied reeds" around Tripoli in present day Lebanon and that the locals made a form "of snow or white salt" from its juices that was "more pleasing than the honey of bees."[17] As more people heard of sugar, the Republic of Venice began importing increasing amounts of sugar. Sugarcane was also introduced into Sicily around 1170 A.D.

An interesting story during this period relates to the Jewish physician, Moses Maimonides, who was born in Spain in 1138. Maimonides left Spain to avoid persecution when he was a young man, and then lived in Morocco and later in Old Cairo in Egypt. One of his observations was that diabetes was absent in Spain and Morocco, whereas it was common in Egypt, where he saw more than 20 cases.[18,22] However, at that time sugar was readily available in Egypt whereas it was still relatively expensive and hard to get in Spain.

While sugar was not available to the commoner in Europe, it was a favorite food in the royal court. Court records, for example, show that the royal household for King Edward I of England ordered 1877 pounds of sugar in 1287 and 6,258 pounds of sugar in 1288.[23] Saint Thomas Aquinas, a famous Catholic priest who lived in Italy during this time, also loved sugar. Since sugar should be considered a medicine, he argued, it is fine to eat sugar during the fast.[23] Perhaps he followed this teaching, for he became very fat.

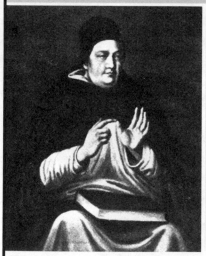

Saint Thomas Aquinas and His Love for Sugar

Saint Thomas Aquinas (1225-1274) was an Italian theologian and Catholic priest who lived in Italy and France. While he made considerable contributions to theology and natural law, he also became extremely fat and loved sugar. In fact, he did not consider sugar a food, and allowed it to be eaten during the fast.
As he wrote, "sugared spices are not eaten with the end in mind of nourishment, but rather for ease of digestion, accordingly, they do not break the fast any more than taking any other medicine."

From Conway P. Saint Thomas Aquinas of the Order of Preachers (1225-1274). London: Longmans, Green and Co.; 1911. Original Portrait in Collegio Angelico, Rome.

The increased intake of sugar, and of sugared-alcohol drinks, is likely why so many kings became obese (the "Adipose Rex" syndrome). William the Conqueror, for example, became so fat during his later years that he was accused of looking like a pregnant woman by King Philip of France. He became so angry at this accusation that he stormed the city of Mantes near Paris in 1087, where he set the city on fire. During the battle, he fell violently upon his saddle, leading to abdominal injury and distention (likely an intestinal perforation). As he lay dying he repented his numerous sins and bequeathed his wealth to the churches and poor. When he was buried in St. Stephen Church in Caen, France, his abdomen became so distended that it ruptured when they laid him in the stone sarcophagus, creating a horrible stench that sent everyone fleeing from the church.

Famous Obese Kings and Religious Leaders: The Adipose Rex Syndrome

Emperor Vitellius of Rome (15-69 A.D.)
Charles the Fat, Holy Roman Emperor (839-888 A.D.)
Sancho the Fat, King of Léon (NW Spain and Portugal) (died 966 A.D.)
Sactius the Fat, King of Spain (around 1000 A.D.)
William the Conqueror (1028 to 1087 A.D.)
Louis VI (Louis the Fat), King of France (1081-1137 A.D.)
King John of England (1167-1216 A.D.)
Saint Thomas Aquinas of Italy (1225-1274 A.D.)
Pope Fat Leo X (1475-1521 A.D.)
King Henry VIII (1491-1547 A.D.)
Louis the XVIII of France (1755-1824 A.D.)
King Fat Frederick I of Württemberg (1754-1816 A.D.)

By the early 1400s the production of sugar in Spain began to compete with the Venetian trade. Portugal also began growing sugar cane in the Madeira Islands, the Azores, and São Tome off the coast of Africa. In 1498 Vasco de Gama circumnavigated Africa, reaching India, opening new routes for trade and bringing additional wealth. An interesting story relates to King Manuel "the Fortunate" of Portugal, who was a religious man and who had become very wealthy from the production of sugar and trade with India. In 1513 the pope died, and there was the coronation of the new pope, Leo X. As a gift, King Manuel sent life sized statues of the cardinals and the pope made of sugar to the Vatican.[24] In addition, he also obtained a young albino elephant from the Kingdom of Cochin (a small Indian kingdom in southern India that fell under Portuguese rule) and gave it to Pope Leo. Pope Leo was famous for luxuriant living and would have lavish parties, and he loved his white elephant, named Hanno. Of interest, Leo became fat and gouty with age.

King Manuel of Portugal and his Gift of Sugar

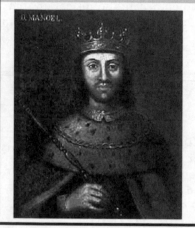

Manuel I of Portugal (1469-1521), a religious king, sent as a gift to Pope Leo on his coronation in 1513 two presents; life sized sugar effigies of the pope and the cardinals, and Hanno, a young white Indian elephant. Pope Leo, who loved luxurious foods, went on to become fat, and to suffer from gout.

Despite the increased production of sugar, sugar remained too expensive for the general populace. According to Galloway, the price of 1 pound of sugar between 1259 and 1400 was equivalent to approximately 28 pounds of cheese or 34 dozen eggs. Contrast this with 1937 when 1 pound of sugar was equivalent to 3 ounces of cheese or 2 eggs.[24] However, this was not long to last, for with the discovery of the Americas, and with the initiation of trade with the East Indies, a major change would occur, one that would have the greatest negative impact on the health of man.

CHAPTER 12

Sugar for the Poor

Increased production made sugar affordable to the common man. Once this happened, obesity and diabetes transitioned from being a disease of the wealthy to being a disease of humankind.

In medieval England, sugar could only be afforded by the wealthy. For the majority of the people, the daily diet was based primarily on cereals, such as unleavened bread made from rye or oats, milk and cheese, vegetables, and chicken or pork. For sweets, there was the rare honey, which when available was often added to wine or used to make beer. According to some linguists, the phrase "honeymoon" originated during this time and referred to the highly desired dowry of honey or honey drinks (such as mead) that the newlyweds would receive and which was to last until the next full moon.

In Portugal and Spain, however, a rapid sugar industry was developing. Sugarcane was introduced into the Madeira islands in the 1420s, in the Canaries in the 1480s, and in Sáo Tome by the mid-1500s.[24] It was on La Gomera, one of the outer Canary Islands, where Columbus stopped on his first voyage to the New World. Here he met Beatriz de Bobadilla, the recently widowed governess who was only 30 years old and renown for her beauty. Whether a true romance ensued is uncertain, but it is known that he stayed there for weeks even though he had originally planned to stay four days. On his second voyage he again stopped at La Gomera to see Beatriz. When he left, Beatriz gave sugar cane cuttings as a present for Columbus to take to the New World. Columbus took the sugarcane to Santo Domingo on the island of Hispaniola (now the Dominican Republic and Haiti) and it was here that the first sugarcane was planted in the Americas.

The first attempts to grow sugar on Santo Domingo were difficult, and initially the Spaniards tried to use the local Indians to work in the sugar plantations. However, Bartholomew de las Casas requested to King Ferdinand of Spain for protection of the local Taino Indians due to high mortality in their population from small pox introduced by the Spaniards. In part, as a consequence, the importation of Africans as slaves began, with the first ship arriving in America in 1505. Spain also sent "sugar masters" from the Canaries to help establish the sugar industry, and by 1516 the first sugar was being shipped back to Europe.[23]

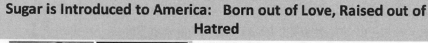

Sugar is Introduced to America: Born out of Love, Raised out of Hatred

Christopher Columbus by Sebastiano del Piombo, 1519

Beatriz Bobadilla by Anonymous (San Sebastian la Gomera, Parador Nacional)

Columbus (1451-1504), on his second trip to America in 1493, stopped at the Canary Islands where he met the beautiful governess of La Gomera, Beatriz de Bobadilla y Ossorio (1462-1501). Romance likely ensued, and Beatriz gave Columbus sugar cane cuttings that he took to Santo Domingo on the island of Hispaniola (currently the Dominican Republic and Haiti). Thus sugar was brought to America as a gift of love, only to be tarnished by centuries in which slavery drove the trade, in what can be considered one of the darkest periods of history.

The Expansion of the Sugar Industry

Spain and Portugal initially controlled most of the sugar trade from the Americas. Much of the sugar was sent from Spain to Antwerp, the largest city in the Low Countries, which was then under the rule of Spain. Here the sugar was traded throughout Europe. During the early 1500s Antwerp became the richest and largest city in Europe, and controlled as much as 40 percent of the world trade.

England countered by developing their own sugar trade, and the first two sugar houses (refineries) were established in London in 1544, which were owned by John Gardiner and Sir William Chester.[16] At first the English could not compete with the less expensive sugar imported from Antwerp. However, the Spanish Empire began to lose its footing, beginning with the Dutch Revolt in the late 1560s. During this period Antwerp lost its prominence as a trading center, and between 1560 and 1590 the population fell from 100,000 to 42,000 people. When Antwerp fell back into the hands of the Spanish in 1585, many of the citizens fled to Amsterdam. The defeat of the Spanish Armada in 1588 by England resulted in the British navy developing an even greater dominating position, with increasing control of the sugar industry in the Americas. This was followed by a rapid expansion of the sugar plantations by the English, in particular in Barbados (1627). The fall of Jamaica to the English in 1655 further reduced Spanish control of the sugar trade.

By the 1600s England had monopolized the West Indies sugar market. In turn, the expansion of the sugar industry drove the slave trade. It is estimated that more than 10 million Africans took the famous "Middle passage" to America to work as slaves in the sugar plantations. In turn, the mostly unrefined sugar was shipped to England where it was processed. England would then ship gunpowder, salt, brass, copper and lead to Africa that was used to buy the slaves, resulting in the infamous "Triangle Trade."

The Triangle Trade Brought Sugar to England

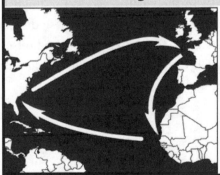

The Triangle Trade lasted three and a half centuries (1500-1850). Ships sailed from Europe to Africa, bringing manufactured goods such as brass, copper, lead, salt, and gunpowder. These goods were used to buy slaves who were taken across the "Middle Passage" to the sugar plantations in the Americas. In turn, sugar, rum and cotton were shipped from America back to Europe. It is estimated that 10 to 20 million Africans were brought to the Americas as slaves during this period.

England and Holland Hoard the Sugar

While sugar had once been only affordable to the wealthy, the marked increase in sugar imports to England led to the general introduction of sugar into drinks and food ("sweetmeats"). One of the more affordable ways to obtain sugar was in drinks. Many wines, especially those brought from Madeira and Portugal, were heavy in sugar content (such as port wines, sherry, and Madeira wines).[16] By the late 1500s, sweet wines were being made more and more with sugar as opposed to honey. This reflected not only the increasing availability of sugar, but also the reduction in the availability of honey due to the progressive closure of the English monasteries (which were major producers of honey) that occurred during the Reformation of the 1540s.[23]

One particularly popular drink in England was *hippocras*, which was wine in which sugar was added, often with cinnamon and nutmeg. *"Sugar and Sack"* was also a popular sweetened wine, and could be combined with boiled milk and eggs to make *"Sack Posset,"* a sweet custard-like dish served at weddings. Rums made from sugar extracts such as molasses were also becoming increasingly popular, especially in the Americas. The British Navy adapted rum as their major liquor following the fall of Jamaica in 1655.

Sugar was also introduced in other drinks. Tea was brought to England from India around 1610, coffee from Africa and Arabia Felix (present day Yemen) around 1615, and cocoa from the Americas in the 1650s. Whereas sugar was not used to flavor these drinks in their native lands, the English had other ideas in mind, and by 1690 the addition of sugar to these drinks had become custom, with a marked increase in teahouses and coffee houses throughout London.[25] By 1700 the English custom of having morning and afternoon tea with sugar had become ritual.[26]

Shakespeare, Falstaff, and "Sack and Sugar"

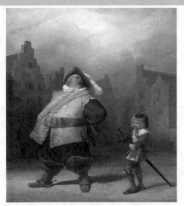

Sir John Falstaff, a braggart and drunk, was a favorite character in several of Shakespeare's plays. Falstaff carried the nickname "Sack and Sugar" after his favorite drink, which was made by combining sweet sherry wine with sugar and nutmeg. Falstaff later developed gout in Henry IVth.

Painting by Adolf Schrödter, 1867

The love of sugar by the English resulted in a dramatic increase in the amount of sugar imported. In 1660 approximately 1200 barrels (termed hogsheads) of sugar were imported to England; by 1700, 50,000 barrels; and by 1753, 110,000 barrels.[23] In contrast, the exportation of sugar fell during the latter half of the eighteenth century as the English kept as much sugar as they could for their people. Whereas the rise in sugar intake per capita increased almost fivefold between 1700 and 1800 in England, it remained flat in France.[26]

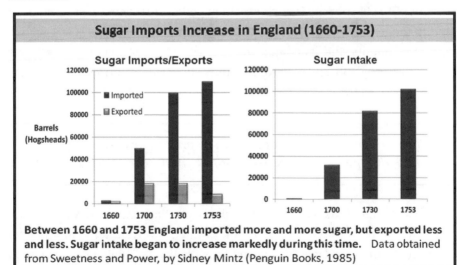

Between 1660 and 1753 England imported more and more sugar, but exported less and less. Sugar intake began to increase markedly during this time. Data obtained from Sweetness and Power, by Sidney Mintz (Penguin Books, 1985)

While England was hoarding most of the sugar from the Americas, the Dutch responded by forming the Dutch East Indies Company in 1602, and began importing sugar from the East Indies. The island of Java rapidly became one of the major sugar producers, with 20 sugar mills in 1650, and 130 sugar mills by 1710. Soon Amsterdam also emerged as a center for sugar trade in Europe.

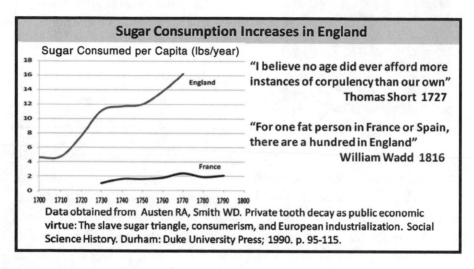

Sugar Consumption Increases in England

Sugar Consumed per Capita (lbs/year)

"I believe no age did ever afford more instances of corpulency than our own"
Thomas Short 1727

"For one fat person in France or Spain, there are a hundred in England"
William Wadd 1816

Data obtained from Austen RA, Smith WD. Private tooth decay as public economic virtue: The slave sugar triangle, consumerism, and European industrialization. Social Science History. Durham: Duke University Press; 1990. p. 95-115.

Obesity Surfaces in England and Holland

Up until 1500, obesity (which was then called corpulency) had been rare among the common people. However, beginning in the early 1600s we see reports of obesity and its complications, with the vast majority of reports being from England and the Netherlands, the two countries where sugar intake increased first.

> *England hoarded sugar and paid the price—for it was England where the epidemic of obesity, diabetes and heart disease began.*

Tobias Venner (1577-1660), a physician from Bath, England, was the first to use the word obesity in his textbook entitled *Via recta ad vitam longam* (*The Right Way to a Long Life*).[27] Stephan Blankaart (1650-1702), a Dutch

Physician from Amsterdam, commented on the marked rise of obesity in Holland in a book written in 1683.[28] The London-based physician Thomas Short starts his book written in 1727 with the phrase "I believe no age did ever afford more instances of corpulency than our own."[29] The Dutch trained physician Malcolm Flemyng (1700-1764), who practiced in England, lectured to the Royal Society of Physicians in 1757 on the increasing prevalence of obesity and suggested it should be considered a disease.[30] Dr. John Fothergill (1712-1780) commented on obesity as "a most singular disease."[1] William Wadd, in his book written in 1816, lamented on the marked rise in obesity in England; "For one fat person in France or Spain, there are a hundred in England."[1]

The Introduction of Sugar Beets and the Spread of the Sugar Industry

The relative hoarding of sugar by the English and Dutch led the rest of Europe to look for other sources of sugar. One promising possibility was the beetroot, which has nearly 12 percent of its weight as sugar. In 1747, Andreas Sigismund Marggraf (1709-1782), a pharmacist from Berlin, extracted sugar from beets by alcohol extraction and crystallization. While he was not interested in commercialization, one of his students developed an economical way to produce sugar from the beet using these principles, and by 1801 the first beet sugar factory opened in Germany. Following the continental blockade by the English in 1806 during the Napoleonic war, a major sugar shortage occurred in Europe. The French began to pay bounties for beet sugar, and soon a marked rise in beet sugar production began throughout Europe. By 1914, world beet sugar production reached 9 million tons and was almost equivalent to that for sugarcane (11.5 million tons).[31]

Sugar consumption also continued to increase in England. According to import and export data, the per capita intake of sugar increased from 4 pounds per year in 1700, to 18 pounds in 1800, and to 90 pounds in 1900.[32] The increasing availability of sugar made it more and more affordable. In addition, the sugar tax, which had been imposed on the English people, was progressively reduced throughout the 19th century, and was finally abolished on the fateful day of April 23, 1874. This led to even more sugar intake. Sugar was rapidly becoming a major component of the English diet.

The Repeal of the Sugar Tax in England in 1874

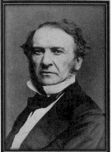 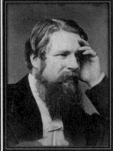

Adam Smith in his famous Wealth of Nations (1776) proposed taxes for luxuries such as sugar, rum and tobacco. The Sugar Tax was operative until April 23rd, 1874 when it was repealed by Prime Minister William Gladstone and Sir Stafford Northcote, Chancellor of the Exchequer.

William Gladstone   Sir Stafford Northcote

Sugar consumption increased in England following the repeal of the sugar tax in 1874.

The Emergence of Obesity, Gout, Diabetes and Heart Disease

As sugar consumption increased in the English and Dutch populations, reports of not only obese individuals, but rather of severe (morbid) obesity began to be observed. Herman Boerhaave (1668-1738), the great Dutch physician, saw a patient who was so obese that he had to wear a sash to hold up his belly and also had to cut out a section of the dining table so he could reach food with his hands.[1] Other individuals with severe obesity were noted from that era, of which the most famous was the Englishman, Daniel Lambert. Lambert was a grocer who was the heaviest human in the world at the time, and who exhibited himself at various fairs as a curiosity. William Wadd, the London-based physician who wrote a book on obesity in 1816, also described over 40 cases of severe obesity (>300 pounds) with approximately 20 cases occurring in children and adolescents.

The Fattest Humans in History

1750 **Edward Bright** of Essex, a grocer, died at age 29 with a weight of 616 pounds reported to be the heaviest man of 18th century England. "He was an active man till a year or two before his death, when his corpulency so overpowered his strength that his life was a burden and death a deliverance" (Wanley, 1806)

1809 **Daniel Lambert** of Leicester, died at age 40 with a weight of 732 pounds. "His waistcoat could easily enclose 7 persons of ordinary size." (Encyclopedia Brittanica, 1890)

1983 **Jon Minnoch** of Bainbridge Island, Washington, reached 1400 pounds before dying of heart failure at age 42. Currently holds the world record for weight.

2010 **Manuel Irbe**, Monterrey, Mexico, currently weighs 1248 pounds and is the heaviest human alive

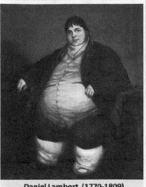

Daniel Lambert (1770-1809)

An increase in the frequency of gout was also observed in England and Holland during this time. As with obesity, gout was originally a disease of the wealthy and royalty, and many kings and famous people suffered from the disease. The "distemper of gentlemen," the "king of diseases and the disease of kings," and the "offspring of luxury and intemperance," were names given to this condition. As the wit, Ambrose Bierce (1842-1913) wrote, "gout is a physician's name for the rheumatism of a rich patient."

Famous Kings, Scientists, and Artists with the Gout

Kings, Popes and Politicians	Scientists, Physicians and Artists
Michael VIII of Constantinople (1223-1282)	Michelangelo (1475-1564)
Pope Leo X (1475-1521)	Galileo of Gallilei (1564-1642)
Henry VIII (1491-1547)	Peter Paul Rubens (1577-1640)
Charles V, Holy Roman Emperor (1500-1558)	William Harvey (1578-1647)
Phillip II of Spain (1527-1598)	John Milton (1608-1674)
Lord Chesterfield (1694-1773)	Thomas Sydenham (1624-1689)
Benjamin Franklin (1706-1790)	Isaac Newton(1643-1727)
Louis XVIII (1755-1824)	Wilhelm Leibniz (1646-1716)
William Pitt the Younger (1759-1806)	Samuel Johnson (1709-1784)
George IV of England (1762-1830)	Alfred Lord Tennyson (1809-1892)
Thomas Jefferson (1743-1826)	

While gout was still primarily a disease of the wealthy, it became increasingly and increasingly frequent, and was highly associated with the drinking of sugared wines and ciders.[33-34] Sugar, by raising uric acid levels, is a known cause of gout, but some experts have suggested these wines may have contributed to the increased risk for gout yet another way. In particular, the physician Gene Ball proposed in the 1960s that some of the wines, especially those shipped from Portugal, may have had very high lead content, as they would be sent in wood barrels that had lead-lined lids or lead fastenings.[35] Lead also raises uric acid and is known to cause gout (termed "saturnine gout"). Ball was able to find four bottles of wine from the 1770 to 1820 period and tested them for their lead content. Two of the bottles, a Port (1805) and a wine from the Canary Islands had extremely high lead content (830-1900 micrograms per liter), representing levels 5 to 10 times higher than modern wines from Portugal or Madeira. Since port was a favorite wine in England during these times (for example, one report showed that 5.5 million gallons of port were imported in 1825), it is possible that lead may have contributed to the increased frequency of gout observed in 18th and 19th century England.[35] Since lead raises uric acid, one might also predict it can increase the risk for obesity similar to sugar. In fact, low levels of lead have been associated not only with gout, but also with obesity, elevated blood pressure, insulin resistance, and kidney disease.[36-38] In a later chapter we will discuss the role of subtle lead poisoning in the epidemic of obesity in more detail.

Diabetes was also "rediscovered" in the 1600s in England, primarily as a condition in which sugar (in this case glucose) had passed into the urine. The urine is "wonderfully sweet [in diabetes], as if imbued with honey or sugar," wrote Thomas Willis (1621-1675), the Sedleian Professor of Natural Philosophy at Oxford.[11,39] Matthew Dobson, a physician in the Liverpool Infirmary, even went so far as to boil 4 pounds of urine from a diabetic patient to obtain 4 ounces, 2 drams (teaspoons), and 2 scruples (like a "pinch") of a whitish sugary cake that "smelt sweet, like brown sugar, and could not be distinguished from sugar, except that the sweetness left a slight sense of coolness on the palate."[11] Dobson also noted that the serum of a soldier dying from acute diabetes also had a sugary taste of the blood.[39] [On a personal note as a practicing physician, I am glad that this part of the physical examination is no longer performed].

Similar to obesity and diabetes, heart attacks from coronary artery disease were first reported in England in the mid-1600s with the description by Edward Hyde (1609–1674) of the recurrent episodes of chest pain his father, the Earl of Clarendon, suffered prior to dying from sudden death in 1632. In 1768 the physician William Heberden described this new type of recurrent chest pain, which he called angina pectoris, to the Royal College of Physicians, and went on to publish 100 cases that he had seen in 1802. Other English physicians were also writing about this peculiar chest pain that could lead to sudden death, including John Fothergill (1774), John Wall (1785), Edward Jenner (1786), Caleb Parry (1788), and James Johnstone (1792) and reports soon emanated from Ireland and Scotland as well.[40]

The cause of the angina was debated during these early days. Some physicians thought it was a disease of the chest wall. Others, such as the famous American physician, Benjamin Rush (1745–1813) (who among other things is credited with bringing golf to the United States) noted the frequent association of angina with gout and obesity and suggested that angina represented an attempt of the body to release its gouty pain elsewhere (which he termed "misplaced gout").[41-42] William Wadd suggested that the heart might be choked by fat. In his book in 1816 on obesity, for example, he told of the case of Dr. Brian Higgins, who died after suffering significant chest pain, and who was found on postmortem to have massive fat encasing his heart.[1] Other physicians, most notably Jenner and Parry, observed the presence of coronary artery disease and suggested this might be the cause.[40] However, it was not until 1880 when the German pathologist, Karl Weigert (1845-1904) documented disease of the coronary arteries in people dying from heart attacks that the cause of ischemic heart disease was established.[43]

Other medical conditions were also being discovered. Richard Bright, a physician at Guy's hospital in London, described the presence of chronic kidney disease in the early 1800s,[44] for which gout and lead poisoning were considered major causes.[34,45] Many of these patients had hypertrophied hearts, suggesting increased pressure in the circulation. This led to the development of methods for measuring blood pressure. Soon the entity of high blood pressure was discovered by a young English physician, Frederick Akbar Mahomed.[46-47] Mahomed noted that individuals with gout frequently developed high blood pressure and suggested that uric acid might be one of its causes. Apoplexy, which is the old medical term for stroke, also became increasingly common in England during this time. The association of obesity with fatigue and sleepiness, which today we call *sleep apnea*, was also increasingly recognized.

The Link of Sugar with Obesity and Diabetes

The possibility that sugar intake may have had a role in these conditions did not escape notice of physicians. One of the earliest to decry sugar as a cause of obesity was Stephan Blankaart (1650-1702) who lived in Amsterdam. In 1683 he wrote a book warning that excessive intake of sugar was likely the cause not only of obesity, but also of gout and dental decay.[28] Later, William Wadd wrote of the relationship of sugar with obesity: "The Chinese slaves in the sugar season get fat without any other substance other than the ripe sugar cane."[1] He commented that the same was true for African slaves working in the West Indies. Benjamin Moseley, who wrote a treatise on the benefits of sugar in 1800, also noted a relationship of sugar intake with obesity. As he wrote, "Taken in tea, milk and beer, sugar has been found not only sufficient to sustain nature, but has caused lean people to grow fat."[16]

Others noted a relationship between the intake of sugar and diabetes. Étienne Lancereaux (1829-1910), noted that diabetes could occur in lean people, which he called *diabetes maigre*, or in fat people, which he called *diabetes gras*, and which we know of today as type 1 diabetes (from loss of pancreatic islet cells) or type 2 diabetes (driven primarily by insulin resistance). Lancereaux suggested that fat diabetes is due to the overconsumption of sugar.[48] Others, such as Sir Dyce Duckworth, noted the frequent association of diabetes with gout.[49]

The association of sugar intake with diabetes was also being observed in other countries. For example, Dr. Thomas Christie, a British Army Physician who was stationed in Colombo, Ceylon (present day Sri Lanka) in the early 1800s, described 10 individuals with diabetes, which interestingly preferentially affected the poorer people. Christie noted that the poor people could not afford the rice which was imported from Bengal, but rather subsisted on local foods such as "yams and sweet potatoes, jack-fruit, plantains or bananas, and particularly coconuts." Importantly, however, the local people also ingested "a great deal of country sugar, or jaggery, prepared from the toddy of the Ritiel Palm, which is cheap and forms an article of export."[50-51] One of his more interesting comments is that the increased frequency of diabetes in Ceylon contrasted with Calcutta where diabetes was less common, based on his physician friend, William Hunter, who was stationed there.[50-51]

Diabetes was increasing in Bengal, however, as well as other countries where sugar production and consumption was increasing. This was highlighted by a series of articles published in 1907 in the British Medical Journal.[14,52-60] Sir Richard Havelock Charles, a Major General based in India, led the conference which focused on the emergence of diabetes in India and several other countries in the world, including Ceylon and Egypt. Charles noted an alarming increase in obesity among the wealthy and sedentary Bengal Indians, whereas it remained uncommon among poorer groups, such as those from the Punjab. Charles noted that the Bengal Indians had significantly increased their intake of carbohydrates, including sugar. Others confirmed this association, not only in India, but in Egypt and China.[14,54-55]

A Rising Storm

While the 1800s and early 1900s were seeing a marked increase in sugar intake associated with increases in obesity, diabetes, and heart disease, the overall frequency of the latter conditions was still relatively low. For example, a study was performed of 12,392 Union veterans from the Civil War, and the frequency of obesity (defined as a BMI > 30) among men between 50 and 59 years old increased from approximately 3.4 percent in 1890 to 5.9 percent in 1900.[61] Likewise, Sir William Osler, the famous physician, was alarmed by increasing rates of diabetes, yet he still projected only 2 to 3 cases per 100,000 population in Europe and America.[62] Indeed, of 35,000 consecutive admissions at the Johns Hopkins hospital in Baltimore in the early 1890s, only 10 cases were due to diabetes.[62] High blood pressure was also being increasingly recognized, in part because of the invention of the blood pressure cuff in 1896 by the Italian physician, Scipione Riva-Rocci. By 1912 the Metropolitan Life Insurance company had data that high blood pressure (using the same definition as today) increased the risk of death. Nevertheless, only 5 to 10 percent of the adult U.S. population was hypertensive.

However, it was just the beginning of a rising storm. One of the more striking reports came from Haven Emerson, the Commissioner of Health for New York City (1915-1917) and a Professor of Public Health and Columbia University. Emerson wrote a landmark paper in 1924 in which he evaluated risk factors for people developing diabetes.[63] He had become concerned because diabetes had increased nearly 10-fold over a 40 year period in New York City. Emerson linked the development of diabetes to being wealthy and sedentary, and especially for merchants working in the food industry. Most notably, Emerson found that diabetes was common in those with a high sugar intake, and he proposed that sugar might be the primary cause of diabetes.[63] Consistent with his hypothesis, he noted that the rates of diabetes were lower in countries where sugar intake was lower, such as Australia.

Haven Emerson, Sugar, and The Rise in Diabetes in New York City

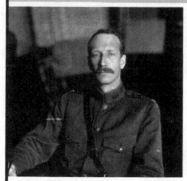

Haven Emerson, the New York Health Commissioner and Director of Public Health at Columbia, noted that diabetes had increased from 2.8 cases/100,000 in 1880 to 19 cases per 100,000 in 1920 in New York City. To better understand why, Dr Haven Emerson performed a study to identify potential risk factors for the development of diabetes. His main finding was that being sedentary, wealthy and over the age of 45 years conferred risk. But one of the greatest risks? Sugar intake.

Haven Emerson (1874-1957)

Emerson was not alone in his concerns for sugar as a cause of diabetes. One of the most vocal was Sir Frederick Banting. Banting had discovered insulin in 1922 for which he received the Nobel prize. However, like others, he had noted a worrisome increase in the frequency of diabetes in Europe and the Americans, and he also became quite concerned that refined sugar might be one of its major causes. Interestingly, he did not think it was sugar-cane itself, for he noted that Panama sugar cane workers would suck on sugar cane much of the day but did not seem to have an increased risk for diabetes.[64] Based on the studies we presented earlier (Chapter 9), this is not surprising, as the ability of fructose to activate the switch is dependent on the concentration of fructose in the liver, and this would be related to both the *rate* and *total amount* of sugar ingestion.

Frederick Banting suggests Sugar is Cause of Diabetes

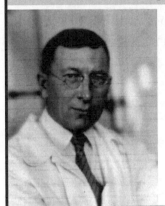

"In the United States the incidence of diabetes has increased proportionately with the per capita consumption of cane sugar. One cannot help but conclude that in the heating and recrystallisation of the natural sugar-cane something is altered which leaves the refined product a dangerous food-stuff."

Sir Frederick Banting, Edinburgh Medical Journal, 1929; 36: 1-18.

Introduction of Sugar in Naive Populations Results in Increased Obesity

As sugar became less and less expensive, it also became a great item for trade when westerners interacted with individuals in their native lands. When James Cook arrived to New Zealand in 1769, the Maori Indian was reported to be stout and muscular and devoid of fat.[65] At that time their diet consisted of the bitter fern root, the sweet potato, and fish and fowl.[65] With the introduction of western culture, sugar became a major staple of the diet, and this was associated with a remarkable increase in both gout and diabetes in this population.[66-67]

Another example is the Pima Indians, who lived in the Gila River Basin in Arizona. When they were first visited by westerners, the Pima were healthy and athletic. Following the discovery of gold in California, a wagon route was built across Pima lands. Gold seekers would stop at the trading posts en route to California for supplies, and one of the favorite trading items for the Pima was sugar.[68-69] By 1900 both obesity and diabetes were already prevalent among the Arizona Pima; interestingly, for the Pima living according to their native traditions and diet in Mexico, obesity and diabetes remained absent.[69]

An epidemic of obesity, diabetes, and heart disease was also observed in the early 1960s by Campbell among the Natal Indians working in the sugarcane fields in the "sugar belt" of South Africa. Sugarcane had been grown in this region since the mid-19th century, and many of the workers had come from India. Unlike their relatives in India, who were eating only about 12 pounds (5.4 kg) of sugar per capita per year, the average Natal Indian was ingesting 77 pounds (35 kg).[70] While the black African was less sensitive to the effects of sugar than the Natal Indian, Campbell noted that they could also get diabetes and obesity if they ate enough sugar. Campbell wrote that the unpopular king of the Zulus, Mpande, whose "chief interests were his large harem and his eating, . . . became so fat that he actually couldn't walk and had to be dragged about on ox-skins."[70]

In another study, Cohen reported that Jewish Yemenites moving from Yemen to Israel after the World War had a remarkable increase in prevalence of diabetes, from near absent among newly arrived Yemenites compared to 7.7 percent among Yemenites age 50 to 60 who had lived in Israel for 20 or 30 years. Cohen further correlated this increased risk with a marked increase in sugar intake (approximating 50 to 60 grams/day) compared to nearly negligible intake of sugar when they lived in Yemen.[71-72]

Others also noted a relationship of sugar intake with the development of diabetes and obesity. For example, Concepcion reported in 1922 that diabetes was rare in the Phillipines except in Manila, where it correlated with sugar consumption.[73] Albertsson reported in the early 1950s that diabetes had been extremely rare in Iceland until the diet started changing from one based on protein and fat to one high in carbohydrates, particularly sugar.[74]

The introduction of western culture and diet, especially sugar, was also associated with remarkable transformations of native American Indians such as the Navaho,[75-77] the Australia Aborigines,[78] Samoans and other Pacific Islanders from healthy populations where diabetes was rare to one where obesity and diabetes were common. Increased rates of gout, hypertension and diabetes were also observed in Japanese and Filipinos following their immigration in the 1950s to the United States and Canada with the adaptation of western diet.[79-80]

An intriguing observation related to the Africans brought to America to work the sugar plantations. Diabetes and hypertension were rare in Africans living in Africa.[81-82] Diabetes was also initially less common in African Americans compared to Caucasians in cities such as New York City in northeastern United States.[63,83] However, it was observed early on that high blood pressure and diabetes were more common in blacks than whites living in southeastern United States and the Caribbean.[63,84-85] In particular, L.I. Dublin, the head statistician of the Metropolitan Life Insurance Company and one of the early leaders in epidemiology, noted that diabetes was already becoming common by the 1920s among African Americans in some urban cities in the South.[63] One possible explanation, which we proposed, relates to the earlier exposure of African Americans to sugar by virtue of their work on the plantations.[86] The slaves were frequently provided the leftover treacle and molasses during the preparation of sugar, and as such molasses became a regular staple in the diet in the early years. While the increased exposure to molasses and sugar likely changed following the abolition of slavery after the Civil War, African Americans still eat more sugar today. The reason, however, may now be different. As sugar has become less expensive, sugar intake has increased, especially among the economically less privileged—and this is true for African Americans, as well as Hispanics, Australia Aborigines, and Samoans—all populations with skyrocketing rates of diabetes and obesity.[87-90]

> *The increased risk for obesity, diabetes and heart disease in African Americans may be due to increased intake of sugar.*

Loss of an Alarm Signal: Fluoride Masks the Rise in Sugar Intake

Excessive sugar intake is also a known cause of caries (dental cavities) and gum disease (gingivitis).[91-92] Not surprisingly, the emergence of caries can be linked with a rise in fructose intake in various populations, whether it be with the introduction of honey among the wealthy and nobility of ancient Egypt,[9] the introduction of sugar among the Eskimo,[93] or with the rise in sugar intake in Ethiopian Jews moving to Israel in the 1960s.[94] Even Blankaart linked sugar intake with dental cavities, as well as obesity and gout, in Amsterdam in the late 17th century.[28] More recently, a study analyzed sugar intake and caries rate in 12-year-old children living in 47 countries, and 6 of the 7 countries with the highest caries rate had an average sugar supply of >120 g/day per person.[7]

Thomas Cleave wrote that a rise in caries within the population acts as an alarm signal to predict the later development of diabetes and obesity, for caries develop within a few years of sugar exposure whereas its systemic effects may not occur until a decade or more later.[95] This relationship was dampened, however, when fluoride was introduced as a means to reduce the rate of caries.[96] Today fluoride has been added to the drinking water of over 200 million people in the United States, and since the early 1950s, fluoride has been commonly added to toothpaste. The benefits of this approach remain debated, for fluoride can also be associated with toxicity, leading to discoloration of teeth and possibly other side effects.[97] Cleave and others such as Phillipe Hujoel from the University of Washington have noted a yet another negative consequence, for it has masked the tell-tale sign that sugar intake is increasing.[92,95] In so doing, fluoride use may have effectively removed this "alarm signal" that tells us we are eating too much sugar.

High Fructose Corn Syrup Enters the World

Sugar intake increased more than 5-fold increase in England during the 1800s, but this increased even more with the introduction of soft drinks. Carbonated lemonade was introduced in the 1830s, and ginger ale and root beer about 40 years later. Dr. John Pemberton, a pharmacist in Atlanta, introduced coca cola at Jacob's pharmacy in 1886. Pepsi-Cola was introduced in 1898 by Caleb Bradham, a pharmacist from North Carolina. Initially soft drinks were sold in 6 to 8 ounce bottles, but by the 1960s the size had increased to 12 ounces, and by the 1990s it had increased to 20 ounce and 1 liter bottles.

One reason that the size of soft drinks increased was because the cost of producing soft drinks fell due to the introduction of a new sweetener, high fructose corn syrup (HFCS). Corn syrup is normally composed primarily of glucose and is not very sweet. While a method had been developed in the late 1960s by which some of the glucose in the corn syrup could be converted to fructose using enzymes from bacteria, the process was expensive and impractical. However, this changed in the early 1970s when two Japanese scientists, Tsumura and Sato, discovered a way to convert the glucose in corn syrup to fructose by running the syrup through a column to which the enzymes had been attached. Since the enzymes were stuck to the column, they could be reused over and over.

> *The introduction of high fructose corn syrup to the American diet resulted in a 30% increase in fructose consumption.*

The HFCS produced represents a mixture of both glucose and fructose, and the concentrations could be varied. The two most common mixtures contain 55 percent fructose and 45 percent glucose (used primarily in soft drinks), or 42 percent fructose and 58 percent glucose (used mainly in pastries and sweets). This contrasts with sucrose, which consists of fructose and glucose bonded together, resulting in a 50 percent mixture.

HFCS rapidly became popular as a sweetener in the United States, for unlike table sugar it was liquid and could be mixed into foods easily. It also had a long shelf life, and did not form crystals in ice cream or candies over time such as can happen with sugar. It also was not taxed as much as sugar, making it less expensive. By the early 1980s both Coca-Cola and Pepsi-Cola began switching the sucrose in soft drinks to HFCS. As more and more HFCS was consumed, the intake of cane and beet sugar began to fall. Unfortunately, however, HFCS did not simply replace sucrose, but the overall effect was to further increase the overall intake of sugars containing fructose. Between 1970 and 2000 there was a 20 to 30 percent increase in the intake of fructose from these two major sources.

Obesity, Diabetes, and Heart Disease become Epidemic

The continued rise in intake of sugars from sucrose and HFCS was associated with a parallel and daunting increase in obesity, with an acceleration in the last 40 years following the introduction of HFCS.[98] For example the prevalence obesity in 60-year-old men increased more than 10-fold over the last century reaching 41.3 percent in 2000.[61] Diabetes also increased, and now affects 10 percent or more of the population in the United States. Hypertension has also increased stepwise, from a prevalence of 5-10 percent to 32 percent of the population. Chronic kidney disease has quadrupled in the last 40 years, and fatty liver disease has become prevalent and now affects 20 percent of our population.

There has also been a remarkable increase in heart disease since the early 1900s. In London Hospital there were only 13 documented deaths due to coronary artery disease confirmed by autopsy between 1907 and 1913, and only three cases at Guy's Hospital during this same period.[43] Following World War I this started to change. The famous American physician, Robert Platt, for example, noted that by 1929 the family physician was commonly seeing people with coronary artery disease.[99] In 1940, the subspecialty of cardiology began in the United States, and by 1950 there were 500 cardiologists in the United States. By the early 1960s the first coronary care units were introduced. Today there are over 20,000 cardiologists performing more than 2.7 million cardiac catheterizations per year in the United States; in 2003 there were also more than 150,000 coronary artery bypass surgeries. One in three deaths in the United States today is from cardiovascular disease. While cardiovascular mortality is decreasing on a per capita basis due to our ability to better treat heart disease with medications, stents and cardiovascular surgery, cardiology will remain an active and lucrative discipline until the underlying mechanisms driving the cardiovascular epidemic are halted.

The figures below show the impressive correlation between sugar intake (which includes HFCS) and rates of obesity in 60-year-old men, and with the rate of diabetes in the United States.[86,100] Dips in intake of sugar did occur during both World Wars, and this was also associated with dips in both the frequency of obesity and the death rate from diabetes. When HFCS was introduced into the American diet in the 1970s, there was a further increase in overall sugar intake by nearly 30 percent in association with an increase in obesity and diabetes.

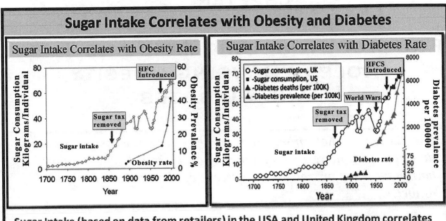

Sugar Intake (based on data from retailers) in the USA and United Kingdom correlates with the obesity rate (60 year old men) and the rate of diabetes in the USA. Adapted from Am J Clin Nutr 2007; 86:899 and Endo Rev 2009; 30:96-116. Copyright 2007, American Society of Nutrition and 2009, The Endocrine Society.

The worldwide increase in obesity, diabetes, and hypertension is staggering. In some countries, such as Kuwait, as many as 75 percent of the Kuwaiti people are overweight or obese, and 25 percent are diabetic. Hypertension is also increasing worldwide, and is predicted to increase to more than 1.5 billion people in the world by 2025. At the current rate of increase in diabetes in the United States, the Centers for Disease Control predicts that one in three children born in the U.S. today will become diabetic.[101]

CHAPTER 13

FRUCTOSE AND URIC ACID AND THEIR ROLE IN CAUSING OBESITY AND DIABETES

> *Associations do not prove cause and effect. In the case of fructose and uric acid, however, experimental and clinical evidence suggest both have a major role in the current epidemic of obesity and diabetes.*

By the early 1900s the association of sugar intake with the development of obesity and diabetes was strong. Whenever and wherever sugar was introduced, one could see an increase in the frequency of obesity and diabetes. Haven Emerson's careful study showing that the rise in diabetes in New York City correlated closely with increasing intake of sugar provided some of the strongest evidence.[63] Frederick Banting, the Nobel Laureate who had been a codiscoverer of insulin, also argued refined sugar was likely the major cause of diabetes.[64]

However, a countering argument was proposed by Elliot Joslin (an expert on diabetes and founder of the Joslin Diabetes Clinic) and Louis Dublin (famed public health statistician from the Metropolitan Life Insurance Company who was one of the first to describe an association of obesity and hypertension with increased risk for death). Joslin and Dublin argued that diabetes and obesity were not the consequence of eating sugar, but that they resulted from simply eating too many calories (which they termed "overnutrition"), coupled with a sedentary lifestyle.[102] According to their argument, sugar was important, but only as a source of calories. To support their argument, they quoted a study by Mills who showed that of the 13 countries with the top sugar production, 11 were countries with the highest diabetes rates, but notably two countries, Cuba and Hawaii, had high sugar production but low diabetes rates.[103]

Joslin's argument was considered convincing, and overnutrition has been viewed as the most likely cause of obesity and diabetes until this day. The concept of overnutrition switched the focus from sugar to fat, since it is the latter food with the highest caloric content (9 calories per gram). By the 1950s many investigators felt that high fat diet was the driving cause of not only obesity, but also of heart disease. The lead proponent was Ancel Keys, a nutritionist from the University of Minnesota. Keys was already famous for developing the "K-rations" in World War II that could provide non-perishable ready-to-eat meals that could be carried during combat. Keys argued quite convincingly that high fat diet was the cause of heart disease. The observation that cholesterol-laden fat was the major component of the atherosclerotic plaque present in diseased blood vessels in the heart and elsewhere supported this hypothesis. Furthermore, the frequency of coronary heart disease in various countries correlated with overall intake of fats.[104]

The possibility that sugar might have a role in obesity, diabetes and heart disease was nevertheless resurrected. Campbell, a South African physician who had observed the association of sugar intake with diabetes in the Natal Indians working in the "Sugar Belt" of South Africa, wrote a paper with Thomas Cleave, a naval surgeon, suggesting that sugar (which he called the "Saccharine disease"), was the cause of obesity and diabetes.[105] They attributed the problem to both refined sugar and flour and suggested that when dietary sugar constituted greater than 10 percent of the diet, that the risk for obesity and diabetes would manifest, with an approximate 20 year delay between the increase in sugar intake and rise in diabetes ("Rule of 20 Years").

Dr. John Yudkin, a physician from the University of London, also proposed that high sugar diets were responsible for heart disease. Yudkin did not deny that fat intake correlated with the development of heart disease.

However, Yudkin noted that countries with high fat intakes also had high sugar intake, and thereby suggested that it was the sugar intake that was responsible for the development of diabetes and heart disease.[106-108] Nevertheless, the debates between Keys and Yudkin usually ended in favor of Keys. After all, why was not coronary artery disease increased in Cuba given its high sugar intake? And is it not obvious that a high fat diet should not be the cause of the fat laden plaques in diseased coronary arteries from patients suffering from heart attacks? Even more importantly, our society is characterized by overnutrition—so many of us are eating too much and exercising too little. Isn't it obvious that this is the reason we are obese and diabetic?

The problem, of course, is that associations do not prove cause and effect, but only linkage. Based on the experimental studies we presented earlier, we *are* becoming obese because we are eating too much and exercising too little, but the driving force is not because we are choosing to eat too much, but rather because our body is asking us to eat more. Hollingshed's suggestion that the introduction of chimneys in houses in the 1500s correlated with sedentary behavior and more obesity may be true, but which behavior is driving the other?

Robert Koch and the Scientific Method to Assess Causality

While epidemiology is wonderful for generating hypotheses, proof that a factor is causing disease requires more. Fortunately, there is a scientific approach to determine causality, and it can be traced to a meeting in Berlin, about 130 years ago. On the evening of March 24th, 1882, a young physician, Robert Koch, gave a lecture to the Berlin Physiological Society that would forever change the science of medicine. Koch had already made an impact a few years earlier by discovering the cause of anthrax, a bacterial disease that was highly transmissible and frequently fatal. He had made that discovery by identifying the bacteria with his microscope in a self-made laboratory in his home in Wöllstein, Germany. For this achievement, he was invited to join the Imperial Health Bureau in Berlin in 1880 where he took on the goal of identifying the cause of tuberculosis.

Tuberculosis is one of the most ravaging diseases of mankind, for which its historic name was "consumption," as it commonly causes high fever, sweats and progressive weight loss. The major site of infection is the lung where it causes a chronic pneumonia, often with the coughing of blood. It can also spread throughout the body where it can infect the liver, kidney, bones and even the fluid bathing the brain.

At the dinner meeting, Koch presented his experimental studies that showed that tuberculosis was due to a bacteria. First, he found bacteria in the lung tissues from patients dying from tuberculosis by using special dyes to stain the tissues and then examining them under the microscope. These experiments established an association of the bacteria with the presence of disease. He then took the infected tissue specimens and placed the macerated contents in a culture dish, and after several days the cultures started growing bacteria. He injected these bacteria into normal rabbits and shortly thereafter the animals contracted tuberculosis. This provided direct experimental evidence that the suspected bacteria were the cause of tuberculosis. As final proof, he isolated the bacteria from the infected lung lesion of the rabbit and showed that it had the same characteristics as the original bacteria isolated from the patient.

During the presentation the audience was spellbound, and even the famous and outspoken professor, Rudolf Virchow, sat speechless.[109] What was striking was not simply the discovery, which was enough to garner Koch the Nobel Prize, but that his lecture provided a conceptual breakthrough of the "scientific method" for proving the cause of disease. Koch's approach are still applied for identifying causes of infectious diseases today, although we now like to see evidence that killing the organism cures the disease, or similarly that removal of the suspected agent can prevent or treat the condition. However, at the time of Koch, antibiotics had not yet been developed and it was not until the late 1940s that the first effective antibiotic treatment for tuberculosis was shown.

The strong deductive reasoning and sound scientific principles used by Koch to prove the cause (or etiology) of tuberculosis became known as Koch's postulates and has provided an approach scientists have used to not only find the causes of other infectious diseases, but also for other diseases and conditions. Today we know that Koch's approach is not perfect, for not everyone reacts the same way to an agent, for example. People are genetically diverse and also have had variable exposures to various things. For example, many of us are exposed to various viruses that can cause nasal and upper respiratory infections ("colds") but not all of us develop symptoms as some of us have better defense systems or have been previously exposed to a related virus and have developed immunity. Nevertheless, Koch's approach still provides one of the best ways to look for the cause of disease.

Fructose in the Causation of Obesity and Metabolic Syndrome

Can we use Koch's postulates to determine if fructose has a role in obesity and metabolic syndrome? First, as noted by the previous chapters, the rise in sugar intake parallels the rise in obesity and metabolic syndrome, both in the United States and throughout the world. Studies within the United States also have repeatedly shown that those individuals who consume the most nondiet soft drinks are at the greatest risk for metabolic syndrome, fatty liver, and diabetes.[110-111]

Second, there is experimental evidence in animals that sugar and fructose may cause obesity and diabetes. Fructose can rapidly induce all features of the metabolic syndrome in rats, including visceral obesity, fatty liver, elevated triglycerides, low HDL cholesterol, and elevated blood pressure.[100] While high doses are needed, these animals make vitamin C and also have uricase, so they are expected to be resistant to fructose (see Chapter 10). As mentioned, when we block uricase, only low doses of fructose are necessary to induce insulin resistance, elevated blood pressure, and elevated serum triglycerides.[112]

Third, we have identified a scientific mechanism by which fructose causes metabolic syndrome. Specifically, we found that fructose increases uric acid in the cell that then alters the mitochondria to preferentially shunt the energy from food into fat. The mitochondrial oxidative stress also has a role in causing insulin resistance and hypertension.[113] Fructose also causes leptin resistance, and blocks ATP production.[114] These data explain why feeding fructose to mice results in increased food intake and decreased physical activity, and why it causes fat accumulation.

Fourth, clinical studies show that giving fructose to people can induce features of metabolic syndrome. One of the best studies was done by Kimberly Stanhope and Peter Havel from the University of California, Davis. They took overweight men and women and provided meals in which 25 per cent of the calories were from glucose or 25 percent from fructose. Individuals took these meals for 10 weeks. Fat accumulation was measured at the beginning and end of the study using special X-rays (computerized tomography or CT scanning). In those individuals that ate a fructose-enriched diet, there was a significant increase in visceral fat compared to those given a glucose-based diet.[115] The fructose fed individuals also developed worse insulin resistance and higher serum triglycerides following their meals.

One of the more impressive studies, however, was performed on the island of Menorca off the coast of Spain by Enrique Perez-Pozo and Julian Lopez-Lillo with our research group. In this study healthy adult men were supplemented with two liters a day of water containing 10 percent fructose, which represents a dose of fructose that is approximately threefold greater than the mean dose of fructose currently ingested in the United States. The remarkable finding was that the ingestion of fructose resulted in an increase in blood pressure, a rise in serum triglycerides, a lowering of HDL cholesterol levels, and worsening pf insulin resistance. At the end of the study, approximately 25 percent of the individuals had newly diagnosed metabolic syndrome using classic criteria.[116] While not part of our study, efforts were made to reverse these findings by placing the individuals on a low fructose diet afterwards, and most people did show significant improvement.

This latter study has been criticized for using doses of fructose that are significantly more than current western diet, but it can also be argued that it acts as a proof of principle of what fructose can do. When one recalls that Cleave and Campbell wrote that it takes 20 years from the time that sugar is introduced into a culture before a rise in diabetes is observed,[105] the fact that high doses of fructose can induce such dramatic changes in only a two week period is impressive.

Koch's Postulates: Sugar as a Cause of Metabolic Syndrome (MS)	
1. Association is strong	Sugar intake increases risk of MS
2. Experimental Evidence	Lab rats develop MS when given sugar
3. Mechanism Identified	Fructose alters Mitochondria
4. Fructose Causes MS in people	Giving fructose to people induces features of MS
5. Reducing fructose improves MS	Pilot studies suggest reducing sugar prevents and improves MS

While the relationship of fructose and sugar intake with metabolic syndrome is impressive, the relationship of fructose intake with weight gain has been more variable. However, it can be explained by understanding the mechanisms. The metabolic syndrome is induced by oxidative stress to the mitochondria that shifts energy from food into fat.[117-118] This does not require increasing energy intake above one's ordinary intake, and in fact one can induce metabolic syndrome in rats with sugar even if overall caloric intake is restricted. In effect, to become diabetic or increase your percentage of body fat one only needs to eat a sugar-rich diet—weight gain is not necessary.

In contrast, to gain weight one has to take in more energy than one spends. The way fructose does this is by inducing leptin resistance,[114] which then encourages more food intake. Since fructose is a low calorie food compared to high caloric foods, such as fat, increasing weight is not always apparent in short-term clinical trials, especially since experimental studies suggests it takes weeks to months to develop the leptin resistance. An experimental study that increases fructose content but then limits the individual from choosing other foods is also likely to be negative. Thus, fructose increases weight by encouraging food intake, by increasing the appetite and blocking the sensation of fullness. The gaining of weight is facilitated by eating high fat foods. This is why the combination of soft drinks with high fat foods like french fries is such a powerful way for gaining weight.

Fructose is the fire; high fat diet is the firewood. Together they drive the obesity epidemic.

Finally, to fulfill Koch's postulates, one would like to see that the reduction of sugar intake translates into less obesity and metabolic syndrome. An opportunity to evaluate this possibility resulted from a public health policy that was passed in 2003 in California in which soft drinks were banned from grade schools and middle schools. This measure was successful in reducing the number of soft drinks that children drank over the next four years. In 2003, over 22 percent of school children between the age of 6 and 11 were drinking more than two soft drinks per day, and by 2007 this had decreased to approximately 10 percent. This change in soft drink consumption translated into a significant reduction in obesity among school children 11-years-old and younger. During this same period of time the percentage of these children who were obese dropped from 13.5 percent to about 11 percent.[119]

> *Fructose is least kind to those who are overweight. In these individuals the effects of fructose are amplified.*

To summarize, excessive intake of sugar, and in particular fructose, can cause metabolic syndrome and diabetes. How, then, can we explain studies that show minimal effects of sugar or fructose on features of metabolic syndrome?[120] Typically the studies that show minimal effects of fructose have been in young healthy individuals, whereas more prominent effects on plasma triglycerides or insulin resistance are seen in individuals who already are overweight or insulin resistant.[121-125]

The observation that young healthy individuals are relatively immune to the effects of sugar is not unexpected. It is known that when we are young that we do not absorb fructose very well.[126] The reason is that fructose is absorbed in the intestines through a special "transporter" and this is normally expressed at low levels. However, we and others have shown that the more an animal is exposed to sugar, the more it will increase the expression of this transporter.[117,127-129]

Evidence for how important this is comes from a study we did with Jillian Sullivan and Shikha Sundaram from Children's Hospital in Denver. Jillian and Shikha wanted to know if obese children with fatty liver would absorb

113

fructose differently from age-matched children who were healthy and lean. The absorption of fructose was made using the "hydrogen breath test," in which the children were given a specific dose of fructose. If fructose is incompletely absorbed, some fructose enters the colon where it is broken down by bacteria, which then release hydrogen and methane that can be detected in the breath. The results were striking. None of the lean children absorbed all of their fructose. In contrast, every one of the fat children absorbed all of the fructose that they were given.

These studies emphasize the danger of thinking that just because you are lean and healthy you can guzzle soft drinks with freedom and impunity. Repeated intake will increase the transporter and increase absorption, resulting not only in more calories being absorbed, but also in activation of the switch. Repeated sugar intake is therefore like a trap, in that it takes an initially healthy individual and slowly alters not only how they absorb the sugar, but also how they respond to it.

What about Fruits and Fruit Juices?

Animals use fruits to increase their fat stores by waiting until the fruit is very ripe or by gorging on as many fruit as possible. One reason for waiting until fruit is ripe is that it increases the amount of fructose and decreases the vitamin C levels.[130] However, the fruits we typically eat are not mushy ripe fruits but rather are more tart and contain less fructose and have high contents of vitamin C, antioxidants, potassium and fiber. As a consequence, high intake of fruits in humans is associated with a reduced frequency of diabetes.[131]

Insights into the role of fruits in metabolic syndrome was shown in a study we performed with Magdalena Madero and which was conducted on obese adults living in Mexico City. The individuals were randomized to receive a low fructose diet for six weeks with or without natural fruit supplements.[132] Both diets also restricted total caloric intake. Both diets caused weight loss and improvements in blood pressure, plasma triglycerides, and insulin resistance, and these latter effects were much greater than expected for the degree of weight loss. However, the low fructose diet with natural fruit supplements was actually superior to the low fructose diet alone in causing weight loss.

These studies suggest that the benefits of vitamin C and other substances in fruits likely outweigh the negative effects of fructose. However, it should be emphasized that the ingestion of large amounts of fruits, especially for those fruits low in vitamin C, is not recommended. Dried fruits, for example, contain high concentrations of fructose and have lost their vitamin C content. Fruit juices and punches are also problematic, for the rapid intake of juice could lead to significant elevations in the concentration of fructose in the liver, which is key for activating the metabolic switch. Drinking fruit juices is associated with an increased risk for obesity and diabetes, especially in children.[131,133-134] This has led to recommendations by the American Pediatric Association to restrict fruit juices in children.[135]

> *Natural fruits contain antioxidants that block fructose effects. In contrast, fruit juices contain more fructose and can overcome any benefits fruits may have.*

Is there a Difference between HFCS and Sucrose?

A common question is whether HFCS and sucrose are different in their ability to cause obesity, fatty liver or insulin resistance. The corn industry has argued that the composition of HFCS, which in soft drinks usually consists of 55 percent fructose and 45 percent glucose, is not too different from sucrose or table sugar, which is 50 percent fructose and 50 percent glucose. It is also known that sucrose is not stable in soft drinks, and that the acids present in the drink will breakdown sucrose over time to fructose and glucose. Hence, if you buy a sucrose-containing soft drink that has been on the shelf for several months, it may actually contain little sucrose, but rather consist primarily of fructose and glucose. This has led the corn industry to promote HFCS as being not different from sucrose, and has resulted in the proposal that HFCS should be called "corn sugar."

However, there are some biological differences between drinks containing HFCS and sucrose. To show this, Myphuong Le led a collaborative study with Dr. Julie Johnson and our group in which 40 healthy individuals were asked to drink 24 ounces of soft drinks that were identical except that one contained HFCS and the other contained sucrose.[136] The individuals then returned a few weeks later and repeated the protocol, but drank the other beverage. This allowed us to compare how the two drinks affected any particular individual.

Because the HFCS-containing beverage had higher fructose content, blood levels were about 20 percent higher overall compared to the sucrose-containing beverage. Not unexpectedly, this resulted in a greater rise in serum uric acid and a higher rise in blood pressure. The individuals receiving HFCS also showed a higher than expected rise in serum glucose, consistent with greater insulin resistance.[136] All of these effects occurred despite the fact that the majority of the sucrose was already broken down before it was ingested.

This study suggests that even the small difference in fructose content with HFCS and sucrose in soft drinks could be clinically significant. This concern is even greater based on a recent study in which the fructose content was measured in various soft drinks. Whereas bottled soft drinks tended to be accurate in stating how much fructose was present in the drink, the authors found that fountain drinks often had substantially higher amounts of fructose than listed, with some containing as much as 65 percent fructose.[137] This suggests that some of the fountain drinks were being spiked with preparations of HFCS that had a higher percentage of fructose.

There is also some evidence that the biological effects of fructose are greater with HFCS compared to sucrose even if the total amount of fructose is kept equal. This is because the absorption of sucrose in the gut first requires that the sucrose be degraded by a gut enzyme, sucrase. Sucrase degrades sucrose to fructose and glucose that then are absorbed. This should result in a delay in absorption. In contrast, drinks containing HFCS already have the fructose and glucose available for immediate absorption. Hence, the fructose should be absorbed more rapidly, likely with higher peak concentrations. This might theoretically lead to worse fatty liver.

Consistent with this possibility, our group found that when rats were fed equal amounts of sucrose or fructose and glucose for four months, the livers from the rats receiving the free fructose and glucose tended to have greater fat in their liver.[138] Nicole Avena's group also found that rats provided drinks with HFCS, as opposed to sucrose, gained more weight and were more obese.[139]

> *HFCS may be slightly worse than sugar in its ability to induce fatty liver and metabolic syndrome. The take-home message, however, is that both sugar and HFCS are driving the obesity epidemic.*

While these studies suggest that HFCS may have greater effects than sucrose to cause fatty liver or obesity, it is important to emphasize that *both* sucrose and HFCS activate the switch to cause obesity and fatty liver. Replacing one with the other is not the best approach if you want to lose weight.

Uric acid as a Cause of Obesity and Insulin Resistance

Koch's postulates can also be applied to the role of uric acid in obesity and metabolic syndrome. First, epidemiological studies repeatedly show that people with an elevated uric acid are at risk for developing obesity, fatty liver, and insulin resistance.[140-141] In one study, 433 healthy Japanese men under the age of 50 were followed for five years. At the end of the study, the 74 people whose initial serum uric acid level averaged 5.5 mg/dl gained 16 pounds compared to a 4-pound weight gain in the 359 individuals whose uric acid levels averaged around 4 mg/dl.[140]

Second, studies in laboratory animals have shown a role for uric acid in causing metabolic syndrome.[118,142] In particular, lowering uric acid partially prevents fructose-induced metabolic syndrome in rats.[118] Importantly, the effect requires high doses of allopurinol that would not be typically used in humans. The reason is that uric acid induces insulin resistance by its effects on mitochondria inside the cell, and higher doses of allopurinol are needed to lower uric acid levels inside the cell as opposed to simply lowering the serum uric acid level.

Third, pilot studies have examined the effect of lowering uric acid on insulin resistance and obesity in humans. For example, our collaborator, Dr. Daniel Feig, performed a study in which he randomized 60 obese children to receive one of two different drugs that lower uric acid (allopurinol or probenecid) or placebo for a period of two months. All of the children had serum uric acid levels that were >5.5 mg/dl. The primary endpoint was blood pressure, which was lowered by both therapies. However, lowering uric acid was also found to have an effect on weight. During the two month period, the obese children on placebo gained 7.5 pounds whereas the probenecid group only gained 3.5 pounds, and the allopurinol-treated group actually lost 1 pound. The reason for the differences between probenecid and allopurinol could relate to their relative effectiveness at lowering uric acid, for the allopurinol was much more effective (lowering the uric acid level to 3.4 mg/dl versus 4.3 mg/dl).

One small pilot study also reported that probenecid could improve insulin resistance in patients with heart failure,[143] and we have unpublished results with Dr. Mehmet Kanbay in Turkey in which allopurinol was given to individuals with asymptomatic elevations in uric acid with similar findings. Nevertheless, in another study, treatment with allopurinol could not prevent the worsening of insulin resistance in response to high doses of fructose (2 liters of a 10 percent solution for two weeks) even though this treatment prevented the rise in serum uric acid and blood pressure that occurred.[116] Since the dose of fructose was exceptionally high, it is possible that the allopurinol was not able to fully block the effects of fructose to raise intracellular uric acid.

Koch's Postulates: Uric acid as a Cause of Metabolic Syndrome (MS)	
1. Association is strong	Elevated uric acid increases risk of MS
2. Experimental Evidence	Lowering uric acid improves MS in animal models
3. Mechanism Identified	Uric acid alters Mitochondria
4. Raising uric acid causes MS	Not done
5. Lowering uric acid improves MS	Pilot studies suggest reducing uric acid may improve MS in humans

Summary

Both fructose and uric acid can be shown to activate the fat switch in cells by acting on the energy factories, or mitochondria, in the cell. There is evidence that both fructose and uric acid are used by animals to increase their fat stores and become insulin resistant. Furthermore, there is increasing evidence that they may have a role in human obesity and diabetes, although more studies are needed. But what about other foods? Could other common foods have a role in triggering the fat switch? What other ways can the fat switch be activated?

SECTION 4

OTHER WAYS TO GET FAT

CHAPTER 14

BEER AND THE FRIAR TUCK SYNDROME

> *While sugar (fructose) is likely the major driver of the obesity epidemic, heavy beer drinking is another cause. Other foods that can raise uric acid are also likely involved, although to a lesser extent. This includes the umami foods.*

Few tales capture the imagination more than that of Robin Hood and the Merry Men of Sherwood Forest, the outlaws that fought for the poor in medieval England. The legend of Robin Hood passed through generations as ballads and rhymes as part of the oral tradition, and by the early 15th century the Robin Hood Games were part of the annual May Day celebrations that were held throughout England.[1-2] One of the favorite stories, and which may have been introduced at the May Games, was that of the meeting of Robin Hood with Friar Tuck, in which Robin Hood forces the Friar to carry Robin on his back across a stream. The Friar then insists on Robin Hood to do the same for him. The problem comes when Robin tells the friar to take him over for a second time, for halfway across the friar dumps Robin into the water. From this a fight ensues, but out of this fight a friendship develops in which the friar joins Robin Hood and his men.

The reason I tell this story is not simply because I love the tales of Robin Hood, but because Friar Tuck is usually depicted as fat, at least from the late 16th century onwards. One of the earliest references, which was shared with me by Allen Wright, an expert on Robin Hood, was from William Shakespeare, who in his first play, *The Two Gentlemen of Verona* (circa 1590), has one of the outlaws in the play exclaim "By the bare scalp of Robin Hood's fat friar."

As noted by Rogers and Waldron[3], Geoffrey Chaucer, in his *Canterbury Tales* written in the late 14th century, also tells of the priest whose "head was bald, and shone like looking glass, and so did his face, as if it had been greased. He was a fat and personable priest." In the *Piers Ploughman*, a poem by William Langland that dates from the same period, the master friar is described as liking to "gobble up countless different dishes—mince meat and puddings, tripes and galantines, and eggs fried in butter."[3] But were these reports of fat friars and monks simply reflecting the literary creativity for these authors, or did obesity occur at a higher frequency in the monasteries?

The Legend of Robin Hood and Friar Tuck of Sherwood Forest

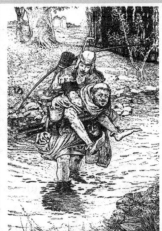

Friar Tuck Meets Robin Hood
Bold Robin Hood And His Outlaw Band by Louis Rhead (1912)

Lightly leapt the fryer off Robin Hoods back;
Robin Hood said to him again,
Carry me over this water, thou curtal frier,
Or it shall breed thy pain.

The frier took Robin Hood on 's back again,
And stept up to the knee;
Till he came at the middle stream,
Neither good nor bad spake he.

And coming to the middle stream,
There he threw Robin in:
'And chuse thee, chuse thee, fine fellow,
Whether thou wilt sink or swim

Robin Hood and the Friar (play, 1560) from *The English and Scottish Popular Ballads* by Francis James Child, 1888. (on web sitehttp://boldoutlaw.com/rhbal/bal123.html)

Work by archeologist Tony Waldron at University College in London has made a strong case that the monks living in the Abbeys likely were fatter than the regular populace. The way Waldron showed this was quite clever. Waldron was aware of a bone disease that can be looked for in skeletons that is strongly associated with obesity, as well as diabetes, gout, and elevated uric acid levels. The lesion is called DISH (for diffuse idiopathic skeletal hyperostosis) and is associated with new bone formation, particularly along the right side of the spine, and especially in the chest (thoracic) area. The extra bone forms on the vertebra, and also along the ligaments that run along the spine, and the sparing of the left side is thought to be due to pulsations of the aorta on that side which keeps the new bone from forming.[3]

Waldron examined skeletons taken from a large cemetery near the Royal Mint in London where victims of the Black Death had been buried, and he examined skeletons from the adjacent Abbey of Saint Mary Graces, both dating to the mid-1300s. While DISH was absent in all of the 301 skeletons from the cemetery for the common people, DISH was present in 6 of 103 skeletons from the Abbey. Waldron also examined skeletons from the Wells Cathedral in London and also found DISH more commonly in the skeletons from the two chapels as opposed to the main cemetery, again suggestive that the monks and bishops were more commonly obese.[3] Philippa Patrick, a colleague of Waldron's, also confirmed that skeletons of monks taken from medieval abbeys including St. Mary Graces Abbey, Tower Hill, and St. Saviour's Abbey, had a threefold greater risk for DISH than the general population at that time.

If monks were indeed fatter, then what is the reason, given what we have learned so far? Living in a monastery was not a life of luxury, and many monks lived very modestly. Early monasteries often allowed only one meal per day in winter, and two meals in the summer.[3] Over time this changed, though, and it became common for monks to eat large meals, often with very high caloric content. For example, records from Westminster Abbey document that the monks were allowed meals that equated to approximately 6200 calories per day, with 5300 calories during the Advent and 4900 calories per day during the Lent.[4] While the monks were expected to donate one third of their food to the poor, this still allowed a significant food intake. Monks also had to pray up to eight times per day, raising the possibility that they may have had less time for exercise than their countrymen. However, between prayers they were often very physically active, for they often spent a lot of time growing vegetables and grain.

Since weight is tightly regulated, one would not expect the monks to have ingested excessive amounts of food unless they had developed some degree of leptin resistance—in other words, that they would have had to activate the fat switch. In this regard, the monasteries were a major place where honey, wine, and beer were made. For many wines, the monks would add sugar or honey, such as the claret and mulberry wines, and beer would sometimes be made from honey (mead).[3] This suggests that the intake of sugar could have played a role in the obesity of these early monks. However, monks were especially famous for drinking beer or ale. The Bury Saint Edmunds Abbey in Suffolk, for example, had three breweries and the monks were entitled to eight pints of beer per day.

In the early 1900s Frederick Allen noted that diabetes was common in the Trappist monks living in Belgium, even though they did not consume a lot of sugar.[5] The diet of the Trappist monks was explored in more detail in a study in the early 1960s.[6] The Trappist monks lived in austere conditions, with minimal heat, only rarely speaking to each other, and with a diet that was strictly vegetarian. Their diet was low in sugar and saturated fat. In contrast, the Benedictine monks ate a western diet with eggs, meat, butter and more sugar. The Trappist monks weighed on average 20 pounds more, and 35 percent were moderately obese compared to 17 percent of the Benedictine monks. The Trappist monks also had higher blood pressure, whereas the Benedictine monks had higher cholesterol levels, the latter likely a consequence of their high fat diet.[6]

One might expect the Benedictine monks to have been fatter since they were eating more butter and sugar. However, I believe the reason why the Trappist monks were fatter is related to the drinking of beer. The Trappist monks drank at least a half liter of home-brewed beer daily, whereas the Benedictine monks drank no beer.[6] Furthermore, the Trappist monks allowed the drinking of the rich brown ale during Lent, and hence beer could be drunk all year long.

Beer, like sugar, is very potent at raising uric acid levels, but this occurs over hours instead of minutes. As you will recall, we have found that uric acid directly causes oxidative stress to the mitochondria and leads to fat accumulation in cells. This suggests that beer should be similar to sugar in its ability to increase fat stores.

Beer is much more effective than other alcohol-containing drinks in its ability to raise uric acid levels.[7] This is why gout is more commonly observed in people who drink beer as opposed to wine.[8-9] While alcohol can raise uric acid levels, the observation that alcohol-free beer raises uric acid to almost the same extent as regular beer shows that alcohol is not the cause.[10] Rather, the primary way by which beer raises uric acid levels is due to the yeast content, which is rich in nucleic acids that stimulate the production of uric acid. Brewer's yeast has the highest RNA content of almost all foods. Recall that RNA is a nucleotide which is metabolized to uric acid in the liver. While yeast is also used to make other types of alcohol, the yeast content in beer is particularly high, especially in unfiltered beers.

Since we found that uric acid has a role in obesity and insulin resistance, it is not surprising that heavy beer drinking is associated with obesity and diabetes. The fact that beer is rich in RNA explains that the "beer belly" is associated with beer drinking and not with the drinking of other alcohol-containing drinks. Excess beer intake is not only associated with abdominal obesity, but also with high serum triglycerides, elevated blood pressure and fatty liver, consistent with beer being another cause of the metabolic syndrome. If uric acid also has a role in leptin resistance, as suggested by some of our studies,[11] it would also explain why the Trappist monks could become obese, as it would stimulate them to eat more without having the sensation of fullness, thereby allowing them to reset their weight.

> *The Beer Belly is associated with high blood pressure, fatty liver and elevated triglycerides—in other words, it is a type of metabolic syndrome.*

Sumo wrestlers also use beer to help them gain weight. These individuals eat an enormous amount of food, amounting to more than 5000 calories each day. While they eat a wide variety of foods, their drink is primarily beer, which they consume in excessive amounts at each meal. One study of 800 sumo wrestlers showed that they not only were markedly obese, but also had elevated serum uric acid and triglyceride levels, as well as higher blood pressure than healthy Japanese. Sumo wrestlers also have an increased risk for diabetes.[12]

> *Sumo wrestlers use beer to help them gain weight.*

Beer is not simply a way humans get fat. The Japanese feed beer to Waygu cattle to make Kobe beef, a beef that is famous for its marbled fat and tenderness. The beer is given to the cattle to stimulate food intake and is given primarily during the summer months. Some cattle have been fed as many as 40 pints of beer a day to help them gain fat.

Beer becomes another food, much like fructose, for raising uric acid and activating the pathways to become fat. Sugar and beer intake likely both have a role in the obesity epidemic, but the former plays a much greater role. What about other foods that can raise uric acid?

Umami Foods Raise Uric acid and Activate the Fat Switch

The earliest primate ancestors ate primarily fruit, and the fructose present in fruit was the major means by which they stored fat. The uricase mutation that occurred during this period served as a way to enhance the accumulation of fat from fructose by amplifying the rise in uric acid within the cell. While primates living in tropical forest environments could continue with fruit as a major food source, ancestral humans had to diversify their diets with changing climates and the move away from tropical forests. As such, there was a gradual shift to a hunter gatherer society. New sources of food became available, of which certain foods, such as organ meats and bone marrow, were rich in nucleotides and could also raise uric acid.

Today there are many foods in the diet that are rich in nucleotides (such as RNA) or their breakdown products (such as purines), and which can serve as a source for making uric acid. Most dieticians do not think about the nucleotide content in foods, but rather focus on the calorie content from the fat, carbohydrate, and protein content. Nevertheless, foods high in purines and nucleotides can raise uric acid and thus could theoretically activate the fat switch in the mitochondria and increase the risk for becoming obese. While the purine and nucleotide content of food can raise uric acid, uric acid can also be made from scratch by amino acids, particularly glycine and glutamine. A related amino acid, glutamate, can also rapidly increase the formation of uric acid and other nucleotide products in the liver of rats and chickens.[13-14]

Given that foods containing nucleotides and glutamate could be important in increasing fat, one might think that the body would have developed a signaling system to stimulate intake of foods rich in these substances. Afterall, there is a sweet receptor in the taste buds that triggers a sensation of pleasure when sugar is ingested, and there are receptors for sour and bitter which likely were originally meant to help avoid noxious foods. There is also a salt receptor in the taste bud, which encourages salt intake which likely had an important role in helping to maintain the circulation and protect us from dehydration.

In fact, the taste buds do sense foods that raise uric acid, and it is called umami (pronounced oo-Ma-mee), or the fifth taste. The source of the umami taste was identified by Kikunae Ikeda, a Tokyo University professor who in 1907 discovered that the savory flavor present in traditional Japanese foods such as kombu (sea kelp) was due to the presence of glutamate. Later, Dr. Shintaro Kodama showed that the savory taste from glutamate was markedly enhanced by foods containing nucleosides, such as IMP (inosine monophosphate), which are present in the dried bonito tuna flakes that are often added to the Japanese soups. Later other nucleotides, such as AMP (adenosine monophosphate) and GMP (guanosine monophosphate), were also shown to enhance the umami taste.[15] This is particularly interesting as our group found that the fat switch consists of a conversion of AMP to IMP by the enzyme AMPD, and the IMP is later broken down to uric acid. In fact, we have some unpublished data that IMP itself may stimulate fat accumulation. Moreover, if AMP or IMP is given orally to volunteers, serum uric acid rises.[16]

The savory flavor of umami has led many food companies to add monosodium glutamate (MSG) to their food as a flavor enhancer. There are also many natural foods that are rich in glutamates or nucleotides, including blue cheese, shiitake mushrooms, fish sauces, and mussels. Perhaps not surprisingly, all foods high in purine content are also rich in umami since they contain nucleotide products such as IMP. Moreover, since glutamate also increases uric acid production in the liver,[14] one can say with relative confidence that all umami foods would be expected to have a role in obesity and insulin resistance if enough is ingested.

The Similarities of High Purine and High Umami Foods	
High Purine Foods	**High Umami Foods**

Meats:
   High: Organ meats, beef extract.
   Medium: Lamb, beef, pork, duck, turkey
Seafood
   High: shellfish, shrimp, crab, lobster, squid
Anchovies, sardines, mackerel, tuna, salmon
   Medium: most fish
Vegetable
   Medium: Soybeans, peas, brussel sprouts, broccoli, spinach
Mushroom:
   Medium: portobella, porcini, chanterelles
Dairy/Cheese
   Medium: Blue Cheese, Roquefort
Drink: Beer
	Meats:
	   High: Organ meats, beef extract.
	   Medium: Lamb, beef, pork, duck, turkey
	Seafood
	   High: shellfish, shrimp, crab, lobster, squid
	Anchovies, sardines, mackerel, tuna, salmon
	   Medium: most fish
	Vegetable
	   Medium: Soybeans, peas, tomatoes, red bell peppers, spinach
	Mushroom:
	   High: shitake, portobella, porcini, chanterelles
	Dairy/Cheese
	   High: Parmesan, Blue Cheese, Roquefort
	Drink: Beer

It should not be surprising, then, that studies have suggested that people who are eating foods high in glutamate content are at increased risk for obesity. For example, one study followed 10,095 healthy Chinese adults for an average of 5.5 years and found that those individuals that ingested high amounts of MSG had a higher risk for developing obesity.[17]

MSG has also been found to induce obesity in mice, particularly if given early in life.[18] In addition to obesity, it can cause insulin resistance, hypertriglyceridemia, and an increase in abdominal girth.[19] Cats given MSG also develop increased body fat and insulin resistance.[20] The role of umami foods could be very important in cats since they cannot taste sweet foods as they lack the sweet taste bud,[21] and they are also resistant to the effects of fructose to stimulate fat accumulation.[20]

The mechanism by which umami foods have been postulated to cause obesity has been attributed to its palatability, and possibly due to its ability to induce leptin resistance.[20] However, we suggest that the effects are due to the ability of glutamates and IMP and related nucleotides to raise uric acid, thus activating the switch to induce leptin and insulin resistance and fat accumulation.

RNA Foods and Obesity in Animals

While fructose is an excellent way to increase fat stores, not all animals have access to fructose, and the ingestion of RNA-rich foods may provide another way. For example, in the Antarctic winter, in which only a few hours of light are present each day, the sea ice expands to five times what it is at the peak of summer, reaching close to 7.7 million square miles (20 million square kilometers). The expansion of the ice blocks the sun, reducing the phytoplankton population to small numbers since they need light to generate energy and reproduce. This severely affects the Antarctic krill population, which are small crustaceans that live on the phytoplankton, and with the reduction in food supply they are forced to reduce their metabolic rate and live off of their fat stores.[22] As spring comes, the ice recedes and the phytoplankton bloom, extending as far as 150 miles (250 kilometers) from the edge of the ice. The bloom of the phytoplankton stimulates a massive increase in the Antarctic krill population, with swarms that have rarely been reported to extend 7.5 miles (12 kilometers) in length. As the krill grow, their RNA content rises dramatically as new proteins are being made.[23-24] The swarms of krill are then ingested by squid, fish and seabirds including some types of penguins. In turn, the Emperor penguin eats the RNA-rich squid and fish, and double their weight in preparation for the winter.

Other animals also eat RNA-rich foods to help them gain weight. The whale, for example, will ingest huge amounts of amphipods (a type of crustacean) in the Arctic, resulting in very high uric acid levels, serum that is yellow from the fat content, and huge fat stores. This allows the whale to fast when it leaves the Arctic for its mating grounds.[25]

The ability to degrade RNA is especially important for ruminants. Ruminants, which include cattle, goats, sheep, giraffes and camels, digest their food in a special compartment of their stomach, and then regurgitate it and rechew it as cud. The cud includes not only the half-digested food, but also bacteria that was present in that part of the stomach. These bacteria are killed when the food is swallowed a second time into a different stomach compartment that contains acid. The released RNA is degraded by the pancreatic RNase as the food is transported into the intestine. This technique allows the animal to obtain RNA not only from food, but from the bacteria that digest the food. This allows a maximal increase in uric acid.

Some animals have also improved their ability to increase their uric acid levels in response to RNA foods through evolutionary adaptations. The uricase mutation would be one way to amplify an increase in uric acid in response to RNA-rich foods. Other animals, such as the hippopotamus, horse, and rat, acquired pancreatic RNases with high activity to help degrade more RNA from foods.[26-27] The leaf eating colobus monkey made a particularly interesting adaptation.[26] Unlike most primates whose diet consists of fructose-rich fruits, the colobus monkey has a diet primarily of leaves, so it needed a different way to increase its fat stores. It did this by duplicating its pancreatic RNase gene. While the original pancreatic RNase in the colobus monkey was mainly designed to inactivate viruses that contain double stranded RNA, the duplicated RNase has increased RNase activity against single stranded RNA such as present in leaves and bacteria, and also has better enzyme activity in the alkaline intestinal environment.[28] This allows the colobus monkey to maximally breakdown the RNA and increase its uric acid levels from the leaves it eats.

Humans also have pancreatic RNase, and this is secreted into the intestinal lumen.[29] However, its activity is 60-fold less than that seen in the colobus monkey.[28] Nevertheless, it remains possible that the human RNase could increase in activity if continuously stimulated by foods rich in RNA. So beer drinkers beware!

While these studies suggest that eating umami foods could be another cause of obesity, it is dwarfed by the effects of sugar. So please do not panic at this point. Nevertheless, for some people, the role of umami foods in causing insulin resistance and fat accumulation should not be underestimated. Currently the mean intake of glutamate is in the range of 550 to 580 mg daily in the United Kingdom and Japan, respectively, but some individuals may be eating as much as 4 to 10 grams of glutamate a day.[17] Umami foods can also be addicting, and indeed, rats will become addicted to both regular beer as well as nonalcoholic beer.[30] There are also genetic differences in how individuals respond to the taste of umami foods.[15] Furthermore, just as with fructose, individuals with high uric acid levels show a greater increase in uric acid levels in response to the administration of foods containing IMP.[16]

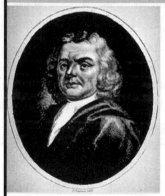

Boerhaave's Syndrome and Death by Umami

On October 30, 1723, the Dutch Grand Admiral, Baron Jan von Wassenaer, a man known for luxuriant living and excessive meals, had a lunch of veal soup and cabbage boiled with mutton, calf sweetbreads, spinach, a large portion of duck, two larks, apple compote, bread, and beer, followed by a dessert of pears, grapes, sweetmeats, and Moselle wine. After a brief ride on his horse, he developed stomach pains and tried to induce vomiting with thistle extract and ipecac. Unfortunately, the large meal caused such distention of his stomach, that the junction with the esophagus ruptured, causing his death. The Dutch physician, Herman Boerhaave, made the diagnosis and forever since this entity has been called Boerhaave's syndrome. As for the admiral, his love of duck and beer led to his obesity and gout, and is a sad example, of "death by umami," although sugar was likely an accomplice.

Herman Boerhaave 1668 -1738   Patton AS. The Curious Case of the Incurable Epicure . Harvard Medicine
http:harvardmedicine.hms.harvard.edu/bulletin/spring2005/
Artist J Chapman 1798 http://ihm.nlm.nih.gov/images/B29694 PD-US

More studies are needed before a verdict is passed, but there are likely some individuals in which umami foods may be the principal factor driving insulin resistance and fat storage. One group for which this is likely important are Asians, as this group has the highest intake of umami foods. In turn,

Asians commonly have high uric acid levels, as well as high frequency of insulin resistance, diabetes and high blood pressure. While they show evidence of mild obesity with an increase in abdominal girth, they typically do not develop severe obesity. I believe this is because, as mentioned in earlier chapters, the increase in uric acid and other RNA products is important in triggering leptin resistance and setting the fat switch, but it is not the sugar or the umami foods that act as the primary fuel for weight gain. Rather, the strongest fuels for weight gain are foods high in fat content, which are less a part of the Asian diet as opposed to the American diet. In the next chapter let's take a closer look at the role of high fat foods in the epidemics of obesity and cardiovascular disease.

CHAPTER 15

HIGH FAT DIET AND LIFE
OF THE ESKIMO

High fat diets provide a fuel for weight gain if the fat switch is turned on. However, if the fat switch is turned off, such as by a low carbohydrate diet, then diets high in fat and protein may result in weight loss.

Of all places humans have survived, there is none more severe or challenging than the Arctic. As the explorer, Vilhjalmur Stefansson, wrote in the early 1920s, it is a land "covered with eternal ice; there is everlasting winter with intense cold; and the corollary of the everlastingness of the winter is the absence of summer and the lack of vegetation. The country, whether land or sea, is a lifeless waste of eternal silence. The stars look down with a cruel glitter, and the depressing effect of the winter darkness upon the spirit of man is heavy beyond words. On the fringes of this desolation live the Eskimos, the filthiest and most benighted people on earth, pushed there by more powerful nations farther south, and eking out a miserable existence amidst hardship."[31]

The life of these people was extraordinary. When winter came the temperature could fall to 30 or 40 degrees below Fahrenheit, and for months the sun would never rise above the horizon, creating only twilight. Yet driven by the need for survival, the men would leave their snow huts and sit by holes in the ice, waiting for hours behind a snow wall for the sound of the seal surfacing for a breath of air, so they could lunge their bone-pointed harpoons or spears blindly through the hole to catch their prize.[32] The seals were critical for existence, not only as food but because the skins could be used for clothing and tents, and their blubber for fuel and light.[33]

In the spring and early summer the men would kayak along the coastal waters where they would harpoon the 40-ton whales returning from their summer migrations, and if they were lucky they might kill one or two for their village. By midsummer and autumn the tribes would move inland to hunt caribou by bow and arrow and to fish for salmon. But other than the rare salmon berry, there were no vegetables or fruit. Furthermore, while they would light stone lamps using seal blubber as their oil, with which they could cook, often they would eat their meat raw. It was for this reason that the Indians to the south referred to these people as the "Ieschimou", which means raw flesh eaters. This name was later transformed by the early French explorers to the Esquimaux, or the Eskimo. Today, however, these brave people are called the Inuit, which is the name they used to refer to themselves and which means, The People.[34]

The diet of the Inuit was almost exclusively from eating sea mammals, such as the seal, white whale, narwhal and walrus, and in the summer there was the caribou. Occasionally they would eat fish, such as the salmon, whitefish, or trout, and at times they would catch birds, such as the eider duck, auk, or murre, but this was never a major part of their diet. For the Inuit, the diet consisted of cooked and uncooked meat and fat, and there were no vegetables, and an absence of salt.[35] As such, the daily diet consisted of fat (50 percent) and protein (35 percent), with the only carbohydrate the glycogen (or animal starch) present in the meat (15 percent), with an average intake of 3000 calories per day.[36]

Survival in the Arctic: Life of the Inuit

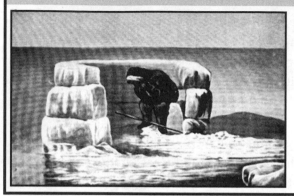

An Eskimo waiting for a seal to surface through a breathing hole.

From: Lewis AJ and Peck EJ. The Life and Work of the Rev. E.J. Peck among the Eskimos. 1905

One could say that the Inuit diet is the extreme of a high fat, high protein, low carbohydrate diet. Given that the energy content of fat is so high (9 calories per gram compared to 4 calories per gram for proteins and carbohydrates), one might wonder if such a high energy diet was needed to survive in the Arctic. On the other hand, I have told you that in the absence of fructose, it is hard to store fat. So this leads to the question—do high fat diets increase our fat stores and weight similar to that which occurs with high sugar diets? Let's look at the evidence.

High Fat Diets and Weight Gain

Contrary to some opinions, a diet that is high in fat can cause *weight gain*, especially if supplemented to the current American diet. James Hill, a Professor of Medicine at the University of Colorado and a leading expert on obesity, performed a study in which 22 healthy non-obese individuals were studied for four days on three different diets containing different contents of fat (26, 34 and 40 percent fat). The total number of calories, or energy intake, increased with higher concentrations of fat in the diet, and on the highest fat intake, the individuals were taking approximately 250 extra calories per day.[37] These observations are consistent with studies in experimental animals in which high fat diets have been found to stimulate weight gain, especially when given as part of a "western diet" that also contains sugar (or fructose).

There are likely at least two reasons why high fat foods cause weight gain. The primary reason relates to the fact that most Americans are eating enough sugar that they likely have mild leptin resistance, so when high fat foods are provided it is like providing high grade fuel for weight gain. The other reason, however, relates to the relative lack of effect of high fat foods to tell the brain to quit eating (satiety response). When we eat carbohydrates, the rise in glucose stimulates insulin release from our pancreas, which causes leptin to be released from the fat tissues that signals the brain that we are full and that we should quit eating. A high protein diet also results in a satiety response,[38] although the mechanism responsible for this effect is not clear. In contrast, high fat diets do not stimulate insulin release as well, and hence the leptin response is weak.[39] This latter mechanism is most important when 40 percent or more of the diet is fat.

While these studies suggest that high fat diets might contribute to obesity, they are not the driving force. Our studies suggest excessive sugar intake remains the dominating way to become fat and insulin resistant. Indeed, there has been a reduction in overall fat intake in the United States between 1971 and 2006 despite the remarkable increase in obesity.[40] This is further supported by the finding that while low fat diets are an effective means for losing weight, weight loss is rarely sustained, likely because the fat switch is still turned on.

High Fat Diets, Cholesterol and Heart Disease

While high fat diets do not cause leptin resistance or metabolic syndrome, high fat diets may increase our risk for heart disease. Recall Ancel Keys, the outspoken nutritionist from Minnesota, who argued that high fat diets were the cause of the dramatic rise in cardiovascular disease that occurred in the 20th century.[41] In the famous "Seven Countries Study," Keys reported that the intake of high fat diets correlated with rising rates of coronary artery disease.[42]

At this point we need to distinguish two different processes that can cause heart disease. One process is *atherosclerosis*, which occurs when cholesterol-enriched plaques build up in blood vessels such as the coronary arteries. These plaques occur in the lining of the blood vessels and can increase to the point where they start to block the blood flow. In the heart this can result in a heart attack (myocardial infarction) or even sudden death. Sometimes the plaques can rupture, and the cholesterol-laden material can be dislodged and enter the blood stream where it may travel to areas such as the brain until it lodges in small vessels, causing the tissue supplied by those small vessels to die, or infarct. This "embolization" can be a cause of stroke. Diseases in which atherosclerosis is important include heart attacks and aortic aneurysms.

The second process is *arteriolosclerosis*, and is due to disease of the smaller arteries, which are known as arterioles. These are the small vessels that constrict and relax in response to changes in blood pressure, and help to maintain the blood flow to the organ. In arteriolosclerosis these small arterioles become abnormally thickened or scarred so they cannot constrict or relax appropriately. Cholesterol is not involved in arteriolosclerosis; rather, this condition is associated with hypertension and metabolic syndrome, and can be induced experimentally by feeding animals fructose or by raising serum uric acid.[43-44] Because the arterioles lose their ability to regulate blood flow, critical tissues such as the brain, kidney and heart can be exposed to varying blood flow and pressures. As such, disease of the small vessels predisposes to stroke, heart failure, heart attacks, and kidney disease.[45]

Atherosclerosis Versus Arteriolosclerosis

	Atherosclerosis	Arteriolosclerosis	
What is it?	Cholesterol plaques in medium-sized blood vessels	Thickening and scarring of the small blood vessels (arterioles)	Atherosclerosis is associated with cholesterol plaques and is driven by high fat diets, high serum cholesterol, smoking and genetics.
What causes it?	High Cholesterol Smoking High fat diet Genetics	High Blood Pressure Sugar (fructose) Uric Acid	For arteriolosclerosis, work by this author suggests a role for uric acid and sugar (fructose), although this has not been accepted by all authorities.
How does it present?	Myocardial Infarction Carotid artery disease Aortic Aneurysm Perifpheral vascular disease	Hypertension Heart Failure Stroke Chronic Kidney Disease	

Diets high in fat do not predispose to arteriolosclerosis, but they increase serum cholesterol and hence may increase the risk for atherosclerosis. An example relates to Vilhjalmur Stefansson, an Arctic explorer, and his friend, K. Andersen, who wanted to show that the Eskimo diet, which is high in fat and protein but low in carbohydrate, was safe and would not cause vitamin deficiencies or other problems. These two individuals decided to eat a diet extremely high in fat (about 80 percent) with 20 percent protein and 1 percent carbohydrate.[46] This is higher in fat content than the typical Eskimo diet which is closer to 50 percent fat.[35-36] Both men took their meals in a metabolic ward at a New York hospital for seven weeks and then continued their diet at home for a period of one year. Both men had an initial loss in weight, but then the weight stabilized and in general the diet was well tolerated. However, both were found to have blood so rich in fat that it would appear milky, with cholesterol levels that at times reached 800 mg/dl.[46]

While Stefansson's diet was exceptionally high in fat, it was not truly representative of the Inuit diet which was closer to 50 percent fat content. Whether the typical diet of the Inuit increases the risk for coronary artery disease remains debatable. One study of Inuit showed that these individuals averaged total cholesterol levels of 220 mg/dl, which while still high is lower than that observed in Stefansson.[36] Autopsy studies in the Inuit have also documented that some individuals (about 10 percent) have mild evidence for atherosclerosis, although this was rarely the cause of death, possibly because they often died earlier from other causes due to living in such a harsh environment.[36] Nevertheless, this is lower than might be expected compared to people eating a western diet. One reason may relate to the type of fat ingested by the Inuit. This is because marine fats tend to be high in fish oils, which contain omega 3 fatty acids (including DHA (docosahexaenoic acid) and EPA (eicosapentaenoic acid)) that may help protect against atherosclerosis. Fats that contain omega 3 fatty acids appear to be safer than those that contain primarily omega 6 fatty acids, the latter which is especially concentrated in various oils from sunflower, corn, canola, and soybeans.

Given that high serum cholesterol increases the risk for atherosclerosis, and that high fat diets may increase serum cholesterol, one might expect low fat diets to reduce heart disease. After all, studies have shown that the lowering total and LDL cholesterol with statins reduce the risk for heart disease. Nevertheless, the benefit of a low fat diet on cardiovascular disease has been difficult to show. For example, in the Women's Health Initiative Study, 48,000 postmenopausal women were randomized to a low fat diet (20 percent fat) or a normal fat diet (35 percent) for eight years. Despite relatively good adherence, there was no benefit on either the frequency of stroke or heart attack.[47] One obvious reason, of course, is that a low fat diet is frequently a high carbohydrate diet, so while it may reduce the risk for cholesterol-rich plaques, one might be increasing the risk for arterioloscle-rosis.

High Fat Diets and Weight Loss

While high fat diets can cause weight gain in the setting of a western diet, high fat diets can also cause weight loss, and this is in the setting where carbohydrate intake is severely restricted. One of the earliest documented cases was that of William Banting, who was so fat that he could not bend over to tie his shoes and he had to walk downstairs backwards so he could decrease the risk for falling. In 1862 Banting went to see an ear specialist, William Harvey, for deafness. Harvey felt that Banting's marked obesity might be contributing to the deafness, and recommended a diet high in fat and protein but low in carbohydrate. His reasoning was a bit obscure, but he had heard the French physiologist, Claude Bernard, speak of his discovery that a sugar-like substance, glucose, could be produced in the liver from starch and this blood sugar and was elevated in the blood in diabetes. Because Harvey recognized that obesity and diabetes were commonly asso-ciated with each other, he reasoned that foods that could reduce this glucose output might benefit both obesity and diabetes, and he was aware that sugar could be used to fatten animals and, conversely, that high protein foods could help control blood glucose levels in diabetic individuals.[48] So Harvey prescribed a diet that only restricted carbohydrate intake. The results were impressive. After one year Mr. Banting had lost 50 pounds with a decrease in his waist girth by 13 inches. He also noted an improvement in his gout.[49]

> *William Banting lost 50 pounds in one year by going on a high fat, high protein, low carbohydrate diet. This diet was later adapted by Robert Atkins and is currently known as the Atkins diet.*

There are at least two reasons why weight loss occurred with Harvey's diet. First, the absence of fructose in the diet may have helped turn off the fat switch and leptin resistance, thereby reducing appetite and increasing energy. Second, when there is minimal carbohydrate content in the diet, the glycogen stores in the liver rapidly become depleted, and this triggers the burning of fat, in association with a rise of ketones in the blood. Thus, the diet should act to reduce appetite, increase energy and stimulate the burning of fat.

How did the Inuit Survive?

Given that the Inuit had minimal carbohydrates other than the glycogen present in their meat, a natural question is how the Inuit could survive. Recent studies suggest that they did acquire a few ways to adapt in this hostile environment. For example, one study found that the Inuit absorbs cholesterol from their diet more effectively than others.[36] The Inuit also lived in a state of relative vitamin C deficiency. As discussed earlier, vitamin C is an antioxidant that acts on mitochondria and likely helps prevent fat formation. Severe vitamin C deficiency causes the disease scurvy (which results in bleeding gums and joints) whereas a mild deficiency of vitamin C is commonly observed in obese and hypertensive individuals and likely contributes to these conditions. The daily intake of vitamin C among the Inuit was low (about 30 mg/day).[50] To avoid developing scurvy, the Inuit would eat some of their meat raw due to the higher content of vitamin C, or perhaps the skin of the whale (*muktuk*) which was one of the only rich sources.[50] Nevertheless, most Inuit had mild vitamin C deficiency and this may have helped the Eskimo increase their fat stores. Some of the foods that the Inuit ate were also RNA-rich , such as the bone marrow of the caribou. This may also have helped increase their fat stores.

Perhaps as a consequence, Inuit women have higher amount of abdominal fat as noted by high waist to hip ratios when compared to other ethnic groups of the same weight.[51] In a study performed in 1994, the mean percentage body fat in women was 32 percent with average BMI of 27.[51] For women with normal body mass index (BMI<25), over 90 percent of Inuit women had high waist to height ratios versus 29 percent in age-matched Canadian women, documenting higher abdominal fat. In contrast, subcutaneous fat, such as measured by skin fold thickness in the arm, was not increased in the Inuit.[52] Given what we have learned, the relative increase in abdominal fat in the Inuit women might have been beneficial for the increased energy demands that occur with pregnancy.

The Inuit also found ways to adapt to the cold environment. For example, cold stimulates brown fat,[53] which generates more heat than regular fat when it is burned. The mitochondria of the Inuit and other American Indians have also been found to generate more heat when compared to other peoples. This adaptation resulted from a mutation and likely occurred during the prehistoric migrations of these peoples through Siberia and the Bering Strait, and would have allowed better adaptation to the cold environment.[54-55]

Despite all of these adaptations, early European explorers commented that starvation was not rare among the Eskimo. Life relied on being able to hunt seal and caribou, but not always could these animals be found.[36] One vulnerable time was in early spring, before the caribou came north from the woodlands to the south.[56] When famines occurred, such as among the Caribou Eskimo between 1917-1921, the Inuit would be forced to eat their dogs,[35] and even then many did not survive. Infanticide was also not uncommon, especially if there were twins, as it was too hard for the mother, although sometimes other women would adopt the second child. Some tribes were also known to abandon the aged or infirm when food became scarce.[33]

> *The Inuit survived in the Arctic on a high fat, high protein and low carbohydrate diet, but maintaining fat stores was difficult and survival was difficult.*

Summary

High fat diets contribute to the obesity epidemic, primarily by acting as fuel once the fat switch has been turned on. Nevertheless, weight loss can be induced with high fat and high protein diets if carbohydrate intake is significantly reduced, as this latter move helps turn off the switch. Unfortunately for the Inuit, the high fat and low carbohydrate diet was not the ideal diet to maintain their fat stores in the harsh environment of the Arctic, but it is what they had. Today the low carbohydrate, high fat diet is one of the most popular ways to lose weight. The knowledge of the fat switch should allow us, however, to develop better ways to lose weight that are safe and do not require having to make such drastic changes to the diet.

CHAPTER 16

STARCH AND THE PILLSBURY DOUGHBOY SYNDROME

The fat "Pillsbury Doughboy" as seen in the television ads has scientific basis! Some of us convert the starch we eat into fructose which is why starch can cause obesity.

When I wrote my book on sugar, *The Sugar Fix*, I promoted the idea that the benefit of the low carbohydrate diet was due to the reduction in the fructose.[57] After all, it made great sense, for we had shown that rats fed starch do not develop obesity whereas rats fed sucrose not only become fat but develop metabolic syndrome.[58] Consistent with this concept, the major benefits of a low carbohydrate diet were not only more rapid weight loss but also relatively greater reductions in blood pressure and serum triglycerides,[59] tell-tale signs consistent with a reduction in fructose intake. As a consequence, I viewed my low fructose diet as an alternative to the low carbohydrate diet that would be just as effective as the low carb diet but would be easier to adapt since a normal intake of carbohydrate (55 percent), protein (15 percent), and fat (30 percent) would be possible. Since a high fat diet increases serum cholesterol and its risk for atherosclerosis, and because there is evidence that diets high in protein can have bad effects on the kidneys,[60] I thought the diet would also be healthier.

However, I remember my interview with Jimmy Moore, who has a blog promoting the low carbohydrate diet (the "Livin' La Vida Low-Carb" blog www.livinlavidalowcarb.com/blog) as well as a podcast website (www.thelivinlowcarbshow.com/shownotes). Jimmy had once weighed over 400 pounds, but lost over 180 pounds on Dr. Atkin's low carbohydrate diet.[61] He liked this diet over other diets not only because it worked but because it also reduced his desire for foods. However, the comment that this veteran dieter told me which struck me deeply was his conviction that reducing sugar was not enough and that to lose weight, and to maintain the weight loss, he had to reduce *all* carbohydrates.

There were other findings that also made me worried about the benefits of a diet that only lowered sugars containing fructose. For example, why was corn so effective at fattening chickens and cattle? Corn contains primarily starch unless it is converted chemically to make high fructose corn syrup. Indeed, a French delicacy is *foie gras*, which is made from the fatty liver of a duck or goose. While the fatty liver was historically made by force-feeding figs (which is a rich source of fructose), today it is commonly made by placing a tube down the mouth of a goose and overfeeding the goose with corn.

While we and others have found that reducing the intake of sugars containing fructose or high fructose corn syrup is beneficial on weight and features of metabolic syndrome,[62-64] a comparison of the low fructose diet with the Atkins diet has not yet been performed, and so we do not yet know which diet is more effective in the short and long run. However, there is a new twist to the story, as it now appears that there is another source of fructose which we had not considered before, and that is the stealth production of fructose generated during the metabolism of carbohydrates by the body.

The Body also makes Fructose

Like the rest of the world, I had always thought that almost all of the fructose in our body comes from the sugar, high fructose corn syrup, and fruits and fruit juices we eat or drink. The idea that the body can make large amounts of fructose was really not considered. While we knew that fructose can be made from glucose by a series of enzymes known as the polyol pathway, these enzymes were thought to be turned on only in diabetes. Diabetic individuals have higher blood and urine levels of fructose than nondiabetic people, and these levels remain elevated even when fructose is removed from the diet.[65] If diabetic patients are given an "oral glucose tolerance test" in which they have to drink a bottle containing glucose water, there is not only a rise in glucose in the blood, but also a rise in fructose levels.[66] While studies such as these show that the diabetic can make fructose, no one thought that nondiabetic individuals were also making significant amounts of fructose.

However, we are making more fructose than we realize. We discovered this when we were studying the special mice that could not metabolize fructose. These mice were generated by mutating the fructokinase enzyme. Since these mice cannot metabolize fructose, their blood levels of fructose increase to a much greater extent than normal mice after being fed fructose. The surprising finding, however, was that these mice had very high levels of fructose in the blood and urine even if they were fasting. Therefore, these mice are making fructose every day even when there is no fructose in the diet. And guess where the fructose is coming from? It is coming from the glucose present in carbohydrates.

Fructose generated from Glucose Drives Obesity

As I mentioned earlier, rats fed either starch or glucose in their food tend not to gain weight or develop features of metabolic syndrome compared to rats on normal diets, whereas rats fed sugars containing fructose develop fatty liver and metabolic syndrome. However, if mice are given glucose in the drinking water, they will increase their weight, abdominal fat, and develop fatty liver. One of the reasons appears to be taste, as mice love the taste of glucose and will drink much more water if it contains glucose as opposed to normal drinking water. Since they are getting a lot of calories by drinking the glucose water, they decrease their intake of solid foods (mouse chow), but they do not decrease the intake of the chow to the degree necessary to maintain their normal body weight. As such, they become progressively fat over time.

When we discovered that even normal animals are generating fructose from glucose in the diet via the polyol pathway, we wondered if the reason glucose water was causing obesity and fatty liver might be due to the glucose being converted to fructose in the body. In this regard, the polyol pathway can be stimulated by a number of ways, but one way is by incubating a cell with high levels of glucose. This, in fact, explains why diabetes is associated with high fructose levels in the blood. We realized that if one ingests foods that would increase glucose levels rapidly in the liver, then this might act as a stimulus for converting the glucose to fructose. One way would be by ingesting drinks high in glucose content, such as glucose water. Perhaps that might explain why glucose in the drinking water was much more effective at causing obesity than glucose that is in starch and which would be released more slowly following ingestion.

To test this hypothesis, Drs. Miguel Lanaspa, Takuji Ishimoto, and Yuri Sautin performed experiments in which mice lacking fructokinase were given glucose water. The findings were exciting. Normal mice given glucose water gained weight and visceral fat, and developed fatty liver and insulin resistance. In contrast, the mice lacking fructokinase still gained weight, but it was much less and they were almost completely protected from developing fatty liver and insulin resistance. This was particularly striking as the mice lacking fructokinase loved the glucose water and drank the same amount of glucose water as did the normal mice. When we examined the livers, we found that the polyol pathway was activated in both groups of mice. However, the mice lacking fructokinase were not able to metabolize the fructose, and as a consequence they were largely protected from developing features of the metabolic syndrome.

> *It is not just the fructose we eat, but the fructose we make, that makes us fat.*

These data show that glucose can also cause obesity, but that the mechanism is driven in part by fructose that is generated within the body. Thus, this explains why starch can cause obesity in some individuals, and why

Jimmy Moore was adamant that it was not enough to just reduce sugar intake to lose weight. Gary Taubes also proposed in *Good Calories, Bad Calories* that obesity is driven primarily by intake of all carbohydrates, but had suggested that it was driven by insulin.[67] Our studies would be consistent with Taube's theory in that the mice lacking fructokinase still gained some weight when given glucose water. However, the major reason glucose causes obesity and fatty liver appears to be due to the conversion of glucose to fructose in the liver. So, in a way we were right in considering fructose as a primary nutrient driving obesity, but we were wrong in thinking you only get fructose from fructose-containing foods.

An important question relates to the level of activity of the polyol pathway, for it will govern how much fructose is produced from the glucose provided by starches and other foods. We had mentioned how this pathway can be activated by rapid rises in glucose in the liver, such as following the drinking of glucose water. This is relevant to soft drinks that contain either sucrose (which is 50 percent glucose and 50 percent fructose) or high fructose corn syrup (which typically contains 55 percent fructose and 45 percent glucose) as both contain significant amounts of glucose in addition to fructose.

The fact that high concentrations of glucose in the blood can generate fructose also explains a nutritional mystery. People who have had extensive surgery on their gut, or who were born with various conditions in which they have problems ingesting food, are sometimes fed by vein for months with solutions that contain high concentrations of glucose, amino acids, and lipids. The administration of nutrients by injecting them directly into the blood is called total parenteral nutrition (TPN), and is life-saving. However, many people who receive total parenteral nutrition, and especially small children, develop fatty liver, and this occasionally progresses to end stage liver disease. In contrast, if patients receive feedings via a tube into the intestine (termed enteral feeding) only rarely does fatty liver develop.[68] Experimental studies have shown that the fatty liver is due to the high glucose concentrations in the TPN, and studies of the liver show the very same changes one observes with fructose.[69] It is therefore very likely that the high glucose solutions are activating the polyol pathway in the liver and the glucose is being converted to fructose. In turn, the fructose causes the fatty liver, while the infusion of lipids likely accelerates the fatty liver by providing fatty acids as fuel.[70] Hence, the fatty liver associated with parenteral nutrition is another fructose-dependent disease.

> *The reason artificial feeding (feeding by vein, or total parenteral nutrition) causes fatty liver is likely because the highly concentrated glucose solution is being converted to fructose.*

The observation that increased concentrations of glucose can activate the polyol pathway and generate fructose could be relevant to the types of starches one eats. For example, certain foods raise blood glucose more effectively than others. These "high glycemic" foods include starchy foods such as breads and potatoes. It seems likely that these foods might be able to activate the polyol pathway more easily than more complex carbohydrates. Intake of white rice, for example, has been associated with increased risk for diabetes in Asian women.[71] However, whether this is due to activation of the polyol pathway or because rice intake in Asians is commonly associated with the ingestion of traditional Japanese umami-rich diets which are also associated with increased risk for diabetes[72] remains unclear.

High Glycemic Foods

Food	Index
Glucose	100
Baked Potato	85
Corn Flakes	84
Waffle	76
Doughnut	76
Corn Chips	74
Watermelon	72
White Bread	70
Table Sugar	65
White Rice	58
Fructose	20

High glycemic foods are carbohydrates that tend to raise serum glucose more than other carbohydrates following ingestion. A score of 100 means that the food has a similar glycemic index as glucose itself. High glycemic foods (defined as an index >70) include sugar, potatoes, chips and pretzels, and to a lesser extent, rice. Pasta tends to have a lower glycemic index. Fructose has a low glycemic index.

> *High glycemic foods, that is, foods that lead to a greater rise in glucose, may be more likely to generate fructose.*

The generation of fructose by the polyol pathway may also be more likely in individuals with insulin resistance and metabolic syndrome, for these individuals will show a greater rise in glucose following meals than normal people. Individuals with metabolic syndrome also frequently have an elevated uric acid level, and Miguel Lanaspa found that uric acid stimulates the polyol pathway to make more fructose from glucose. This might explain why individuals with obesity or metabolic syndrome may find it harder to lose weight, for in these individuals the ingestion of carbohydrates generates more fructose than would be observed in a lean, healthy individual. This is likely why Jimmy Moore found that he had to restrict all carbohydrates to lose weight.

> *Starch causes obesity most easily in those who are insulin resistant, fat, or have high uric acid levels.*

This could also explain why it is so easy to induce fatty liver in geese with corn, and why birds in general develop fatty liver so easily, as they have the uricase mutation and hence have higher uric acid levels and may be more susceptible to the fattening role of carbohydrates. In contrast, this could also explain why laboratory rats that have low uric acid levels are relatively resistant to the effects of starch.

Summary

Intake of added sugars remains the major cause of the epidemic of obesity and metabolic syndrome, but it is not the only cause. Fructose can be generated other ways, including from simple carbohydrates. This latter way of becoming fat is most important when people are drinking liquids containing glucose (such as soft drinks and juices), when they have impaired glucose tolerance or diabetes (in which blood glucose levels are high), or when their serum uric acid is elevated. So there are at least two sources of fructose, one from the sugars we eat, and one from the fructose we make. But alas, there is another, even more sneaky way our body can get fructose, and it relates to other life forms that live within us.

CHAPTER 17

STEALTH SOURCES OF FRUCTOSE AND URIC ACID

> *There is a stealth source of fructose–which is the fructose generated by the bacteria in our gut.*

On May 5, 1973, the American Thoroughbred racehorse, Secretariat, shattered all previous records at Churchill Downs by running the one and a quarter mile Kentucky Derby in under two minutes. In the beginning he was in last place, but with each quarter mile he accelerated, and in the final stretch he passed the leader, Sham, winning by two and one-half lengths. Secretariat went on to win the U.S. Triple Crown, which was the first time this had been done in more than 25 years, and his records at both the Kentucky Derby and the Belmont Stakes continue to this day. The champion racehorse retired to the rich pastures of Kentucky, but later developed laminitis (Founder disease), a painful condition in his hooves that crippled him. On October 4, 1989, he was put to sleep at the age of 19 years, and the world lost one of its most famous American Thoroughbreds. Ironically, laminitis, which is the second most common cause of death in racehorses, is likely due to a stealth form of fructose which might also have a role in human obesity and health.

"Tell me what you eat, I'll tell you who you are," wrote the French writer Anthelme Brillat-Savin in the early 1800s. However, in the last decade we have discovered that this statement may need to be modified. We are not just what we eat, but we are also what the bacteria inside of us eat and produce. We had, in fact, learned about this earlier. Animals such as camels generate food not just from the grasses they eat, but when they regurgitate their food, they also digest the gut bacteria that are mixed with the food, and this provides another source of food. In fact, we suggested that the DNA and RNA in the bacteria are important for these animals so they can generate uric acid which they use to help make fat. However, there is another way gut bacteria can provide calories. Some bacteria are resourceful in that they can digest components of plants that we cannot, and in so doing they can produce foods inside our gut. One of the foods they produce is fructose.

Fructans: A Stealth Source of Fructose

Plants use photosynthesis to produce carbohydrates that they use as food. One of the major carbohydrates they produce is starch, but some plants, like the sugarcane and sorghum, produce sucrose. Most tropical plants use starch as their major energy source, and since they are producing starch daily, they only store small amounts.[73] However, plants living in cold zones, or in areas in which droughts are common, developed a better way to store carbohydrates. These plants, which include grasses called C3 grasses, as well as some flowering plants such as the daisy and aster, store their carbohydrates as polymers of fructose, which are known as fructans. In essence, fructans consist of multiple fructose molecules bound together. They are then transported to the stems or root of the plant where they are stored as food. When the plant is in need of nutrition yet the environment does not allow adequate production, they breakdown the fructans to produce fructose which they use as a food source.[74] This is particularly true for perennial plants that live in the north and die off except for the roots that keep the plant alive over winter. The fructans not only provide a food source but also help protect the plant from the harsh conditions of winter by acting like an antifreeze.[74-76]

Not only do plants make fructans as a way to store food, but so do some bacteria. One of the best examples is *Streptococcus mutans*, which lives in the human mouth and is largely responsible for causing caries (cavities). Its favorite food is sugar, and especially fructose. In fact, individuals who eat little sugar (or fructose) almost never get caries.[77] However, the *Streptococcus* has a problem, in that they would like to have food available during periods when humans are not actively eating. To do this, the bacteria produce their own fructans from the fructose we eat, and then store them in the crevices of teeth which often become the sites of cavity formation.[78] If the ability for *Streptococcus* to generate fructans is interrupted, caries formation is reduced in laboratory rats in which sugar solutions are provided intermittently.[79]

Fructans as a Mechanism for Causing Obesity

As mentioned, plants and bacteria that make fructans have developed ways to convert the fructans back to fructose. They do this by producing enzymes called fructanases. Humans and other mammals do not have fructanases, so for us fructans are indigestible. However, this is not the case if we have bacteria in our gut that produce fructanases.

Much of our understanding of the role of gut bacteria in obesity comes from the work of Jeffrey Gordon, a scientist from Washington University in Saint Louis.[80-83] Gordon discovered that the gut bacteria of obese animals tended to be different from that of lean animals, and when he would transfer the bacteria from an obese to a lean animal, the animal would spontaneously gain weight and fat. He also documented that obese humans have the same types of bacteria as obese laboratory animals. When he looked at the characteristics of the bacteria from fat animals, he found that they commonly belonged to a particular type of bacteria called Firmicutes (which are primarily "gram positive" bacteria meaning that they stain blue with a particular stain) and that they had the ability to degrade sugar polymers such as fructans. While he attributed the ability of the bacteria to increase weight and fat to the production of additional calories generated from breaking down these sugar polymers, it seems likely that one of the major mechanisms by which these bacteria increase weight is by the generation of fructose.

> *Fructans are polymers of fructose made by certain plants, particularly wheat. While humans cannot metabolize fructans, some gut bacteria can convert the fructans to fructose. This can be another source of fructose.*

The primary sources of fructans in the human diet are wheat, rye, onions, artichokes, and green beans. Whether this could provide an additional reason for why wheat flour may increase the risk for obesity is not yet known. Importantly, in the current American diet the greatest source of fructose is from added sugars such as sucrose and high fructose corn syrup, and it seems likely that this remains the major food item driving the obesity epidemic. Indeed, the finding that obese people tend to carry fructan-degrading bacteria does not mean that the fructans are driving obesity, as these bacteria typically like fructose from sugar as well.

For those of you who love evolution, the ability of plants to make fructans as a way to store food began in the Miocene during the same period of global cooling in which the uricase mutation occurred among ancestral apes, and these early fructan producing plants mainly occurred in the northern latitudes such as Europe.[76] It is known that during the mid- to late Miocene that the apes in Europe were undergoing periodic starvation,[84] likely from the gradual loss of tropical rainforests and less availability of fructose-rich fruit.[85] There is some evidence that this was a period of rapid evolution, including the development of stronger teeth that allowed eating harder foods, changes in the skeleton that favored knuckle-walking, and the first development of primitive tools to allow the extraction of food.[86-87] Some studies suggest that the apes had to eat "fallback" foods to compensate for the loss of fruits, and it is thought that one of the key foods were plant tubers and roots.[88] While speculative, one wonders if these fallback foods might have been an additional source of fructose under these extreme conditions.

High Fructan Foods

Wheat
Rye
Onions
Garlic
Artichoke
Jerusalem Artichoke
Chocolate
Pasta
Cheese spread

High fructan foods are foods that contain polymers of fructose called fructans. Normally these are not digested. However, certain gut bacteria can convert fructans to fructose. The major source of fructans in the American diet is from wheat. Other sources include onions, artichokes, green beans, and chocolate.

Fructans and Secretariat

While fructans may not be a major cause of obesity in humans, they likely have a role in obesity in horses. Fructans are highly concentrated in the pasture grasses in northern latitudes, such as in Kentucky and Virginia. Horses that eat fructan-rich grasses are known to be at risk for developing the "equine metabolic syndrome" in which they develop obesity, insulin resistance, elevated serum triglycerides and occasionally high blood pressure. The increased fat in horses accumulates in their neck ("cresty neck") and in the tailhead. In collaboration with Tanja Hess, a horse nutritionist in the Equine Sciences Department at Colorado State University, we have hypothesized that this occurs because the horses are generating fructose daily from the fructan-rich grasses and that over time it causes obesity and metabolic syndrome similar to the way it does in humans.[89]

A Horse with Obesity and Insulin Resistance

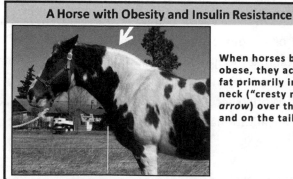

When horses become obese, they accumulate fat primarily in their neck ("cresty neck" *see arrow*) over their ribs, and on the tailhead.

Horses that eat pasture grasses rich in fructans are also at risk for developing laminitis, or Founder. This is an extremely painful condition in which the attachments between the bone (distal phalanx) and the hoof are separated in association with inflammation. Once laminitis develops, it is hard to reverse, and it leaves the horse lame and in pain. Often the only kind thing one can do is to put the horse to sleep with a lethal injection. Sadly, laminitis is very common among thoroughbred racehorses, and several famous horses including Secretariat died this way.

Recently it has been shown that fructans present in pasture grasses are a major cause of laminitis. Specifically, if a horse is given a large dose of fructans, laminitis develops within 24 to 48 hours.[90] This syndrome is associated with the development of a colitis, in which there is diarrhea, often with the presence of bacterial products (such as endotoxin) and lactic acid in the blood. Usually the main bacteria isolated from the gut are Streptococci which, as we mentioned earlier, is an organism that can both make and break down fructans.

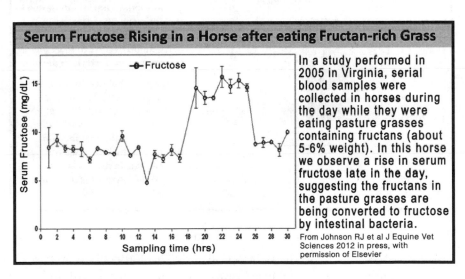

Serum Fructose Rising in a Horse after eating Fructan-rich Grass

In a study performed in 2005 in Virginia, serial blood samples were collected in horses during the day while they were eating pasture grasses containing fructans (about 5-6% weight). In this horse we observe a rise in serum fructose late in the day, suggesting the fructans in the pasture grasses are being converted to fructose by intestinal bacteria.

From Johnson RJ et al J Equine Vet Sciences 2012 in press, with permission of Elsevier

Founder likely results when a horse eats a very large amount of fructans at one time. It is known that the fructan content of grasses can vary as much as 10-fold, and can occasionally approach 30 to 40 percent of the overall weight of the grasses during certain times of the season, such as in the late afternoons in late spring and summer.[73] Since a horse weighing 1200 pounds (500 kg) can ingest up to 33 pounds (15 kg) of grass in a day, it is possible that a horse could eat as much as 15 pounds (7 kg) of fructans in one day. In addition, pasture grasses contain smaller amounts of fructose, glucose and sucrose that could also become significant source of sugars for a horse that eats a lot of grass, and could add up to another 4 to 7 pounds (2 to 3 kg) of sugar per day.[73]

The generation of this amount of fructose will result in some being absorbed where it is metabolized by the liver, and some of it passing into the colon where it will be further degraded, generating acids and gas from the breakdown of fructose and causing the overgrowth of bacteria.

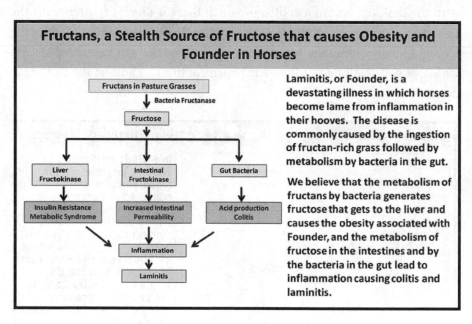

Fructans, a Stealth Source of Fructose that causes Obesity and Founder in Horses

Laminitis, or Founder, is a devastating illness in which horses become lame from inflammation in their hooves. The disease is commonly caused by the ingestion of fructan-rich grass followed by metabolism by bacteria in the gut.

We believe that the metabolism of fructans by bacteria generates fructose that gets to the liver and causes the obesity associated with Founder, and the metabolism of fructose in the intestines and by the bacteria in the gut lead to inflammation causing colitis and laminitis.

Recall that the primary enzyme that metabolizes fructose is fructokinase, which is not only in the liver, but is in high concentrations in the wall of the small intestines. Some fructokinase is also present in the cecum and large intestines, at least in the mouse. Since fructokinase is present in the intestinal wall, some fructose will be metabolized here. As we discussed earlier, the breakdown of fructose by fructokinase is rapid and results in a brief period in which the cells become depleted of energy (ATP), causing "cell shock" and leading to the production of uric acid and oxidants. We have proposed, with Tanja Hess, that this inflammation in the intestines likely has a major role in causing the abdominal pain and colitis and at the same time increases the risk for bacterial products to get into the blood. The systemic inflammation that results may have a role in causing the inflammation in the hooves, and may not be too dissimilar from an episode of gout that can also occur in humans following a meal of fructose. The latter, however, is thought to be driven primarily by crystals of uric acid whereas in laminitis there are no uric acid crystals present.

Fructose generated from fructans may have a role in causing metabolic syndrome in horses as well as laminitis (Founder).

While fructans are considered the most common cause of laminitis, there are examples where laminitis can be induced by high doses of starch.[91] The classical teaching is that this is due to unabsorbed starch reaching the hindgut where it is metabolized by bacteria to generate acids and gas that cause intestinal inflammation and the absorption of bacterial products (such as endotoxin) into the blood. Given our observation from the previous chapter that some starch may be converted into fructose, it remains possible that this also involves a fructose-dependent pathway. In the next few years we hope to do studies where we will be able to determine if equine metabolic syndrome and Founder are diseases driven by fructose and intestinal fructokinase. If they are, then prevention, treatment, and cure may not be far away.

Antibiotics in Animal Feed

In the 1950s it was discovered that the addition of antibiotics to chicken feed could result in larger chickens. Soon the addition of antibiotics to animal feed became common practice, and it is estimated that between 3 and 25 million pounds of antibiotics are used yearly in the United States for this purpose.[92] Not surprisingly, the mechanism by which antibiotics work involves altering the gut bacteria, as it is known that antibiotics do not stimulate the growth of chickens that have no gut bacteria.[93-94]

One difference from the previous discussion is that some antibiotics increase weight without increasing fat, whereas other antibiotics stimulate both weight and fat accumulation. For example, in one study the administration of the antibiotic streptomycin made larger and fatter chickens, whereas the use of penicillin made larger and leaner chickens.[95] This is particularly interesting as streptomycin kills gram negative bacteria and hence would stimulate fructanase producing gram positive bacteria, whereas penicillin would be more likely reduce the fructanase-producing bacteria since this drugs mainly kills Streptococcus and gram positive bacteria.

> *Antibiotics promote growth and, in some case, fattening, of chickens, by altering the types of bacteria in the gut.*

While it has been thought that most of the increased weight in chickens over the last decades is from an increase in muscle and lean mass, a recent study suggests that chickens are getting fatter, not unlike humans.[96] Whether this is due to the forced inactivity, the type of feed, or the use of antibiotics is not known. It likely involves a combination of these factors. However, the concept that the chicken you are eating today is the same as the chicken your parents ate years ago is likely not true.

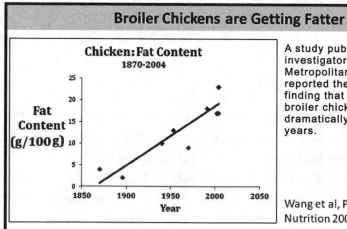

Broiler Chickens are Getting Fatter

Chicken: Fat Content
1870-2004

Fat Content (g/100g)

Year

A study published by investigators from London Metropolitan University reported the sombering finding that the fat content of broiler chickens has increased dramatically over the last 150 years.

Wang et al, Public Health Nutrition 2009; 13:400-408

The use of antibiotics in animal feed has led to public health concern since it increases the risk for the emergence of antibiotic-resistant bacteria. This has led to the use of prebiotics and probiotics. Perhaps not surprisingly, prebiotics tend to be spores of fructanase producing bacteria such as Bacillus subtilis, whereas probiotics are often fructans. However, what is interesting is that trials using these agents have tended to show that these agents increase lean mass and, if anything, protect from obesity, including in short term human trials. Why we are seeing this paradox is unknown. It may relate to the fact that individuals taking these substances are reducing their intake of added sugars, and in some of the studies the control groups were given sucrose. It is also possible that the administration of a probiotic, for example, acts more like fiber in the absence of bacteria that can degrade fructans. Clearly more studies are needed to understand this better.

Lead, Uric acid and the Roman Empire

Just as there are ways to take in fructose without knowing it, there are also stealth ways to raise uric acid. One of the more sinister ways may be from low grade exposure to lead. Lead increases serum uric acid by blocking its excretion by the kidney. It has therefore been known for over 100 years that lead poisoning can cause gout.[97] However, the presence of lead in the blood, even at relatively low levels, has also been associated with increased risk for obesity, insulin resistance, chronic kidney disease and elevated blood pressure.[98] Whether the reason that lead poisoning is associated with these conditions is due to the increase in uric acid has not yet been proven, although our group did report that lead associated hypertension in laboratory rats with kidney disease could be improved by decreasing uric acid levels. Similar to the fructan story, we are at the beginning of our understanding of this area of science, but there is suggestive evidence that low levels of lead might have some contributory role of obesity and metabolic syndrome.

In the past, lead poisoning was much more common than today. For example, lead often contaminated the sweetened grape drinks (*sapa*) that the Romans used to use as their source for sugar. Some Romans insisted on lead pots being used to store *sapa* as the lead acetate which leached off these pots was also sweet (lead sugar) and enhanced the taste.[97] Lead poisoning was also common in the 17th and 18th centuries in England, in part due to the shipping of port and other wines from Portugal in wooden barrels with lead lined lids. Lead was also historically used in presses to make cider (an alcoholic drink made from apples), and this was the cause of widespread lead poisoning in the 1760s in Devonshire, England that resulted in gout and abdominal pain (The Devonshire Colic).[99] Lead was also common among painters as it was originally a component in paints. Indeed, the French physician Lancereaux, who described lean and fat diabetes, also was the first to recognize the risk of lead poisoning in painters when he diagnosed gout in a painter who liked to lick his brush between paint strokes.[100] More recently lead poisoning has been observed in bootleggers who distill their own liquor in the Appalachians, and in children who ingest lead-based paints.[101]

> *Many people may have low levels of lead in their body without knowing it. In turn, the low concentrations of lead can increase serum uric acid and increase the risk for high blood pressure, kidney disease, and possibly metabolic syndrome and obesity.*

Today frank lead poisoning is rare, but low levels are common in some populations and are associated with increased risk for high blood pressure and kidney disease.[102-103] Currently major sources for exposure in children include being in old houses where there is lead-based paint that is flaking off the walls and ceiling that children may inadvertently ingest, and toys that have been contaminated with lead (such as recently occurred with toys originating from China). Other potential exposures include environmental exposures from local foundries, smelters or factories that make lead acid batteries or process lead in which the lead leeches into the water supply or in which lead particles get into the air. Occupational exposures include working with lead such as lead miners, plumbers or welders. It is interesting that Haven Emerson, the Public Health Commissioner whose seminal paper in the 1920s linked sugar intake with diabetes, also commented that miners were protected from diabetes except for those working in lead mines.[104]

Summary

In our opinion, intake of fructose-containing sugars remains the major reason for the epidemic of obesity throughout the world, but it is not the only mechanism. Fructose can be generated other ways, including from fructans in the diet and also from simple carbohydrates. Uric acid can also be generated from other foods, such as from beer and umami foods, and also by low grade intoxication with lead. Even high fat foods, if given in large amounts, increase body fat. In the next section we will address the diseases driven by the fructose and uric acid pathways. While you will be able to guess some of these, a few will catch you by surprise.

SECTION 5

OTHER BIOLOGICAL EFFECTS OF FRUCTOSE AND URIC ACID

CHAPTER 18

HIGH BLOOD PRESSURE AND HEART DISEASE

> *Fructose, and its messenger, uric acid, likely have a major role in driving the epidemic of high blood pressure and heart disease.*

The discovery of high blood pressure occurred in mid-nineteenth century England, during an unprecedented era of increasing sugar intake. The discoverer, Frederick Akbar Mahomed (1849-1884), was only a resident in training at Guy's Hospital in London.[1] A man of Indian descent, he was the grandson of Sake Mahomed, an Indian who had become wealthy by establishing Indian bathhouses in London, and who was the royal shampooer for the King. Early in his life Akbar had wanted to be a physician, and in 1869, at the age of 20, he began his medical training at Guy's Hospital. Many medical residents had research projects, and Mahomed was interested in measuring blood pressure. Mahomed was aware of the work of the French physician, Étienne-Jules Marey (1830-1904), who reported in 1863 that he could measure blood pressure using a portable, spring-loaded machine that attached to the wrist and would measure the tension of the pulse in the radial artery. Working with a local watchmaker, Mahomed made a lightweight version of Marey's blood pressure device and began measuring the blood pressure in both hospitalized patients and healthy individuals in the general population. While it had been known that patients with chronic kidney disease often had high blood pressure, Mahomed discovered that high blood pressure could occur in people with no clinical evidence of kidney disease as noted by the absence of protein in the urine.[2] In retrospect, this was the first report of primary hypertension, which is also known as essential hypertension.

Frederick Akbar Mahomed and the Discovery of High Blood Pressure

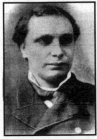

Mahomed, a medical resident at Guy's Hospital, used a spring-loaded instrument to measure the pressure of the radial pulse. In so doing, he discovered that some people, especially those with gout, had high blood pressure. This was one of the first reports of hypertension in the general population.

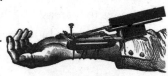

"People who are subject to high blood pressure, frequently belong to gouty families, or have themselves suffered from this disease."

Frederick Akbar Mahomed

Portrait with permission of King's College London; Figure from Verdin, Charles. Catalogue des instruments de précision servant en physiologie et en médecine construits par Charles Verdin. 1882. Chateauroux

---

The spring-loaded sphygmograph was an impractical way to measure blood pressure, but with the introduction of the blood pressure cuff in the late 1890s, it was possible for the practicing physician to measure blood pressure in their patients. Soon a definition of hypertension was defined as a pressure in which the systolic pressure (the pressure during the contraction of the heart) was 140 mm Hg or higher, or in which the diastolic blood pressure (the pressure during the relaxation of the heart) was 90 mm Hg or higher. By 1912 the Metropolitan Life Insurance company reported that the presence of high blood pressure conferred a twofold increase risk for death,[3] and from that day forward the blood pressure cuff became a companion of the physician, a key equipment in his black bag, and one that would be used routinely in the physical examination.

The development of standardized ways to measure blood pressure allowed studies to evaluate how common hypertension was in the population. Perhaps not surprisingly, high blood pressure was present in about 5 to 10 percent of the adult population—but only in two areas of the world, that being Europe, and especially England, and the southeastern United States.

These, of course, were the two regions where sugar intake was increasing markedly. In other populations less than 1 percent had high blood pressure, including among Africans, Chinese, Arabs, Eskimos, Native American Indians and Australian Aborigines.[4]

During the twentieth century, the frequency of hypertension progressively increased throughout the world, not only in the United States but in all countries. Today approximately one third of adults in the United States have high blood pressure. High blood pressure is now common in all populations, and it continues to increase. By 2025 there are expected to be more than 1.5 billion people with high blood pressure in the world.[5]

A White Crystalline Substance Linked with Blood Pressure—Salt

As the frequency of high blood pressure increased, so did strokes, heart failure, heart attacks and kidney disease. It became critical to find both the cause and treatments. The first major breakthrough was the discovery of the importance of salt in blood pressure. The practice of lowering salt in the diet as a treatment of high blood pressure has been in use since the early 1920s.[6] Further studies showed that populations with higher salt intake tended to have higher blood pressure.[7-8] Moreover, Arthur Guyton proposed that the way a high salt diet caused high blood pressure was because people with high blood pressure could not rid the excess salt from their kidneys as well as others, and blood pressure rose to "push" the salt out of the kidneys.[9] Giving diuretics, which are drugs that increase the excretion of salt, became the standard practice to treat high blood pressure, and were soon shown to improve survival.[10]

The Yanomamö Indians: Fierce but with Normal Blood Pressure

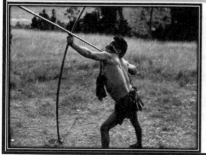

The Yanomamö Indians live in southern Venezuela and are known as the Fierce people. Studies conducted by Bill Oliver and Jim Neel in the 1970s showed that these people have normal blood pressure. One reason may relate to their salt intake, which was minimal. Studies of these Indians gave support to the importance of salt in blood pressure.

Photo provided by the late Bill Oliver.

Studies then shifted to identify what was causing the kidney defect in patients with high blood pressure. Genetic mechanisms alone could not account for the rapid rise in the frequency of high blood pressure over only a few generations. Genetics also fail to explain studies of identical twins in which high blood pressure was found to affect only one of the twins. For example, a survey performed between 1983 and 1985 of white male identical twins born between 1917 and 1927 reported that of 635 twins who were hypertensive, that 60 percent of them had an identical twin who had normal blood pressure.[11]

A second, and still popular, theory is that high blood pressure results from changes that occur to the fetus during pregnancy. Babies born with low birth weight have an increased risk for developing high blood pressure as adults.[12] Since the kidneys are one of the last organs to develop, low birth weight infants often have kidneys with fewer filtering units. In turn, a reduction in the number of these filtering units, or nephrons, could reduce the ability of the person to be able to excrete salt.[13] Unfortunately, while birth weight does influence future blood pressure, it is more of a risk factor than a cause. Many large babies still get hypertension, and studies have also not always been able to link a low number of filtering units with blood pressure.[14]

In the last decade, a third theory emerged to explain how high blood pressure develops. Recall that patients with high blood pressure typically have arteriolosclerosis, or disease of their small blood vessels. Studies from the 1930s showed that these vascular lesions are especially common in the kidneys of patients with high blood pressure.[15] Theoretically, this vascular disease could result in impairing blood flow to the kidney, and the kidney might interpret this as not enough blood volume and respond by holding onto salt. To test this hypothesis, we collaborated with Bernardo Rodriguez-Iturbe and the late Jaime Herrera-Acosta and were able to demonstrate that subtle damage to the blood vessels in the kidney could result in high blood pressure in animals in association with a defect in the ability to excrete salt.[16] Further studies led by Bernardo showed that the primary way this happened was by causing low grade inflammation in the kidneys.[17]

These studies left open the question—what was responsible for causing the vascular lesions in the kidney that could explain why high blood pressure was increasing so rapidly in the world population?

Uric acid and its Role in High Blood Pressure

A relationship of uric acid with high blood pressure was known since the 1800s. Even Frederick Akbar Mahomed, who discovered high blood pressure, wrote that uric acid might be one of the causes, since many of the individuals that he identified as having high blood pressure also had gout.[18] Nathan Davis, the President of the American Medical Association, proposed uric acid as causing high blood pressure through its effects on the kidneys in 1897.[19] Others, such as the French cardiologist Henri Huchard, suggested that the cause of arteriolosclerosis was likely from gout, lead poisoning, or the eating of red meats.[20] One of the most vocal was Alexander Haig, a London physician who claimed uric acid might not only cause high blood pressure, but obesity and diabetes.[21] Unfortunately, these ideas were largely forgotten since there were no treatments at that time to test the hypothesis, as well as little understanding of how uric acid could raise blood pressure.

We became interested in uric acid a little over 10 years ago when we realized that no one had actually tested whether raising uric acid in animals might affect blood pressure. One reason this had not happened was because it is difficult to raise uric acid levels in animals that contain uricase. However, there are drugs that can be given that can inhibit uricase and raise uric acid levels. You can imagine the excitement when Marilda Mazzali, a Brazilian physician who was a visiting scientist in my laboratory, found that the animals who received these inhibitors developed hypertension.[22]

As we studied this model, it became apparent that there were two phases. In the first phase the elevated uric acid was responsible for the high blood pressure. However, over time the rats started to develop vascular lesions in their kidney that resembled arteriolosclerosis along with kidney inflammation. Once this happened, the blood pressure became dependent on salt intake and was driven by the kidney.[23] What was exciting is that high blood pressure in humans follows the same pattern, in which early hypertension is often not responsive to changes in salt intake, but in which the blood pressure becomes increasingly responsive to salt intake over time.[16]

Subsequent studies suggest that an elevated uric acid may be a cause of high blood pressure in humans. For example, people who have an elevated serum uric acid (defined as > 6 m/dl in women and >7 mg/dl in men) have been consistently shown to be at increased risk for developing high blood pressure.[24-25] People with high blood pressure, especially those who have had hypertension for only a short time, also frequently have high uric acid levels. For example, my collaborator, Daniel Feig, and I found that nearly 90 percent of adolescents with newly diagnosed high blood pressure had elevated uric acid levels.[26] Dan and I then performed a pilot trial in which 30 adolescents with newly diagnosed and never treated hypertension were randomized to receive allopurinol (which lowers uric acid) or placebo in a double-blind cross over design. Amazingly, the lowering of uric acid resulted in the blood pressure becoming normal in two-thirds of the adolescents, whereas when the same individuals received placebo pills, only 1 of 30 had their blood pressure fall back to the normal range. In those adolescents whose uric acid was lowered to less than 5 mg/dl, nearly 86 percent had their blood pressure return to normal.[27]

Since then other studies led by Dan and others, including our collaborator, Mehmet Kanbay, have provided more evidence that lowering uric acid can reduce blood pressure, especially in younger people with high blood pressure and normal kidney function.[28] One exception was a study we performed in African Americans with hypertension in which we determined if lowering uric acid provided additional benefit to diuretic therapy. In this study, diuretics alone reduced BP to approximately 120 mm Hg/76 mm Hg, which is ideal blood pressure, and the addition of allopurinol tended to improve blood pressure more but it was not significant. However, one might not expect further blood pressure lowering if levels are already reduced to normal.

Serum Uric acid as a Cause of the Epidemic of Hypertension

Could uric acid be responsible for the epidemic of high blood pressure in this country? Serum uric acid has increased in the United States over the last century along with an increasing frequency of hypertension. Average serum uric acid levels were around 3 or 4 mg/dl in the 1920s but now average 4.6 and 6.1 mg/dl in women and men, respectively.[29] This suggests that something in the western diet could be driving up the uric acid levels.

To get a better understanding of what normal uric acid levels might be, I contacted Bill Oliver, who had been on the field trips with Jim Neel to southern Venezuela where they studied the Yanomamö Indians. These Indians are fierce and aggressive, and at the time Bill visited them in the 1970s and 1980s, were still living in their native way and with minimal western influence. Bill had found that these Indians had very little salt in their diet and maintained normal blood pressure;[30] however, he had not mentioned what their serum uric acid levels were. Bill had since retired from the University of Michigan, and while they had not measured uric acid levels on these individuals, he told me he still had a freezer filled with serum samples from a medical expedition in 1987 to Kedebaböwei-teri, a Yanomamö village near the Mavaca River, a major tributary of the Orinoco River. After performing some cross-checks to make sure that the uric acid measurements would be valid, we tested the samples and found that the uric acid levels in the Indians were around 3 mg/dl and substantially less than that of Oliver and his co-expedition members.[31] The lower levels of uric acid in the Yanomamö Indians likely reflected their vegetarian-based diet, which consist primarily of plantain, manioc and tubers, with rare wild game and fish.

I also contacted Bruce Rideout, who is a Research Scientist at the San Diego zoo, which is one of the largest and best zoos in the United States. Bruce had serum samples from a wide range of primates, including monkeys that expressed uricase and apes that had the same mutation as humans and had no functional uricase. Whereas the monkeys expressing uricase had uric acid levels in the range of 1-2 mg/dl, the gorillas, orangutans, and bonobos (a type of chimpanzee) had uric acid levels around 3 mg/dl, similar to the Yanomamö Indians.[4] Thus, it seemed evident that the blood levels of uric acid in humans and apes are normally around 3 mg/dl if the diet were primarily vegetarian and fruit-based (prior to the introduction of sugar).

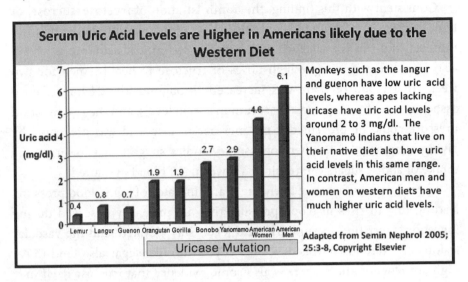

Serum Uric Acid Levels are Higher in Americans likely due to the Western Diet

Monkeys such as the langur and guenon have low uric acid levels, whereas apes lacking uricase have uric acid levels around 2 to 3 mg/dl. The Yanomamö Indians that live on their native diet also have uric acid levels in this same range. In contrast, American men and women on western diets have much higher uric acid levels.

Adapted from Semin Nephrol 2005; 25:3-8, Copyright Elsevier

Another White Crystalline Substance Involved in High Blood Pressure?

Uric acid can be raised by consuming red meats and umami-rich foods, but meat intake has been falling in the country. However, sugar also raises uric acid levels and thus becomes a major candidate for the progressive rise in uric acid levels over the last century. Fructose increases uric acid in the first few minutes of ingestion due to the activation of the fat switch (see Chapter 9), but fructose also turns on the body to synthesize uric acid.[32] Individuals drinking soft drinks have an increase in serum uric acid level during the first hour after ingestion,[33-34] but also will tend to have higher fasting uric acid levels over time.[35] The ingestion of sugary soft drinks is also associated with an increase in serum uric acid levels and the development of hypertension.[36-37]

To evaluate this in more detail, our group gave fructose in high doses to rats, and found that it raised blood pressure acutely in association with a rise in uric acid. Over time the rats also developed arteriolosclerosis-like lesions in their kidney. Most importantly, lowering the uric acid could prevent the development of high blood pressure as well as the vascular lesions. These studies suggest that fructose raises blood pressure by raising uric acid levels.[38]

Consistent with this finding, the administration of fructose, sucrose, or high fructose corn syrup to people also raises blood pressure in the first few minutes, and this is associated with a rise in serum uric acid levels.[34, 39] We also found that if we gave high doses of fructose to healthy men for two weeks that blood pressure was increased throughout the 24-hour day in association with a rise in fasting serum uric acid levels, and the rise in blood pressure could be prevented if the increase in uric acid was prevented by giving allopurinol.[40] Furthermore, some studies suggest that lowering the intake of added sugars can result in a lowering of blood pressure.[41-42]

Sugar intake is therefore likely the grand initiator of high blood pressure, leading first to rises in blood pressure that are primarily observed during ingestion. Over time, serum uric acid levels stay elevated, and the vascular lesions of arteriolosclerosis develop. People who like sugar also tend to eat high amounts of salt.[43] There is also some evidence that fructose itself may stimulate the absorption of salt in the intestines.[44] Suddenly we have the "perfect storm" for the development of persistent hypertension, as the sugar-induced lesions in the kidney result in the kidney holding onto salt.

Cerebral Vascular Accidents (CVAs, Strokes)

Since high blood pressure is the main cause of strokes, it is likely that excessive sugar intake may also have a role in this disease. To date there have not been many studies that have looked at this relationship, but there is now strong evidence that people with an elevated serum uric acid are at increased risk for strokes, including silent strokes.[45-46] One way uric acid may increase the risk for strokes is not simply by raising blood pressure, but rather by its ability to cause arteriolosclerosis. The cerebral arterioles have an important role in controlling blood flow to the brain, and will dilate or constrict as needed to help maintain normal pressures and flows. When the arterioles become diseased the ability to regulate blood flow is impaired. In the kidney, for example, our group showed that uric acid caused the arterioles to become diseased and this impaired the ability of the kidney to regulate its blood flow.

In turn, if the cerebral arterioles cannot regulate blood flow very well, then sudden changes in blood pressure could lead to dangerous alterations in blood flow to the brain, thereby predisposing to strokes.[47]

While people with a high uric acid are at increased risk for stroke, the role of uric acid during a stroke is more controversial. Some studies suggest that those who have a stroke may do better if their uric acid levels are elevated.[48] This may fall back to the survival properties of uric acid, such as the ability to block oxidative stress outside the cell. Nevertheless, lowering of uric acid in the post-stroke period is associated with improvement in systemic inflammation and vascular function.[49-50]

Congestive Heart Failure

Since high blood pressure is the major cause of heart failure, it is not surprising that an elevated uric acid has been found to predict both the development of heart failure and its severity.[51-52] Unfortunately, once people develop heart failure, it has been hard to show clinical benefit with drugs that lower uric acid, with possible exception for those with very high (>9.5 mg/dl) uric acid levels.[53] To date no studies have linked sugar intake with heart failure.

Aortic Aneurysms and Peripheral Vascular Disease

While uric acid and sugar are primarily associated with arteriolosclerosis, and not atherosclerosis, there is some evidence that uric acid may have a role in aortic aneurysms. For example, an elevated uric acid is associated with aortic aneurysms, carotid disease, and peripheral vascular disease.[54-55] Uric acid is also present in the cholesterol-rich plaques that occur in these conditions.[56-57]

A well-known puzzle has been that aortic aneurysms typically occur in the abdominal portion of the aorta as opposed to the thoracic (chest) part of the aorta. To my knowledge, no one has ever explained this. However, recently we found that the abdominal aorta of rats can take up uric acid into the vessel wall where it causes inflammation, whereas the vascular cells from the thoracic aorta are protected. The reason appears to be that the transporter that helps uric acid to enter cells is present in the abdominal aortic cells, but not in those from the thoracic aorta.

Heart Attacks (Myocardial Infarction)

An elevated serum uric acid is also associated with angina (heart pain) and heart attacks (myocardial infarction).[58] Because there is a relationship between uric acid and obesity, high blood pressure, and insulin resistance, the association of uric acid with heart disease often becomes muddled, as it is often impossible to separate uric acid from these other variables.[58] This has led some scientists to remain unconvinced that uric acid is a true risk factor. For me, this argument is a bit superficial, as it is not critical to me whether uric acid causes heart disease through a direct effect, or indirectly by causing high blood pressure or obesity. Either way uric acid has a role in heart disease. Indeed, recent studies suggest that lowering uric acid can reduce chest pain episodes in patients with angina and improve their exercise tolerance.[59] In another study lowering uric acid was found to reduce cardiovascular events, such as sudden death and heart attacks, in individuals with chronic kidney disease.[60] More studies need to be performed, but it is my opinion that uric acid will eventually be recognized as important a risk factor for heart disease as cholesterol.

Sleep Apnea and Pulmonary Hypertension

Obese individuals have long been known to be prone to fall asleep, often at inappropriate times during the day. They also, not infrequently, have episodes where they may quit breathing for a half minute or more ("sleep apnea"). One of the more famous stories is of Dionysus of Heraclea who lived in ancient Greece around 400 B.C. Dionysus was an extremely obese man (from excessive feeding and a "voluptuous life'") who not only would continuously fall asleep during the day, but was also worried that he would suffocate from his fat during sleep. To prevent this from happening, he had his physicians embed needles in his chair so they would pierce him if would try to lean back in his chair for a rest! Charles Dickens also was aware of obesity and its relationship with narcolepsy. In his first novel, *The Pickwick Papers*, which was published in 1836, he describes not only a number of overweight individuals, including Mr. Pickwick himself, but also a fat boy named Joe who was constantly falling asleep during the day.

While there are many reasons for sleep disturbances, both daytime sleepiness and nighttime sleep apnea are commonly associated with obesity. One reason this may occur is because obesity can be associated with some blockage of the upper airways during sleep. During the periods when an individual does not breathe, the lack of oxygen causes a loss of energy (ATP) in the cells that, in turn, stimulates production of uric acid. As a consequence, some patients with sleep apnea may present with gout as their earliest symptom before they realize there is a sleep disturbance present.[61] Some studies suggest that as many as 60 percent of people with metabolic syndrome have some degree of obstructive sleep apnea.[62] In turn, sleep disturbances can be disruptive both at work and in the home. Both obesity and sleep apnea are also associated with the development of pulmonary hypertension that over time can result in heart failure. An elevated uric acid may contribute to the pulmonary hypertension in a way not dissimilar to how uric acid affects systemic blood vessels.[63]

Preeclampsia

Another disease for which sugar and uric acid may be involved is preeclampsia. Preeclampsia is a disease that occurs in pregnant women, usually in the second half of pregnancy (after 20 weeks). It usually presents with high blood pressure and protein in the urine and can rarely progress to seizures. Some patients also develop insulin resistance and fatty liver. Successful treatment usually consists of early delivery, and even then the mother or baby may die.

The cause of preeclampsia appears to result when the blood supply to the placenta does not develop normally. The placenta, of course, has a central role in providing oxygen and nutrients to the fetus, and as a result the fetus may not get enough nutrients. As the fetus grows its nutrient demands increase, and this may explain why the signs of preeclampsia are most likely to manifest during the second half of pregnancy. As fetal growth is impaired in preeclampsia, the babies are usually small at delivery, even when taking into account the number of weeks of gestation.

Beautiful work by Ananth Karumanchi from Harvard Medical School has shown that many of the maternal symptoms of preeclampsia are due to the release of factors from the sick placenta that raise blood pressure and cause kidney damage.[64] However, there is also some evidence that uric acid may play a contributory role. For example, an increase in serum uric acid in the mother is characteristic in this condition and has been found to predict the severity of the preeclampsia.[65-66] A high uric acid level also predicts the development of insulin resistance which frequently accompanies the preeclamptic state.[67-69] This has led several investigators, including our group, to suggest that some of the manifestations of preeclampsia in the mother and baby may be due to the effects of the high uric acid levels.[70-71]

If a high uric acid has a role in driving insulin resistance, fatty liver, and preeclampsia of pregnancy then, theoretically, maneuvers that increase uric acid could increase the risk or severity of preeclampsia. One way might be from excessive sugar intake. To look at this, Torun Clausen from the University of Oslo conducted a food questionnaire in 3110 pregnant women to determine if certain foods might predispose to the development of preeclampsia. The major finding was that diets high in sugar (sucrose) were strongly associated with the development of preeclampsia, especially if the preeclampsia occurred less than 37 weeks gestation. The risk for preeclampsia in this latter group was more than tenfold in those individuals who had more than 25 percent of their diet from sugar.[72] Additional analysis showed that the intake of soft drinks during pregnancy also conferred a major risk for preeclampsia.

Summary

Intake of fructose from added sugars is likely important in causing high blood pressure, probably due to the ability of fructose to raise uric acid levels. In turn, increasing evidence suggests uric acid has an important role in stroke, heart failure, and heart and vascular disease. Obesity driven by sugar and uric acid may also have a role in sleep disturbances. But this, I am afraid, is only the beginning.

CHAPTER 19

SUGAR ADDICTION AND OBESITY

> Sugar (and fructose) can cause addiction-like symptoms and can affect the ability to control one's food intake. Sugar addiction may play a role in causing obesity.

You know how many sugarholics there are in this country? There are millions and millions of them. As you go around the schoolyard, you watch the young boys and girls in this country, see how many of these children with their soft weak muscles, they are out of condition, they don't have the energy and vitality they should have. They look like sugar; they do not look husky and robust and healthy the way they should because their bodies are being made of the sugar they are eating, so they look soft and weak.
—Jack Lalanne (1914-2011) American Fitness Leader and Teacher, TV show host, 1961

"Life is uncertain, eat dessert first," wrote author Ernestine Ulmer years ago, and certainly it rings true for many of us. The love for sweets is part of being human, and can be shown even in infancy.[73] Infants will instinctively choose a drink containing sugar over milk. Desserts are special, and for children often represent the "reward" for eating dinner. Sugar and honey are loved so much that we refer to people we love with words like "sweetie," "sweetheart," "honey pie," or "sugar." In the Middle Ages sugar and honey were important gifts. The word "honeymoon," for example, may have resulted from the custom of the bride's father to give a lunar month's supply of honey and honey-based alcohol (known as mead) as the dowry to the wedding couple.

Sugar is Addicting

The sensation of sweetness is conveyed to the brain by "sweet" receptors in the taste buds that become activated along with receptors in the gut. The sweetness is converted to a pleasure response triggered by the release of dopamine in the center of the brain called the striatum (part of a system known as the basal ganglia). These "pleasure centers" are also activated by sexual arousal or narcotics. Not surprisingly, sugar elicits the same responses, noted by specialized imaging of the brain, as can be induced by narcotics.[74]

The Pleasure Centers of the Brain

frontal lobe
basal ganglia
dopamine pathways

In the center of the brain is the striatum, which is part of the basal ganglia and is the location of the pleasure centers. Certain stimuli can increase dopamine and the pleasure response in these centers, such as sexual arousal, cocaine, and sugar. Repeated stimulation can in some cases result in a reduction in dopamine receptors and a blunted response. Over time this can lead to addiction-like behavior.

There is widespread belief among the general public that sugar might have addictive properties, creating "sugarholics" as proposed in the early 1960s by the late Jack Lalanne in his health show on television. The love for sweets and its addictive potential, which is sometimes referred to as the hedonic drive, may be as important as metabolic mechanisms such as leptin

176

resistance in driving obesity.[74-75] "Breaking the sugar habit" can be one of the most difficult challenges and requires modification of behaviors and counseling.[76]

Much of the key work investigating sugar addiction has been led by Nicole Avena and the late Bart Hoebel from Princeton University, who performed studies in which laboratory animals were given sugar water intermittently.[75,77] Laboratory rats, like humans, love sugar and will wait eagerly for it, and then drink as much as they can as soon as it is brought to them. The bingeing response is associated with the release of dopamine in the striatum that creates pleasure for these rats. The rats become focused on getting more sucrose, and resist other distractions if sugar is present. An interesting feature is that they show a greater "desire response" as opposed to a greater "liking" response for sugar.[78]

Unfortunately, repeated bingeing on sugar takes a toll, and the receptors for dopamine in the brain become effectively exhausted and over time start to decrease in number.[79-80] Dopamine responses may also decrease with time. The animals now must ingest more sugar to get the same response, and this is a classic feature of addiction.[80] At this point the withdrawal of sugar is associated with shaking, teeth chattering, forepaw tremors, agitation, and increased activity, and has similarities to narcotic withdrawal in humans. This withdrawal syndrome to sugar can also be induced by administering drugs that block the dopamine or opiate (opioid) receptors, similar to that which occurs in cocaine-addicted rats.[74-75,81]

> *Rats given sugar intermittently will become addicted to sugar and will undergo withdrawal symptoms if the sugar is withheld.*

The reduction in the dopamine pathway affects behavior. In one study, rats administered a sucrose-rich diet for 40 days showed a reduction in their dopamine receptors and subsequently increased their food intake with the development of obesity.[82] Using electrode stimulation, it was possible to show that these rats had to eat a more sucrose-rich diet to achieve the same pleasure response, and they also became resistant to punishment stimuli (foot shock) to stop eating. Thus chronic sugar intake has the ability to cause food addiction in laboratory animals.

A worrisome finding is that obese humans show the same "dopamine signature" in the brain as rats chronically fed sugar. Using a special imaging process known as functional magnetic resonance imaging (fMRI), the status of the dopamine D2 receptors in the striatum can be measured noninvasively. Studies led by Nora Volkow, Gene Jack Wang, and others have found that there is a lower dopamine response, or lower dopamine receptors, in obese people provided an appetizing meal.[83] Special scans, such as the positron emission (PET) scan, have also confirmed low numbers of dopamine receptors in the striatum in obese individuals.[84-85]

Behavior is largely controlled by the frontal lobe region of the brain, and this region responds to changes that occur in the pleasure centers in the striatum. Volkow and colleagues showed in obese humans that the reduction in dopamine receptors in the striatum was associated with less activity in the frontal lobe (as measured by PET scanning) and less emotional control.[84] This leads to impulsiveness, reduces the ability to control behavior, and is likely responsible for the development of food addiction.

Since sugar causes a reduction of dopamine receptors in the striatum, sugar not only causes sugar addiction but may also have a role in food addiction. Genetic factors also likely contribute. For example, individuals who are born with low dopamine receptors in the striatum are at increased risk for addiction.[86] Obese people also more commonly have the genes associated with low D2 receptors (the gene polymorphism *DRD2-TAQ-IA*) and this is associated with less emotional control.[86-87]

Sugar therefore increases the risk for obesity not simply by causing leptin resistance, but also by effects on the pleasure response. The reduction in dopamine receptors that occurs with chronic intake of sugar results in the need to eat more sugar for the same response, and to lose the ability to say no in response to the sight of appetizing foods. By blocking the ability to say "no" when appetizing foods are present, chronic ingestion of sugar may increase food intake and cause obesity.

Role of Sweetness and of Fructose in the Pleasure Response

One of the more important questions is: What is it about sugar that causes the pleasure response? If it is the sweetness, then theoretically all sweet substances, including glucose and artificial sugars such as sucralose, might cause food addiction. In fact, sweet substances, such as glucose, fructose and sucralose, do stimulate dopamine responses in the brain.[75,88-89] However, the dopamine response to sucralose is much less than is observed with sugar and disappears in mice that lack the sweet taste receptor. In contrast, mice crave sucrose even when the sweet receptors are absent.[88] This suggests sucrose has the ability to cause "stealth" addiction, in that you do not have to taste the sweetness of sugar water to have the desire to drink it.

What about the role of fructose versus glucose in addiction? While both fructose and glucose stimulate dopamine in the brain, there do appear to be differences. For example, one study reported that the infusion of glucose in humans generated a feeling of warmth and increased activity in the brain cortex when measured by a functional (BOLD) MRI, whereas the infusion of fructose generated a sensation of coldness and resulted in opposite effects on the brain.[90] Another study reported that the injection of fructose in the hypothalamus of rats stimulates hunger whereas the injection of glucose does not.[91] These studies suggest fructose and glucose could have different effects.

In contrast, when glucose is given intermittently in the drinking water, mice develop bingeing behavior, withdrawal-like symptoms in response to opiate antagonists, and a decrease in dopamine receptors in the striatum.[81,92] Furthermore, mice given glucose water also become obese. While this may seem paradoxical, recall that we found that mice given glucose water were making fructose from the glucose, and that mice that were unable to metabolize the fructose were partially protected from glucose-induced obesity. These studies raise the possibility that the reason glucose water induces addiction might be from the conversion of glucose to fructose in the body.

One interesting finding is that mice that cannot metabolize fructose do not care for fructose, but they still love glucose water, and in fact drink more glucose water than normal mice. They also like sucrose water, although less than normal mice. It seems that they like the glucose content but not fructose content in this water. These studies suggest that if a drug is developed that can block fructokinase, that it would not block the liking of sugar (sucrose) even though it would largely block the development of obesity. This is good news for the sugar industry.

Mood Disorders and other Conditions

While the emphasis of the book is on what triggers the development of obesity and diabetes, we would like to briefly mention the potential role of excessive sugar intake in mood disorders, and especially attention deficit hyperactivity syndrome, or ADHD. ADHD typically affects children and is characterized by hyperactivity, inability to focus, inattention, excessive talking, becoming easily distracted, and making careless mistakes. ADHD can adversely affect learning and result in poor school performance. Once a child has ADHD, it is hard to cure, and many continue to have ADHD as adults. In adults it may manifest as mood disorders and increases the risk for anti-social behavior and drug or alcohol addiction.[93]

ADHD was originally considered uncommon, but has been increasing over the last several decades, with recent estimates that it affects 13 percent of boys and 5.6 percent of girls in the United States.[94] The cause of ADHD is unknown. Parents commonly report that sugar intake cause their children to be transiently hyperactive, often followed by becoming tired and inactive ("crashing").[95] As such, sugar intake was commonly viewed by parents, and even some physicians, as the cause of ADHD.[96] Nevertheless, numerous clinical studies performed in the 1980s and 1990s by Wolraich and others could not demonstrate a role for sugar in causing symptoms of ADHD.[97-98]

Unfortunately, Wolraich assumed that the effects of sugar to cause ADHD had to be acute. However, the way sugar causes addiction-like symptoms is not immediate but requires chronic intake so that the dopamine receptors become reduced in the pleasure centers of the brain. Once dopamine receptors are decreased, the frontal lobe region of the brain that controls behavior gets turned off, and this results in the inability to concentrate or control behavior. This had been most elegantly shown in individuals with a hereditary reduction of dopamine receptors in the pleasure centers, but it was also consistent with what one observes in rats fed sugar and in humans with obesity.

This led our group to propose that some cases of ADHD result from chronic and excessive sugar intake.[99] Consistent with this hypothesis, people with ADHD have low dopamine (D2) receptors in the pleasure centers of the brain[100] with reduced electrical activity in the frontal lobe[101] in a pattern that is identical to that observed in rats fed sugar chronically. Furthermore, the rise in ADHD parallels the rise in sugar intake in the United States, and the higher frequency of ADHD in the south, among the poor, and in blacks is consistent with these groups having the greatest relative sugar intake. ADHD is also associated with binge eating, consistent with a chronic sugar effect. [102] Children and adults with ADHD are also more obese than people without ADHD. In individuals with severe obesity, ADHD is especially common. For example, in a study of children hospitalized for obesity, ADHD was diagnosed in more than 50 percent.[103] ADHD was also present in 40 percent of adults referred for bariatric surgery to treat obesity.[104]

We believe some cases of ADHD result from the chronic effects of sugar. Children with ADHD have higher serum uric acid levels and the uric acid correlates with the degree of hyperactivity, short attention span, impulsivity, and anger control.[105] Low level lead intoxication also increases serum uric acid and is associated with ADHD.[106] ADHD is also more common in boys than girls, and boys have higher uric acid levels than girls.[105] Some studies have found that raising uric acid can increase dopamine levels in certain regions of the brain, and to stimulate movement in rats.[107-108] While more studies are needed, it seems likely that the dramatic rise in ADHD may be related to the worldwide increase in sugar intake.

It is possible that the loss of the normal control mechanisms from chronic sugar intake may have a role in other mood disorders. Hudson and Pope have suggested that ADHD, generalized anxiety, obsessive/compulsive disorder, panic, and posttraumatic stress syndrome have a similar underlying basis and should be called "affective spectrum disorders."[109] It is worrisome that a study of 17,000 individuals living in the United Kingdom reported that increased sugar ingestion at age 10 correlated with increased

181

risk for violence at age 34 years. Those who were violent ate more than one sweet per day at age 10 compared to those who were not (69 versus 42 percent).[110] At this point, these associations remain highly speculative, and more studies are needed before any verdict can be made.

Genius and Insanity

There is also some evidence that excessive sugar intake, and/or elevated uric acid levels, may increase the risk for dementia. Early reports suggested the opposite. For example, Havelock Ellis, the author of *A Study of British Genius* (1903),[111] wrote that gout was more common among the wealthy and educated in 18th and 19th century England, and that many famous intellects throughout history suffered from gout, including Newton, Galileo, Milton, Franklin, and Harvey. One potential explanation was the fact that uric acid had similarities to caffeine, the latter which is a known stimulant.[112]

Several studies were subsequently performed to see if a higher uric acid was associated with greater intelligence or performance. One study found that an elevated uric acid was associated with statistically significant but biologically minimal increases in IQ in 817 U.S. Army trainees.[113] Another reported that medical students with higher uric acid levels achieved slightly better grades,[114] while yet another reported that gifted children had a higher uric acid level.[115] Some studies examined the relationship of uric acid with motivation, achievement and drive. Here an elevated uric acid also tended to predict motivation and achievement among high school students and college professors.[116-118] Other studies, however, were negative.[119]

The important aspect to remember is that the effects of uric acid on intelligence, motivation, and achievement are mild if present at all, and I do not recommend trying to raise your uric acid to increase your performance on exams. My belief is that, while the raising of uric acid may have some stimulation of the flight and fight mechanisms as we observed in animals foraging for food, the association of gout with the highly educated in the 17th through 19th centuries was because this was the time that only the wealthy could afford sugar.

Genius and Gout

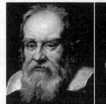
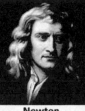
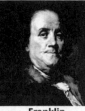

Many intellects and royalty suffered from gout, including Galileo, Newton, Harvey and Franklin, leading some authors to suggest gout has a role in genius. Others, viewed it more a sign of wealth. The wit, Ambrose Bierce, wrote, "Gout is a physician's name for the rheumatism of a rich person."

| Galileo | Newton | Franklin |

Galileo- painted by Justus Sustermans, 1636; Isaac Newton, painted by Godfrey Kneller, 1689, and Ben Franklin, painted by Joseph Duplessis, 1785

In contrast, there is some evidence that fructose and elevated uric acid may have a role in dementia. One type of dementia is called "vascular dementia" and results from multiple small strokes. It most commonly occurs in people with chronically elevated blood pressure and has also been linked with disease of the arterioles that control the pressure and blood flow to the brain. Since both fructose and uric acid can raise blood pressure and also cause disease of the kidney arterioles, it is possible that they might increase the risk for vascular dementia.[120] Several studies have linked elevated serum uric acid levels with increased risk for dementia.[121-122] The presence of "white matter lesions" by MRI scan, which is the hallmark sign in vascular dementia, has also been reported to be increased in older adults with high uric acid levels.[123] We also found evidence for mild cognitive impairment in individuals with chronic kidney disease who had higher uric acid levels.[124]

The most common form of dementia is Alzheimer's disease, which results when proteins known as amyloid accumulate among the brain cells (neurons) and disrupt neurological function. Trying to identify why this amyloid protein is produced is key to understanding how to prevent this important disease. While the cause of this dementia is not well understood, people with the metabolic syndrome are at increased risk for Alzheimer's disease,[125] and recent studies suggest fructose may have a contributory role.[120] The first evidence relates to the discovery that individuals who carry a gene variant for apolioprotein E (ApoE) are at increased risk for developing Alzheimer's disease. ApoE is a type of fat protein (called lipoprotein) that circulates in the blood. Importantly, high sugar diets increase brain ApoE levels and amyloid protein in a mouse model of Alzheimer's disease in association with worsening of memory.[126] Thus, high sugar diets might predispose to the development of Alzheimers by stimulating the production of the amyloid proteins in the brain.

While sugar may increase the production of amyloid proteins in Alzheimers, it may also have a role in blocking the removal of amyloid proteins. Amyloid protein can be broken down by an insulin degrading enzyme but the action of this enzyme is impaired in the setting of insulin resistance.[127] Many patients with Alzheimer's disease have evidence for insulin resistance in the brain, and some groups are even treating patients with intranasal or subcutaneous insulin with the hope that it will improve the dementia.[128] While the cause of the insulin resistance in Alzheimer's disease is not known, one can induce insulin resistance in the brain of hamsters with high doses of fructose.[129] Studies in rats using a water maze test have also suggested negative effects of sugar on memory. For example, rats fed sugar or high fructose corn syrup develop memory and learning defects and have trouble returning through a water maze.[130-131] Obese rats also show short-term and long-term memory defects if they are fed high sugar diets, but not high fat diets.[132] These data raise the scary possibility that excessive sugar intake may increase the risk for Alzheimer's disease.

CHAPTER 20

A KILLER ENZYME THAT DRIVES MODERN DISEASES

Fructokinase C is the killer enzyme that is responsible for fructose effects. Its major role is in the liver and fat where it drives obesity and insulin resistance. However, it may also have roles in food allergy, celiac disease, and kidney disease.

There is an area of Nicaragua known as the "Isla de las Viudas," or land of the widows, for it is here that young men are dying every day from a mysterious kidney disease. Deaths are so common that the land is filled with widows having to raise their children alone. Most of the men are working in sugarcane fields in the intense tropical heat, and hence the name of the mysterious kidney disease is sometimes called Sugar Cane Kidney Disease, or Sugar Cane Nephropathy.[133] The disease is not limited to workers in the sugarcane fields, however, as it also occurs with other agricultural workers. The only common denominator is working long days under intense heat, and it is not uncommon for the men to sweat so much that they can lose 5 to 6 pounds a day. To date all attempts to identify the cause of this mysterious disease that is affecting up to one-third of young men living in this area have been unsuccessful. Tests that have looked for poisoning from heavy metals or from pesticides have been negative.

As more studies have been performed, it has become apparent that Sugar Cane Kidney Disease is not just in Nicaragua, but also in countries such as Costa Rica and Salvador. A similar outbreak is occurring in Sri Lanka.[134] While the cause is still not definite, our studies suggest that the cause, of all things, is likely fructose. Furthermore, fructose may have a role in other diseases that we have not yet discussed. Because these diseases are all likely triggered by the toxic products generated when fructose is metabolized, I have included them in this chapter.

Fructokinase: The Killer Enzyme

Recall that there is a major distinction between fructose and glucose in how they are metabolized. When glucose is metabolized via its *normal* routes, through an enzyme called glucose kinase (or glucokinase), the cell is happy and healthy, as it generates energy for its daily needs. In contrast, when fructose is metabolized by fructokinase, the fructose is so rapidly metabolized that there is an initial loss of energy in the cell before energy is produced. The loss of energy occurs because both glucose and fructose require some energy to be metabolized before they generate energy. However, for glucose the metabolism is very well controlled, and there are all kinds of checks and balances that prevent the cell from metabolizing the glucose too fast. Hence, energy levels never fall. However, when fructose is metabolized, it occurs in an unchecked manner, and this leads to a transient loss in energy, or ATP, prior to more ATP being generated. Fructokinase is like a run-away train, or a speeding truck coming down the mountain that is out of control. The degree of cell shock induced by fructokinase will relate to the amount of fructose it sees and the level of fructokinase present in the cell. When you drink a soft drink, the load of fructose is large and rapid, which is why soft drinks are so dangerous. As one eats more sugar, the levels of fructokinase slowly rise, which is why sugar is more dangerous in individuals who are already overweight or obese.

The danger in fructose is not so much in its calories, but in its special ability to transiently reduce energy inside the cell. When the energy, or ATP levels, plummet, there is the production of uric acid and oxidants inside the cell. These changes are used by the organism to help it store fat. This happens because the uric acid acts on the energy factories (mitochondria) to preferentially increase fat instead of energy (ATP). The low ATP produced actually encourages the animal to eat more, thereby generating more ATP and further increasing its fat stores. This process appears to be why sugar increases fat so effectively.

> *Fructokinase C is faster than a speeding bullet or a runaway train, and when activated causes a local holocaust inside the cell.*

Fructokinase exists in two forms, but one of them, fructokinase C, is the main enzyme responsible for causing the depletion of ATP in the cell. Since fructokinase C is such a powerful enzyme, our group was interested in where it is expressed in the body, for it could theoretically have important roles in these organs. Perhaps not surprisingly, fructokinase C is heavily expressed in the liver, where it has a role in causing fatty liver and insulin resistance. Fructokinase C is also expressed in our fat, and studies by our collaborator, Yuri Sautin, has shown that fructose has similar effects here as in the liver. Fructokinase C is also present in the islets of the pancreas, and it seems likely that this accounts for our observation that sugar can eventually cause type 2 diabetes in which there is not only insulin resistance but a reduction in insulin production from the islet cells.[135] Fructokinase is also present in the hypothalamus and other brain regions where it may regulate food intake, but it is not yet known if this is fructokinase C. Finally, fructokinase C is expressed in the intestines and in the kidney, where we also think it is driving various diseases.

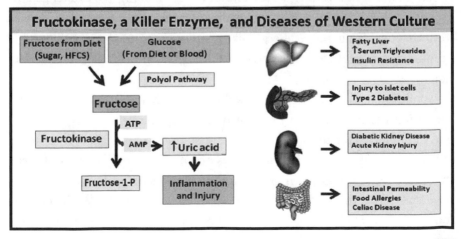

Fructokinase, a Killer Enzyme, and Diseases of Western Culture

Food Allergy

Like obesity, there has been a major increase in food allergies in the United States over the last several decades. In some cases the reactions are mild, and may consist of abdominal pain or discomfort. In other cases it can be severe, resulting in hives or trouble breathing with asthma-like symptoms. I have a good friend who is so allergic to fish and shellfish that he once had such a severe reaction that when he awoke he found himself in a hospital bed with a breathing tube down his throat. Life threatening reactions to food are not that common, but are increasing, and some individuals like my friend have to always carry a kit of adrenaline (epinephrine) in their back pocket in the event that they are inadvertently exposed.

Today between 3 and 6 percent of American children and 2 percent of adults have food allergies. In every classroom there are one or two children who have a significant allergy to food. The most common food allergies are to peanuts, eggs, milk, and fish and shellfish. Since these are common foods, food allergies can have major effects on lifestyle. For example, some children have to bring their own food to birthday parties to assure they will not be exposed to something to which they are allergic.

The cause of the worldwide increase in food allergy is unknown. Since the increase in food allergies was primarily observed in western countries, a common hypothesis was that it is a disease of better hygiene. According to this theory, the reduction in infections that resulted from vaccines and more effective antibiotics resulted in our immune system being less challenged. As a consequence, our immune system did not fully mature, and is skewed towards generating more allergic-like immune responses as opposed to immune responses to foreign proteins such as present in foods or from infectious agents.

While I cannot discard the possibility that better hygiene may have surprising consequences to increase our susceptibility to allergy, there is likely another factor that had not been considered. This is the role of sugar. When food is digested in the gut, there is normally a strong intestinal barrier that prevents the absorption of unwanted components of the food. Studies have shown that this intestinal barrier is broken down in people who develop food allergies. The increase in intestinal permeability allows the absorption of peanut proteins into the circulation where they stimulate the production of antibodies. If the antibody produced is of the IgE class, a serious allergic reaction such as anaphylaxis (hives and breathing trouble) can occur. The important point is that in order for serious food allergy to develop, there has to be an increase in intestinal permeability that allows these components of food to enter the circulation. If these components (called antigens) do not enter the circulation, then no allergic response will develop.

As we mentioned, fructokinase C is expressed in the intestinal wall. Its heaviest expression is in the small intestine (especially the duodenum and jejunum). We hypothesized that if these cells are exposed to fructose that its rapid metabolism might cause local inflammation that could increase intestinal permeability. In so doing, it might increase the risk for food allergy.

To study this, we joined forces with Dr. Stephen Dreskin, a noted expert on food allergy. Steve had developed a model of severe peanut allergy in a strain of mice in which the ingestion of peanuts results in a full-blown anaphylactic reactions that manifests as a fall in body temperature and the development of symptoms (reduction in activity, ruffling of fur) in association with the production of IgE antibodies to the peanuts. However, in order for the mice to develop the allergic response to the peanuts, he would have to also administer a low dose of cholera toxin which acts to increase the intestinal permeability and hence allow the peanut antigens to enter the circulation.

We reasoned that it might be possible to either reduce the cholera toxin, or eliminate it completely, if the mice were given high doses of fructose. To test this hypothesis, we first determined if fructose would increase intestinal permeability. When we gave fructose water to normal mice, we found that the intestinal cells in the duodenum had a reduction in proteins that hold the cells tightly together ("tight junction" proteins) and are important in maintaining the intestinal barrier. Furthermore, when mice that lacked fructokinase were given the same amounts of fructose water, they did not show this loss of tight junction proteins. These studies showed that fructose is likely increasing intestinal permeability and that it is driven by fructokinase in the intestine.

Steve then performed experiments to determine if the administration of fructose would increase the risk for peanut allergy in his mice. To do this, he reduced the dose of cholera toxin to a minimal level. When he did this, the mice given peanuts and low dose cholera toxin developed very mild allergic reactions. However, the mice given fructose with the peanuts and low dose cholera toxin showed a much greater IgE response, worse symptom score, and a greater fall in temperature.

These studies make it likely that the worldwide increase in food allergy is likely driven in part by the worldwide increase in fructose intake, especially from sucrose (table sugar) and high fructose corn syrup. By increasing intestinal permeability, it allows the greater access of food components into the circulation and thereby increases the risk for developing an allergic reaction.

Celiac Disease and Inflammatory Bowel Disease

The observation that sugar can increase intestinal permeability is likely important in a wide variety of diseases. One important condition is celiac disease. Like food allergy, celiac disease is increasing in alarming proportions in our country. This disease is caused by a different type of allergic response to proteins known as glutens that are present in wheat. Unlike serious food allergies, which are driven by IgE antibodies, celiac disease is driven by IgA antibodies. IgA is the principal antibody that fights infections that enter through the gut, but it can be produced both in the intestines as well as in the circulation.

Celiac disease is a disease of the small bowel in which the lining becomes mildly inflamed. While some patients have minimal symptoms, others develop bloating, diarrhea, and occasionally severe malabsorption. Treatment requires avoiding foods with glutens. While celiac disease was once rare, it is also increasing at an alarming rate, doubling every 15 years, and this cannot be accounted simply by better diagnosis.[136] Today 1 to 3 percent of the population is expected to develop celiac disease at some point in their lives.[137]

Like food allergy, patients with celiac disease have evidence for increased intestinal permeability, particularly in the duodenum and jejunum where fructokinase C is most heavily expressed.[138] This is also the site where the low grade inflammation is present. While not proven, we believe it is likely that sugar intake is facilitating the development of celiac disease by increasing the intestinal permeability, thus allowing increased access of glutens into the circulation where the IgA response then develops.

> *Sugars containing fructose increase intestinal permeability and likely have an important role in driving food allergy, celiac disease, and Crohn's disease.*

Similarly, Crohn's disease is a type of inflammatory bowel disease that is also increasing at alarming rates. In this disease the cause remains unknown, and unlike celiac disease it often prefers the more distant regions of the small bowel, especially the ileum. Repeated studies have reported that patients with Crohn's disease eat more sugar than normal, but it has been difficult to show any benefit when dietary restriction of sugar is imposed.[139] Interestingly, patients with Crohn's disease also have increased intestinal permeability. The increased intestinal permeability is likely important since it precedes the condition and also predicts the risk for relapse.[140] Indeed, there is some evidence that blocking the intestinal permeability may be a useful treatment of the disease.[141]

We believe that Crohn's disease may also be triggered by the absorption of some protein for which we still do not know the cause, and that the risk increases in those who have lost their intestinal barrier. Since fructose acts like a mini-bomb inside cells expressing fructokinase C, it may well have an underlying role in facilitating the development of this serious disease.

Other Diseases associated with Increased Intestinal Permeability

There are likely other diseases driven in part by the increased permeability of the intestine driven by the intestinal fructokinase system. For example, in Chapter 17 we discussed how horses develop laminitis (also known as Founder) from eating fructans in grasses that are then converted to fructose in the gut. In this disease a dramatic increase in intestinal permeability develops in which bacterial products such as endotoxin enter the blood. It is thought that this increase in intestinal permeability is responsible for the disease. Since the fructan-rich grasses can contain up to 25 or 40 percent of their content in fructans, a horse that ingests 22 pounds (10 kg) of these grasses in one day could have an enormous amount of fructose generated in their gut from fructan degrading bacteria. Hence, it seems likely that this disease is also driven by intestinal fructokinase.

> *Fructokinase may have a role in causing Founder, the painful arthritis that afflicted Secretariat and is a major health disease observed in race horses.*

Bariatric Surgery and Reversal of Diabetes

As people are becoming more obese, surgery is becoming an increasingly common treatment. This "bariatric" surgery, which refers to surgery designed for weight loss, involves measures to either reduce food intake or food absorption. Different types of surgery have been used, such as reducing the size of the stomach (banding or stapling the stomach), or bypassing portions of the gut involved in the absorption of food. Today bariatric surgery is reserved primarily for those who have severe or morbid obesity, as defined as a BMI >40.

An exciting finding has been that the bypassing of the duodenum results not only in weight loss, but can also be associated with resolution or improvement in diabetes. These benefits are not seen with bariatric surgeries that only involve reducing the stomach size (simple gastric banding).[142] Rather, studies suggest that it is the specific bypassing of the duodenum that is important, as the benefits on diabetes occurs if the duodenum is bypassed without banding the stomach.[143] Furthermore, it is not related to weight loss, as the benefits occur earlier.[144]

The reason why bypassing the duodenum is so beneficial remains unclear. One thought is that the bypassing of the duodenum results in more rapid delivery of food to the distal areas of the bowel where it may stimulate hormones such as glucagon-like peptide-1 (GLP-1) that stimulate insulin release. However, bypassing the duodenum acts to block the development of insulin resistance rather than to enhance insulin secretion. This had led physicians to realize that bypassing the duodenum must have other benefits.

Recall that fructose increases fats (triglycerides) and causes insulin resistance through its effects on the liver. Recently it has been recognized that the gut is also a major player in the production of triglycerides and insulin resistance.[145] Since fructokinase is so important in the development of insulin resistance, it seems likely that it is the fructokinase in the duodenum that is driving the gut response. We believe the benefit of duodenal bypass on diabetes is because one is bypassing this fructokinase-rich segment of bowel. Once fructokinase inhibitors are available, one will be able to accomplish the same effect without having to undergo surgery.

Kidney Diseases

The other major site of fructokinase is the kidney. As you may recall from your days taking biology at school, each kidney consists of a million little filtering units that filter the blood, keeping the blood cells and proteins but allowing the liquid filtrate to enter many tiny tubules that eventually join up with each other and then drain into the bladder where it is excreted as urine. The initial filtrate has the same concentrations of glucose and electrolytes as the plasma in the blood, but all of the glucose and most of the electrolytes are reabsorbed by the tubules as the urine flows through the kidney. Indeed, in the end only 1 percent of what is filtered is excreted, and almost all of the water and electrolytes are reabsorbed back into the blood. However, the waste products from the body, such as acids and urea, are retained in the urine. The kidneys are thus a very sophisticated system for cleansing our blood.

When one ingests fructose, most of it is taken up in the liver and intestines where it is metabolized. However, some fructose enters into the circulation where it is filtered in the kidney and ends up in the filtrate. Here much of the fructose is taken up by the tubules, while some fructose escapes into the urine. Studies have shown that urinary fructose increases in both animals and humans after ingesting a fructose-rich diet, so the tubules are exposed to fructose with each meal. In the proximal tubule which expresses fructokinase, the absorption of fructose can cause injury with the release of oxidants and inflammation.[146] Indeed, we found that rats fed high doses of fructose developed tubular damage.[147] A study in humans has also linked soft drink intake with kidney disease.[148] We have also reported that chronic kidney disease in rats is accelerated when animals are fed a diet high in fructose.[149] These findings raise the alarming possibility that high fructose diets may cause low grade kidney damage.

While our earlier studies focused on dietary fructose as triggering kidney disease, in recent years we have identified a more sinister way kidney fructokinase can cause kidney damage. As you recall, glucose can be converted to fructose in the body by an enzyme system called the polyol pathway. Normally the polyol pathway is not present in the kidney tubules where fructokinase C is expressed, and so most of the time the only exposure the tubules have to fructose is that which comes from the diet. However, under conditions such as diabetes or dehydration the polyol pathway is activated. Since these tubules are reabsorbing a lot of the glucose that is filtered from the blood, there is a lot of glucose that can be converted to fructose when this pathway is activated. When this happens there is a surge in fructose inside the cell that provides the ammunition for fructokinase to produce oxidants and uric acid. Depending on how much fructose is generated, the injury may be low grade, resulting in inflammation and scarring, or high grade in which the tubular cells die.

Recent studies by our group show that diabetic kidney disease is likely driven in part by the conversion of glucose to fructose in the tubules, for animals that cannot metabolize the fructose are partially protected from developing kidney damage. Other kidney diseases may also be driven by the generation of fructose, including acute kidney damage that can occur following cardiovascular surgery or in patients receiving dyes (radiocontrast) for x-ray procedures.

We believe the kidney fructokinase system is also responsible for why thousands of young men are dying from Sugar Cane Kidney Disease. As we mentioned earlier, the young men that are typically affected spend much of the day in the hot tropical sun where they are sweating excessively. As they become dehydrated, the polyol pathway is activated in their kidney tubules and converts glucose to fructose. In turn, many of the workers are rehydrating themselves with mango or pineapple juice to which they add sugar, or with soft drinks rich in sugar. The increase in fructose in the tubule is like an arsenal, releasing inflammatory mediators and causing local holocaust.

Recently we have received generous funding from Danone to investigate if the cause of Sugar Cane Kidney Disease is due to recurrent dehydration and activation of fructokinase. The studies represent a group effort that has brought together scientists from all over the world, including Stockholm, Australia, Mexico, Costa Rica and Nicaragua. For more information, please visit Jason Glaser's web site laislafoundation.org

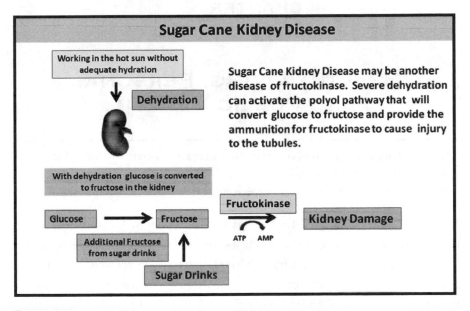

Summary

The worldwide increase in dietary fructose is likely having an effect much greater than simply driving obesity, diabetes, and heart disease. Sugar may have a role in food allergy, celiac disease, and even kidney diseases. But for those of you who are now worried about every sugar cube you place in your coffee, and for the risk of eating some high fructose corn syrup that has been snuck in the package of food you are opening, please hold on. For when we understand the basis of what causes a disease, then cures are often around the corner. So stay tuned.

Section 6

Prevention, Treatment, and Cure of Obesity

chapter 21

Healthy Living: Personal and Public Health

> *Preventing obesity involves avoiding excessive intake of sugar and umami foods coupled with exercise.*

Some of us have struggled to maintain normal weight for all of our lives, but for many of us, there was a long period where it seemed we could eat anything without fear of gaining weight. However, this period of "immunity" is actually an incubation period. As many as two-thirds of young healthy individuals do not absorb fructose very well. Excellent endothelial function and low uric acid levels, which are so common in young people, also help combat the effects of sugar. Over time, however, the continued intake of sugar leads to more and more sugar being absorbed for the same dose, due to the increased expression of the proteins in the gut that aid in the absorption of fructose. A gradual but continued increase in the levels of fructokinase occurs in the liver, and elsewhere, in response to the continued assault of sugar. Slowly the body's defense systems break down. Leptin resistance develops, and the mitochondrial switch gets turned on that helps convert the energy we eat into fat. The sleeping giant has awakened, stimulating hunger, increasing our body fat, and knocking down our energy.

By the time we reach our thirties and forties, the average person is gaining 1 or 2 pounds per year.[1] Studies have shown that this equates to eating only 100 or so calories per day (less than the calories in a single apple) more than we need to maintain our normal weight.[1-2] This emphasizes how obesity results from subtle increases in food intake. More importantly, it demonstrates that minor defects in our ability to match intake with energy expenditure can have long-term effects on body weight. Recall that all animals "know" what weight they should be at any time and will rapidly return to that weight even if it is transiently disrupted, such as by force feeding or starvation.[3-4] This suggests that the change in "metabolism" that occurs as we get older likely involves activation of the fat switch.

In this chapter we discuss how to keep the switch off, or at least minimally activated, so one can maintain good health. In the next chapter we will attack the problem of what to do when one is already overweight or obese.

General Principles

Maintain a normal balance of carbohydrates, protein and fat. For thousands of years humans have maintained a balanced diet consisting of approximately 50-55 percent carbohydrates, 30 percent fat, and 15 percent protein, and it is my opinion that this balance in nutrients has become entrenched in our culture and biology. I therefore believe that a successful long-term dietary plan will likely require maintaining these relative ratios of nutrients. It may be possible for some individuals to permanently reduce overall carbohydrate intake to 25 to 30 percent of the diet, with relative increases in fat and protein. These types of diets are effective at preventing the development of obesity. Nevertheless, low carbohydrate diets, such as Paleolithic diets, hunter-gatherer diets, Inuit diets, and the Atkins diet, are hard to maintain and most people can follow these diets for only a few months. This is why I believe it is better to alter the diet to protect against obesity without changing our current balance of carbohydrate, protein and fat.

Exercise daily. Maintaining a healthy exercise program, consisting of at least 30 minutes per day, provides numerous health benefits. Exercise helps burn fat and prevent weight gain. It has also been shown to help maintain weight loss in animals.[5] Exercise may be of benefit by helping keep the fat switch from being turned on, as chronic exercise has been shown to lower uric acid levels and to improve mitochondrial function, and even to stimulate the regeneration of mitochondria, which is called mitochondria biogenesis. However, extreme exercise that can result in muscle breakdown, such as from marathon running, is not healthy. In addition to causing the depletion of blood volume from loss of water and salt, it can also generate high levels of lactic acid in the muscles and raise uric acid levels in the blood.

Get adequate sleep. Sleeping at least 8 hours a day has many health benefits. Getting to bed early and having the room dark is important. During sleep the biological systems associated with stress are turned off, including a decrease in the sympathetic nervous system and a fall in uric acid levels. At the same time beneficial hormones, such as the anti-oxidant, melatonin, are released from the brain. This allows the body to relax, resulting in a dilation of the blood vessels and a fall in blood pressure. Other hormones are also turned on or off, like clockwork. These "circadian" changes, which occur every night during sleep, have an important role in allowing the body to recover in preparation for the next day of activities. Individuals with obesity or metabolic syndrome often show a disruption of these normal circadian rhythms. Preliminary data from our laboratory also suggests that fructose and uric acid may also alter melatonin secretion in laboratory animals. As such, I do not recommend eating sweets immediately prior to going to bed. Developing healthy sleep patterns are key to good health.

Reduce Intake of Foods that Turn the Fat Switch On

Reduce Intake of Added Sugars. The most common way to turn on the fat switch is by ingesting added sugars that contain fructose, which consists primarily of sucrose and HFCS. The average intake of added sugars in the United States is approximately 22 teaspoons a day, equating to 345 calories, of which one-third can be attributed to soft drinks or energy drinks.[6] The American Heart Association recommends restricting the intake of added sugars to approximately 100 calories per day in women and 150 calories in men, which converts to 6 and 9 teaspoons of sugar per day, respectively.[6-7]

However, this society still views added sugar as simply a source of calories with little nutritional value, and have not considered the strong effect of fructose to turn on the fat switch.

Healthy and Unhealthy Sugars		
Fructose-Containing Sugars		Safe Sugars
Agave	Maple Syrup	Galactose
Beet Sugar	Molasses	Lactose
Cane Sugar	Muscovado Sugar	Maltose
Corn Sugar	Palm Sugar	
Date Sugar	Raw Sugar	
Demerara Sugar	Sucrose	
Fruit Juice and Punch	Syrup	
Granulated Sugar	Table Sugar	
High Fructose Corn Syrup	Tagatose	
Honey Sweetened Drinks	Turbinado Sugar	
Invert Sugar		

Given what we have learned, I recommend reducing overall intake of added sugars to an average of 4 to 5 teaspoons per day. The first step is to eliminate soft drinks and fruit punches with added sugars, as the effects of fructose relate to the concentration that the liver is exposed to, and this relates not only to the amount ingested but also the rate. Desserts should be eaten on special occasions, such as birthdays, holidays, and weddings, and not be a routine. Candy should be significantly restricted. It is not that I am against sugar; in fact, I love the taste of sugar. However, the problem is that we are eating too much sugar and HFCS, and we have to reduce the intake to keep our bodies healthy and to live a long life. One way to do this is to get in the habit of reading food labels. Try to avoid foods with HFCS or sucrose added if there are other alternatives, and learn to recognize the different types of sugars that contain fructose (see table).

What about Fruits, Fruit Juices, and Honey? Fruits and honey contain fructose, raising the question of whether they should also be restricted. While natural fruits contain fructose, most have only 6 to 8 grams per fruit, and hence are much less than in an average dessert or soft drink. More importantly, natural fruits are rich in vitamin C, antioxidants, flavonols, and other substances that combat the metabolic effects of fructose. Cherries may be particularly healthy as they contain substances that lower uric acid.[8] Hence, most natural fruits are safe despite their fructose content.[9]

SELECTING FRUITS			
Fruits Low in Fructose (<4 g/serving)		**Fruits Modest in Fructose (4-8 g/serving)**	
Limes	0 g/lime	Cherries, sour	4.0 g/cup[b]
Lemons	0.6 g/lemon[a]	Pineapple	4.0 g/slice[a]
Cranberries	0.7 g/cup	Grapefruit, pink	4.3 g/ ½ medium[a]
Passion fruit	0.9 g/fruit	Boysenberries	4.6 g/cup
Prunes	1.2 g/ prune	Tangerines	4.8 g/ tangerine[a]
Apricot	1.3 g/apricot	Mandarin	4.8 g/ mandarin[a]
Guava	2.2 g/ 2 fruits	Nectarine	5.4 g/ nectarine
Date (Deglet Noor)	2.6 g/ date	Peach	5.9 g/ peach
Plums	2.6 g/plum[a]	Orange (navel)	6.1 g/ orange[a]
Cantaloupe	2.8 g/1/8 melon	Papaya	6.3 g/½ medium[a]
Raspberries	3.0 g/cup[a]	Honeydew	6.7 g/slice[a]
Clementine	3.4 g/ fruit	Banana	7.1 g/banana
Kiwi	3.4 g/ fruit[a]	Blueberries	7.4 g/ cup[a]
Blackberries	3.5 g/ cup[a]	Date (Medjool)	7.7 g/ medium
Star fruit	3.6 g/ fruit		
Cherries, sweet	3.8 g/ 10 cherries		
Strawberries	3.8 g/cup[a]		
Fruits High in Fructose (>8 g/serving)		[a]Fruits High in Antioxidants [b]May also lower uric acid	
Apple	9.5 g/ apple		
Persimmon	10.6 g/ fruit	Adapted from Johnson RJ and Gower T. *The Sugar Fix.* Rodale, New York, 2008	
Watermelon	11.3 g/ slice		
Pear	11.8 g/ pear		
Raisins	12.3g/ ¼ cup		
Grapes (green/red)	12.4 g/cup		
Mango	16.2 g/½ mango[a]		
Dried apricot	16.4 g/cup		
Figs, dried	23.0 g/cup		

Nevertheless, there are some fruits that are relatively low in antioxidants and may confer some risk for activating the fat switch (see table). Likewise dried fruits are less safe, as the drying process tends to concentrate the fructose while at the same time remove many of the antioxidants. Eating bowls of fruit can also provide a high fructose load despite the benefits of the antioxidants, and fruit juices remain dangerous due to the rapid ingestion with its effect to rapidly raise fructose concentrations in the liver. The strong association of fruit juices with obesity in children has led the American Pediatric Association to recommend restricting fruit juices in children,[10] and I recommend no more than 4 ounces per day in children under the age of six, and 6 ounces per day in children over this age. Finally, despite the widespread belief that honey is healthy, I recommend treating honey like sucrose, and to use it sparingly in foods or to limit it to special occasions.

Keep the Fat Switch Turned Off	
Reduce Fructose-containing sugars	Avoid Soft Drinks and Fruit Juices Read Labels Eat Slowly
Reduce High Glycemic Foods	Avoid drinks containing glucose (dextrose) water Reduce high glycemic foods if you are insulin resistant, have an elevated uric acid, or are predisposed to obesity
Reduce Umami Foods	Limit Beer Intake Limit intake of Lobster, Shrimp, Shellfish Reduce intake of certain fish (sardines, anchovies, mackerel)

Starches and High Glycemic Foods. Lean animals do not develop obesity when fed starch, which suggests that foods such as rice, potatoes and pasta might be safe for those individuals who are not overweight. However, our studies have found that glucose can cause obesity when it is administered in the drinking water. While some of this weight gain may be from stimulation of insulin, much of the weight gain is due to conversion of the glucose to fructose in the body. At this time we do not know how much starch is being converted to fructose in humans, and it likely varies among individuals. We do have indirect evidence that the conversion of glucose to fructose may be increased in those who are overweight, those with some insulin resistance, and those with high serum uric acid levels. Given these findings, my recommendations for those who are at normal weight are to avoid drinks containing high amounts (>10 grams) of glucose-containing liquids, such as your typical soft drink, and to avoid large portions of high glycemic foods such as white rice, bread, and potatoes. If weight does not remain stable with the simple measures of reducing added sugars containing fructose and avoidance of eating excessive amounts of high glycemic index containing carbohydrates, then it remains possible that more significant restrictions of high glycemic foods may be necessary (see next Chapter).

Use of Sugar Substitutes. In my previous book, *The Sugar Fix*, I had concerns about sugar substitutes, but in general favored their use over sugar and hence recommended them as an alternative for those who had a desire for sweet foods. However, I have become less enamored with sugar substitutes after reading Dr. Mercola's excellent book, *Sweet Deception*.[11] One of the more enlightening aspects of his book is that most of these substitute sugars have had limited testing for toxicity, and there is ample concern that toxicity may exist. For example, when aspartame is metabolized in the body, there is the generation of methanol (wood alcohol) and formaldehyde, substances that can be extremely toxic to the body. Sucralose is an organochlorine and was originally made with the thought it would be an effective insecticide like the related organochlorine compound, DDT. Saccharin has also been associated with bladder cancer in mice, although this has not been reported in humans. Aspartame, in addition to its toxic metabolites, can cause life-threatening reactions in children with the rare disease, phenylketonuria, and has also been reported to cause brain tumors in rodents. Hence, while these artificial sweeteners may not activate the fat switch, there are other concerns about their effects on health that are worrisome.

Sugar substitutes may also encourage the development of obesity. This is because the stimulation of the taste buds for sweetness elicits a release of dopamine from the pleasure centers of the brain. While the stimulation of dopamine is much less with sucralose than with sucrose[12], it remains possible that this pleasure response could stimulate the intake of more food.

Finally, some artificial sugars can be converted to fructose, or can act as a substitute for fructose in reaction with the killer enzyme, fructokinase. For example, tagatose is a relatively uncommon sugar substitute, but it is even worse than fructose as it reacts vigorously with fructokinase. Another sugar substitute is sorbitol, which is commonly used in syrups. Unfortunately, sorbitol is rapidly absorbed in humans[13] where it is metabolized to fructose by the polyol pathway, so it is no safer than sugar. Xylitol is another sugar alcohol that is safer than sorbitol as only a small fraction of xylitol is metabolized by fructokinase.[14] This likely accounts for why xylitol is better at preventing caries than sorbitol.[15] Nevertheless, xylitol reduces vitamin C levels in the liver[16] and can raise serum triglycerides and uric acid in humans when given intravenously.[17] Hence, xylitol is also not an ideal sugar substitute.

Avoiding sugar substitutes is wise. If you desire something sweet, have a natural fruit.

Reducing Umami Foods. Most umami foods are rich in purines and may be able to stimulate the production of fat by increasing uric acid levels. As such, reducing intake of umami foods may also be of benefit in reducing obesity and the development of insulin resistance. The primary culprit in western society is beer, which often contains high amounts of RNA due to the presence of yeast. For those who love beer, it is best to gradually reduce intake to only a few beers each week. Other natural sources of umami foods include organ meats, shellfish, and gravies (see Table in Chapter 14). These latter foods are not commonly ingested on a daily basis, and hence simply being aware of the list and trying to be modest in intake is all that is key. It may also be beneficial to read food labels and to reduce foods to which monosodium glutamate have been added if there are alternatives.

Role of Fatty Foods and Trans Fats. The fat switch, activated by sugar and umami foods, acts primarily to change body composition to increase fat stores, and to make one leptin resistant so one is predisposed to gain weight. If one is eating a lot of sugar, then high fat diets will have a role in weight gain. However, by restricting foods containing added sugar and umami foods, the effects of high fat diets to increase weight are mild or absent. Furthermore, the Atkins diet has shown that when carbohydrates are restricted, weight loss can occur even when a person is eating a diet high in fat. As such, it is not important to restrict fats if one is on a diet low in added sugars and HFCS. However, some studies suggest one should avoid eating foods containing trans fats, as these can increase serum cholesterol and risk for heart disease.

Increase Your Intake of Foods that Help Keep the Fat Switch Off

Dairy. There are also foods that have beneficial effects on obesity and metabolic syndrome. Diets high in dairy products, such as milk and cheese, are associated with reduced risk for obesity, diabetes and gout.[18] The exact reason for the benefit is not known, but may be due in part to the fortification of dairy products with vitamin D, coupled with the ability of dairy foods to reduce serum uric acid levels.[19-20] Unfortunately, some people cannot tolerate dairy products due to the presence of lactose intolerance, in which they develop abdominal pain, gas or diarrhea with dairy products. Nevertheless, for those who do tolerate dairy, increasing ones intake of milk and cheese is likely beneficial to overall health.

> *Dairy products are healthy and should be encouraged.*

Coffee. Coffee is a stimulant and is one of the most favored drinks in the world. While coffee drinking can be associated with some undesirable side effects, such as diarrhea, reflux, and benign cysts in the breast, coffee also has some health benefits. The greatest benefit appears to be to decrease the risk for diabetes.[21-23] Numerous studies have shown that heavy coffee drinkers, who drink four to five cups of coffee a day or more, reduce their risk for developing diabetes by 50 percent, which is a quite remarkable feat. The reason why coffee prevents diabetes is not known. However, a likely explanation is that heavy coffee drinking reduces uric acid levels. Heavy coffee drinking is associated with lower serum uric acid levels,[24-26] likely because one of the metabolites of coffee is 1-methyl xanthine that competitively inhibits the enzyme (xanthine oxidase) that produces uric acid.[27]

Dietary Supplements. There are many over-the-counter supplements that likely have benefit on obesity and metabolic syndrome, but few would I recommend for routine daily intake. The first recommendation is to take vitamin C, 250 milligrams twice per day. Vitamin C is an antioxidant that combats many effects of fructose, and it also lowers uric acid.[28] As such, it helps turn off the fat switch. The only problem with vitamin C is that there is some data that at high doses (1 gram daily) interferes with the recovery of mitochondria that occurs with exercise.[29] This is why I would limit the dose to 500 mg daily (which is sufficient to bring the blood concentration to levels associated with obesity (typically 40 or 50 micromol/L) to levels associated with being lean (typically levels of 100-140 micromol/L). For the performance athlete, I would avoid vitamin C entirely and rely on diets rich in fruits.

I also recommend taking 1000 IU (or 25 micrograms) of vitamin D daily. A lack of vitamin D may not only affect the health of our bones, but also increase our risk for high blood pressure and heart disease. Some studies suggest that as many as 5 to 10 percent of adults are deficient in vitamin D.[30] Some of this is due to reduced exposure to the sun, since sunlight can stimulate vitamin D synthesis in the skin. However, vitamin D deficiency is more common in people who are obese or have metabolic syndrome, occurring in up to 75 percent of these children or adults.[30-32] One reason may be that fatty liver interferes with the production of 25-Vitamin D levels, which is one of the active forms of vitamin D, as 25-Vitamin D levels are low in these patients.[33] However, the most active form of vitamin D, which is 1,25 Vitamin D, is reduced in animals fed fructose.[34] The reason was shown by our collaborator, Dr. Diana Jalal, who found that uric acid can inhibit the production of this active form of vitamin D.[35] While supplementing with this active form (1,25 Vitamin D) makes intuitive sense, the dose of regular vitamin D that I recommend is less expensive and should lead to sufficient levels of active vitamin D.

Salt and Water

High salt diets are known to increase the risk for high blood pressure, kidney and heart disease, and consequently, reducing salt intake to 4 grams a day has become a standard health recommendation. Recent work from our group suggests that it is not the amount of salt one eats, but the saltiness of the food that may count. Ironically, some of our data suggests that very salty foods might activate not only the pathways leading to high blood pressure, but also some of the enzymes involved in turning on the fat switch. Hence, drinking plenty of water is important to counteract the effects of high salt foods.

Coming up with health recommendations here must be based on the status of the individual. If you are dehydrated, such as from diarrhea, extensive sweating, or working in the hot fields all day, then salty broths (like the famed chicken noodle soup) with water provides an important way to rehydrate you. However, for the normal individual, I recommend drinking at least 3 or 4 glasses of water a day, and to reduce your intake of very salty foods.

Psychological Adjustments and Counseling

Jack Lalanne once said, "If it tastes good, spit it out," and he is also famous for stating that the "only good thing about a doughnut is the hole." At one level, this is because our taste buds encourage foods that are sweet, savory (umami), or salty and warn us for tastes that are bitter and sour. This love for these types of foods occurred because they all have the ability, at some level, to turn on the fat switch, and hence encouraging an animal to seek these types of foods was beneficial for survival. Today, this creates a battle between what we like (sugar, beer and salted pretzels) and the risk for developing obesity.

So the question is how best to approach this from a day-to-day basis. Clearly, the most effective way would be to turn off the switch, so that the calories we eat act only as calories and do not activate processes that cause weight gain or fat accumulation. This approach will be discussed in a later chapter.

In the absence of turning off the fat switch, we must rely on some of the classical methods, which can work, although imperfectly. One way is via *education*, that being to learn what foods are good for you and which ones are not, and to help guide you when you decide what to eat. A second approach is to work with a *behavioral* program, such as groups like Weight Watchers or Amway's Nutrilite Program. This may involve developing approaches to fight desire, or to develop replacement strategies (such as taking a piece of fruit when you want a piece of cake). Some clinicians, such as Dr. Bill Wilson (carbsyndrome.com), recommend glutamine as a supplement to fight sugar addiction. (Note that this is glutamine and not glutamate, the latter which is the active ingredient in umami foods). Maintaining an active exercise program and getting good sleep also help counter the effects of the fat switch. However, one of the most promising ways of the future is by encouraging better *public health* measures.

Public Health Measures

According to recent studies, sugar intake peaked in the United States in 1999.[36] Data based on sugar dispersed for sales (disappearance data) suggests a per capita intake that hit a maximum of 158 lbs of sugar intake per person that year. This data does not accurately measure the amount of sugar consumed, but rather the sugar that went to the markets and disappeared from the shelves. In contrast, survey data based on questionnaires shows that the average American currently ingests 64 pounds of sugar per year, and that the average teenage boy ingests 109 pounds per year. Intake is higher in certain ethnic groups within the United States, such as the African American and Hispanic, and also varies throughout the world.

The reduction in overall sugar intake in the United States is a victory and is consistent with increasing awareness by the public and medical community to the perils of excessive sugar intake. Consistent with this observation, obesity is now leveling off.[37] We have a long way to go, though, as one-third of the adult population remains obese.[37] As such, several approaches to further reduce sugar intake have been proposed. One way would be to better label the fructose content in foods.

An important approach is to reduce the intake of soft drinks. Soft drinks represent a major source of sugar for adolescents and adults and current intake averages 175 calories per day, which equates to 22 grams of fructose.[38] Repeated analyses also confirm that soft drink intake strongly predicts the development of diabetes and obesity.[39] Soft drinks are more dangerous than other sources of fructose as they are often ingested rapidly, resulting in a rapid rise in the levels of fructose in the liver. Since it is the concentration of fructose that is important in activating the fat switch, soft drinks are more likely to cause obesity than solid foods with similar sugar content.

One approach to reduce intake of soft drinks would be to have warning labels, not unlike that seen on cigarette packages, that state that these drinks increase the risk for obesity and diabetes. Eliminating the frequent practice of providing free refills would also be beneficial. A third approach is to eliminate soft drinks from schools. In 2003, for example, a bill was passed in the California Senate (Bill 677) that banned the sale of soft drinks in elementary and middle schools, and limited their sale in high schools. In 2007 an analysis showed that this approach was effective at reducing both sugar intake by two- to threefold in children under age 11 with a reduction in obesity. However, while some sugar intake was reduced in adolescents over the age 11, one quarter continued to drink at least one soft drink per day and as a consequence, these older kids had no significant reduction in obesity.[40] This emphasizes the possibility that adolescents, who often have money to buy soft drinks, might wait till after class, creating the same bingeing type of drinking that has been shown in rats in which intermittent withholding of sugar water results in a rebound phenomenon.[41-42]

It is for this reason that I would support a sugar tax, or a tax on sugary soft drinks, to reduce sugar intake. Sugar taxes are effective at reducing sugar intake. England, for example, had a sugar tax that was gradually reduced in the 19th century until it was eliminated in 1883 by Northcote and Gladstone. As the sugar tax was reduced, sugar intake increased markedly.[43] Kelly Brownell, a nutritionist from Yale, has performed careful analyses of the impact of a 1 penny per ounce tax on soft drinks. Such a tax would increase the cost of a 20 ounce soda by 15 to 20 percent and would generate 15 billion dollars of revenue in the first year.[38,44] Soft drink intake would be expected to decrease by 10 percent.[38] This would have a major impact as soft drinks currently provide 10 to 15 percent of overall calories in children and young adults, and because each soft drink increases the risk for obesity by 60 percent.[45]

When Sugar is Good

While reading my book might lead to the conclusion that one should not eat sugar; this is definitely not the case. Like all people, I love sugar, and the delight of eating a chocolate cake with whipped cream frosting is something I do not believe we should give up. The trick is to limit our sugar intake, or to find ways to block the switch. There are also times when encouraging sugar intake is good, especially in anorexic individuals or those with no appetite due to cancer or other wasting diseases. Honey has also been commonly used to add to tea or to take in food to aid in combating colds and infections. While data is sparse on whether this is beneficial, the fact that fructose can induce low grade inflammation might theoretically provide a basis for why honey might be helpful in the setting of infection.

Sports Drinks and the Athlete

Sports drinks also contain added sugars containing fructose, raising the question of whether they also constitute risk for obesity and diabetes. The amount of fructose present in most sports drinks, however, is only 4 to 8 grams and is much less than present in soft drinks. More importantly, when a person is exercising, they primarily are burning glucose for fuel. Numerous studies have shown that performance can be increased by providing glucose in replacement fluids. Adding small amounts of fructose has been shown to help increase the glucose absorption, and this translates into more glucose being oxidized. As such, including small amounts of fructose has been shown to increase athletic performance whereas drinks either lacking in fructose or only made of fructose result in poorer performance.[46-48] Hence, sports drinks provide benefit to the individual who is actively engaged in sports, but is not the ideal drink for the person sitting on the sofa and watching television.

> *Sports drinks contain small amounts of fructose and can enhance performance.*

CHAPTER 22

LOSING WEIGHT: REVISITING THE LOW CARBOHYDRATE DIET

Obese people and those desiring to lose weight should perform hard work before food . . . Their meals should be of a fatty nature as people get thus satiated with little food. They should, moreover, eat only once a day and take no baths and sleep on a hard bed and walk naked as long as possible.
— Hippocrates (from Procope J. *Hippocrates on Diet and Hygiene*, Zeno, London, 1952).

> *Losing weight requires both blocking the fat switch and reducing glycogen stores so one can burn fat.*

Losing weight is much more challenging than preventing weight gain. One of the major reasons is due to the "energy gap" which is a concept developed by Dr. James Hill of the University of Colorado. The energy gap is defined as the calories ingested per day above one's metabolic needs.[1] The striking aspect of the energy gap is that very small amounts of excess calories will translate into significant weight gain over time. Let us assume that we have been eating enough sugar to have induced mild leptin resistance. As we stated in the previous chapter, if one ingests only 100 extra calories per day, or the amount present in a slice of toast with butter, this will translate into an extra pound of weight per year. Over years this turns into significant weight gain.[1]

However, while it takes only 100 extra calories per day to gain a pound each year, the opposite is not true. This is because that when an animal "resets" to a higher weight, it must then eat more to stay in metabolic balance. Once this new balance has been attained, it is difficult to lose weight as one has to generate a negative energy balance that is significantly greater than before. For example, let us say a subject weighs 155 pounds (70 kg) and is in balance with an intake of 2000 calories per day, but he is ingesting an extra 200 calories per day due to mild leptin resistance. After five years he has gained 10 pounds. However, as his weight increases his metabolic needs also increase, and as such his daily intake has increased to 2300 calories per day, plus the extra intake of 100 calories per day due to his leptin resistance. Now he would like to lose the 10 pounds and get back to his original weight. To lose weight he must now reduce his intake by many more calories each day, for to be in balance at his lower weight he must go back to 2000 calories per day. Thus, the energy gap concept shows why it is easier to gain weight than to lose weight.

Suppressing the Switch and Burning the Fat: Keep Glycogen Stores Low

We have discussed the importance of turning off the switch in order to minimize weight gain, and it is equally important when we want to lose weight. As such, the general rules for reducing fructose-laden sweets and beer are critical for successful weight loss. Diets rich in dairy and cheese, drinking water and reducing salty foods, and supplements of vitamin C and vitamin D are all encouraged. However, while these measures will help prevent further weight gain, a more aggressive approach needs to be done to induce weight loss. Specifically, you need to do measures to burn the excess fat.

Recall that with fasting, one initially burns the excess carbohydrates in the body, which is stored as glycogen in the liver. Once the glycogen stores are low, the body switches to burning fat. As such, the key to successful weight loss is to learn how to maximize the burning of fat, and the first step is to reduce the glycogen stores in the liver. This is especially important since obese people tend to have high levels of glycogen in their liver.[49]

One of the simplest ways to reduce glycogen in the liver is by fasting, and sleeping is a time when we fast. Glycogen is rapidly depleted during sleep, and after an eight-hour sleep the stores of glycogen are low. This is likely why exercising in the morning on a fasting stomach is more effective at burning fat than later in the day.[50-51] This also suggests that one does not want to snack late at night, and why eating early in the evening may be another way to maximize the reduction of glycogen stores during sleep and hence allow the burning of fat.

Glycogen stores are replenished from carbohydrates in the diet.[52] When starch or sugar is ingested, blood glucose rises and stimulates insulin, which increases glycogen storage in the liver. Fructose is even more effective at increasing glycogen content as it generates uric acid which blocks the breakdown of glycogen to keep glycogen stores high.[53-54] The ability of fructose to block both the breakdown of fat and glycogen is one reason it is so effective at causing weight gain.

The Low Carbohydrate Diet and Weight Loss

It is my opinion that long-term dietary success requires a diet balanced in carbohydrates (50-55 percent), fat (30 percent), and protein (15 percent). In the short-term, however, one can and probably should use other methods. One way, which is common in some religions, is to fast either during the day or for 24 hours. However, this is not easy to do for any sustained period of time. Hence, the best approach for a diet that can be done for weeks to several months is the low carbohydrate diet. As we mentioned in Chapter 15, this diet is similar to the one originally used in the mid-19th century by William Banting in which he lost 50 pounds in one year,[55] and is also similar to the Inuit or Eskimo diet. Most recently it has been promoted as the Atkins diet.[56]

The essence of the diet is to strictly reduce carbohydrates for two weeks, and then to proceed with a modest carbohydrate restriction for the rest of the time on the diet. No restriction in calorie intake is necessary. The severe reduction in carbohydrates during the first two weeks has several benefits. First, it allows the glycogen stores to be rapidly depleted and thereby place the individual in a state where fuels are being generated from fat. Second, it allows the resetting of the fructose enzymes, such as fructokinase, to lower levels, and thereby reduce one's sensitivity to sugar. Most importantly, by removing excessive fructose and beer from the diet, it is helping you turn off the switch.

The reduction of diet rich in carbohydrates is replaced by diets that are high in fat and protein. My suggestion, however, is to keep the high fat component to approximately 50 percent of the total diet, as I remain concerned that higher levels of fat can lead to elevated cholesterol levels and risk for atherosclerotic plaque over the long-term (see Chapter 15). Furthermore, there may be some benefits to higher protein content in the diet in terms of the ability of the diet to quench appetite. However, one does not want to eat large amounts of protein-rich food high in umami, such as organ meats or shellfish.

> *A low carbohydrate diet coupled with exercise is the best way to lose weight.*

The diet has benefits over other diets, as it is tends to result in greater weight loss than most other diets, and also has benefits on features of metabolic syndrome, including on triglycerides, HDL cholesterol, and blood pressure.[57-58] We have seen similar benefits with a diet low in added sugars with or without fruit supplements, but this diet also restricted total calorie intake.[9]

There are some tricks with adhering to this diet, as noted by Volek and Phinney.[59] First, during the first two weeks of a low carbohydrate diet, there is often a significant loss of water and salt.[60] This can result in fatigue, dizziness, and headaches. As such, drinking lots of water is important, and this is also a time when relaxing on the restriction of salt is fine and can even be encouraged.

The reason why a low carbohydrate diet causes this brisk loss of water and salt is not entirely known. Carbohydrates, and especially glycogen, are known to retain water.[61] Studies in human volunteers have also shown that fructose preferentially causes water retention when compared to glucose.[62] It seems possible that, just as fructose aids the animal to store fat, that it may also help the animal hold onto water, which would also be a desirable trait as the animal prepares for a period of food shortage.

A second factor that might make adherence to a low carb diet difficult relates to the not uncommon desire for sugar and sweets during the first several weeks. My recommendation, should this happen, is to have a natural fruit that is relatively low in fructose and high in antioxidants (see Table, previous chapter). The natural fruit will provide the sweetness that is so highly desired, while at the same time the antioxidants will protect the individual from activating the fat switch. Another approach, which was suggested to me by Dr. Mercola, is to try butter from grass-fed cows. The butter can help suppress the desire for sweets and also help stimulate a sense of fullness (satiety). It is also contains a lot of vitamins (such as vitamin A) and healthy fatty acids (such as omega-3 fatty acids and conjugated linoleic acid).

There are some individuals who have stayed on a low carbohydrate diet for a year or more. However, it is my experience that this diet is not tolerated for more than several months. As such, I view this diet as a temporary but effective way to cause weight loss.

The Essentials of a Low Carb Diet	
Phase I Two Weeks	Eat Foods consisting of mainly Fat or Protein Reduce Carbohydrate Intake to 20 g per day Vegetables and Green Salads are Preferable as Carbohydrates Sugar Substitutes may be used during this Phase Avoid Shellfish or Organ meats
Phase 2 Six to 16 Weeks	Eat Foods consisting of mainly Fat or Protein Reduce Carbohydrate Intake to 40 to 50 g per day Avoid High Glycemic Foods Vegetables and Green Salads are Preferable as Carbohydrates Fruits high in Vitamin C and low in Fructose are preferred

Exercise and its Role in Weight Loss

No weight loss program should omit the major importance of exercise. Almost all studies have found that exercise is critical if individuals wish to maintain weight loss.[2,63] While originally this was attributed simply to the burning of calories, experimental studies have shown that exercise blocks both the drive to eat and also helps reverse the defect in fat oxidation.[5] In other words, exercise may be one way to help reverse the fat switch.

The reason exercise is so effective likely relates to its ability to stimulate the production of new mitochondria and the generation of ATP.[64] Recall that the fat switch acts to preferentially convert energy from food to fat rather than to ATP. This is associated with oxidative stress in the mitochondria. Over time, the oxidative stress takes its toll, reducing the number of mitochondria which further decreases energy production.[65-67] ATP levels fall in the tissues of fat people and correlate with the development of fatigue and lack of energy.[68] The fall in ATP also encourages increased food intake as a means to help reverse the loss of energy,[69-71] and weight gain increases.

By stimulating new mitochondria, exercise helps to reverse these effects. With more ATP produced, there is more energy, and this may have a feedback to reduce food intake. If the mitochondria number returns to normal, the individual will have the best chance to reduce their weight and keep it off.

> *Exercise in the morning, or in a fasting state, burns fat faster.*

Therefore, daily exercise is key to success. We recommend a minimum amount of 30 minutes per day. It is important not to do such strenuous exercise that there is muscle breakdown, however, as this reverses any benefit. It is also possible for exercise fanatics to reduce their fat content to dangerously low levels, which is also not encouraged. Having some fat stores is a good thing, particularly if one gets sick.

A common question is whether one can exercise effectively on a low carbohydrate diet. Exercising muscle is often dependent on the glycogen to provide energy, especially for short term, high intensity exercising such as sprinting. However, studies suggest that people on a low carbohydrate diet are able to maintain their exercise capacity by relying on ketones generated from the burning of fat to help fuel the muscle.[72] Nevertheless, I would not recommend a low carbohydrate diet for the competitive athlete who may benefit from having good muscle glycogen stores for intense exercise.

Counseling and Behavior

There is increasing evidence that intensive counseling can also help people lose weight. In one recent study, it was shown that weight loss is much more likely achievable with regular counseling sessions, either remotely by telephone, email or web-based, or by direct contact with counselors on a regular basis, as opposed to no counseling.[73] As such, joining a program in which there are group and personal counseling sessions can improve the ability to lose weight.

Other Approaches to Weight Loss

There are other approaches to weight loss that have been tried. For example, there are some medications that have been administered for weight loss. Stilbutramine (Meridia®) is a selective serotonin reuptake inhibitor that was effective in causing weight loss and an improvement in insulin resistance and serum uric acid levels, but was associated with an increased risk for hypertension and strokes and was taken off the market. Orlistat (Xenical) blocks fat absorption and while effective, can cause abdominal cramps, diarrhea, and a reduction in absorption of fat soluble vitamins such as vitamin D. As such, I am not fond of either drug.

Newer medications may also be soon available, such as Qnexa (phenteramine/topiramide) and Lorcaserin. These agents act primarily by suppressing appetite due to their effects on the central nervous system. There remain some concerns about their safety profile; for example, Qnexa may increase the risk for heart disease, memory problems, and birth defects. Additional studies are ongoing to determine if the benefits of treatment outweigh the potential side-effects.

Finally, mention should be made for bariatric surgery, which is usually reserved for those individuals with severe, or morbid, obesity, as defined as a BMI > 40. Several different surgical procedures have been done, all which are aimed at reducing the amount of food ingested and absorbed. The simplest procedure, which is when the stomach is banded, is not as effective as other procedures for causing weight loss. This has led more and more surgeries to involve bypassing the small bowel, either by doing a gastric bypass or a Roux-en-Y surgery.[63] One of the more remarkable aspects of this latter surgery is that this procedure not only results in weight loss, but can also result in improvement, and sometimes reversal, of insulin resistance and type 2 diabetes.[64] The reason why there is a benefit on bypassing the small bowel is not known, but this is a major site of fructokinase expression (see Chapter 20). It seems likely that some of the benefit of surgery may be to prevent fructose from being metabolized at this intestinal site.

Summary

To lose weight, one has to reduce foods that activate the fat switch and at the same time to deplete liver glycogen stores so one can burn fat. The most effective approach is to combine exercise with a low carbohydrate diet, coupled with counseling. This approach has a great chance for causing significant weight loss.

Nevertheless, there are weaknesses with this approach. Maintaining a low carbohydrate diet is nearly impossible and may not be entirely safe. It also does not get at the underlying basis of the problem, which is the mitochondria. When one activates the fat switch, there is a progressive loss of mitochondria. The loss of mitochondria results in less energy production and has an important role in the resetting of weight to higher levels. While exercise can help reverse this defect, it is only partially effective. Due to the inability to maintain the low carbohydrate diet, and because the underlying defect is not fixed, relapse is common and obesity usually returns. Treatment of obesity becomes like a broken record that keeps replaying and replaying.

It would be good if there was a cure, and there should be. The biggest problem is that we are continuously exposed to foods such as sugar that are activating our switch. We need to figure out how to turn off the switch such that the calories we get from sugar are simply calories and nothing more. We need to find ways in addition to exercise to replenish our dwindling numbers of mitochondria. The future, however, is bright. In the next chapter we enter the new frontier in which the aim is to cure obesity and not simply to treat it.

CHAPTER 23

THE NEXT FRONTIER:
CURING OBESITY

> *To cure obesity, we will need to turn off the fat switch AND*
> *stimulate the repair and growth of mitochondria.*

To date, almost all treatments for obesity are aimed at reducing fat and weight, but not at getting at the basis of what is causing the underlying problem. If the underlying problem is not fixed, it will be very difficult to maintain weight loss. As we have shown, to become obese one needs to activate a "program" in which certain foods such as fructose and purines cause changes in the mitochondria that result in the shunting of energy to fat. When this happens, the individual loses control of their appetite (due to leptin resistance), develops the metabolic syndrome characterized by insulin resistance and increased fat stores, and reduces their overall energy from reduced ATP production. It is as if we are preparing for hibernation, but we do not stop and keep getting bigger and fatter. This all occurs at the expense of continued oxidative stress to our mitochondria. Eventually, the mitochondria decrease in number and we become "locked in" to our new weight, and in some people our islets give out and we become diabetic. It all sounds bleak, and this is why obesity has been so hard to cure. Is there anything we can do?

The great news is that there is a lot of hope, and it is just around the corner. We believe that the approach in the future will be to focus on the mitochondria, with some drugs aimed at preventing the mitochondrial injury that triggers the fat switch, and the other aimed at stimulating the repair and regrowth of mitochondria that have been injured or lost. The combination of blocking injury and stimulating repair will allow the mitochondria to return to their baseline state, and will allow the individual to return to complete health once more.

Blocking the Fat Switch is Critical for Curing Obesity

We predict there will be four major approaches to blocking the switch. We will briefly discuss each approach and the current status on their development and testing.

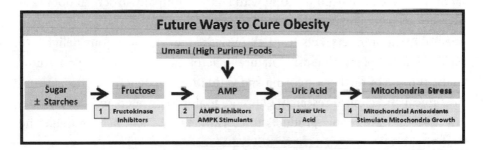

Blocking the Metabolism of Fructose (*Approach 1*). As we discussed in earlier chapters, the key enzyme that is responsible for obesity from carbohydrates is fructokinase. Fructokinase is the first enzyme that metabolizes fructose. Unlike other enzymes in carbohydrate metabolism, the fructokinase enzyme causes a depletion of energy in the cell (ATP), resulting in the activation of processes to make the cell generate fat and become insulin resistant. Activation of fructokinase causes injury wherever the enzyme is present, including in the fat tissues, the liver, and the islets of the pancreas (where it likely contributes to obesity and diabetes), and in the intestines and kidney (where it likely contributes to celiac disease, food allergies, and kidney damage). This enzyme is the single most important target for obesity.

We also know that we do not need this enzyme. Humans who are genetically lacking in fructokinase live a normal life (known as the condition of essential fructosuria).[74] There has yet to be a person with fructokinase deficiency who has been reported to be obese or to have type 2 diabetes. Furthermore, mice that lack fructokinase are exceptionally healthy. One of the more exciting aspects that came from our studies of mice lacking fructokinase is that, while they no longer care for fructose, they still like sucrose, but eat less than a normal mouse. This suggests that they still like sweets but have a more controlled intake. Furthermore, when fructokinase is inhibited, as many as 10 to 30 percent of the fructose calories are excreted harmlessly in the urine. Overall, blocking fructokinase is one of our most promising ways for preventing and treating obesity.

Not surprisingly, several groups are actively developing fructokinase inhibitors. One of the most exciting developments is coming from our own laboratory. We have been working with a large company to screen botanical extracts for fructokinase inhibitors. Using a very sensitive assay, we screened over 1000 different extracts from all over the world, and to our delight we have identified plants that carry natural fructokinase inhibitors. We are now in the process of further exploring and validating the beneficial effects using preclinical and clinical research. Our end goal is to develop and deliver safe, effective, and affordable products to consumers that will help mitigate the undesirable effects of dietary sugar.

Fructokinase Inhibitors are likely to be one of the best treatments for obesity.

Turning the Fat Switch Off (*Approach 2*). During the metabolism of fructose, AMP is generated, and this sits on a fulcrum where it can be a fuel for AMPD to stimulate fat accumulation, or to be a fuel for AMPK where it leads to the burning of fat. Fructose not only generates AMP but also activates AMPD, and this is how fructose causes obesity. Other foods, such as beer, provide increased purines as fuel that also promotes fat accumulation.

Blocking AMPD or stimulating AMPK would therefore be another effective way for reversing the switch and curing obesity.

Currently the major AMPD inhibitor that is clinically available is metformin.[75] This drug is the most commonly used treatment for diabetes, but it has also been successfully used to stimulate weight loss and prevent diabetes. In the Diabetes Prevention Program, individuals with impaired fasting glucose (equivalent of insulin resistance) were randomized to receive weekly intense in-person counseling for six months to lose weight (lifestyle intervention) or to receive metformin 850 milligrams twice daily with a brochure about the importance of diet and exercise. A third group just received the brochures. The average BMI in the group was 34, showing that the individuals were significantly obese. Both the lifestyle and metformin groups reduced the development of diabetes and resulted in a weight loss at a mean of 2.8 years, with the lifestyle program being superior.[76] Specifically, weight loss was greater (12 versus 4.5 pounds) and the reduction in development of diabetes was also better (58 versus 31 percent).[76] The placebo group only lost 0.2 pounds (0.1 kg) of body weight. The study was then continued for an average of 5.8 more years. At this time all three groups were offered a group counseling session every week or two for six months, while the intensive lifestyle group continued to receive group sessions every three months afterwards. The main finding was that the metformin group maintained their original weight loss of 5.5 pounds (2.5 kg) throughout the 10 years, whereas the intensive lifestyle group regained weight and ended up with similar 4.5 pound (2.0 kg) weight loss. In contrast, the placebo group showed no change in weight over the entire period. The net effect at 10 years was a reduction in diabetes by 34 percent in the lifestyle group and 18 percent in the metformin group.[77]

The importance of this study is that it shows the benefit of both intensive counseling as well as metformin in reducing weight and slowing diabetes. Since metformin is a relatively weak AMPD inhibitor and AMPK stimulant, it provides promise for the future development of similar but more potent drugs.

One such drug may be AICAR, which is a purine product that is similar to metformin in that it both stimulates AMPK and blocks AMPD.[78] AICAR may represent the natural AMPD inhibitor. It has also been shown to reduce fat and improve blood sugar in mice with diabetes or metabolic syndrome.[79-81] Moreover, AICAR was found to markedly enhance the running endurance of sedentary rats by 44 percent,[82] creating a stir in the general public that it may act like an "exercise pill." The benefit on the skeletal muscle was shown to involve an improvement in mitochondrial function and the stimulation of mitochondrial growth. Currently AICAR is being considered for clinical trial, but the problem is that high doses are required, it is quite expensive, and at least in our hands, it is also a relatively weak AMPD inhibitor.

Another promising drug is resveratrol, which is a natural compound present in mulberries, peanuts, grapes and red wine. Resveratrol is also an AMPK stimulant and experimentally has been shown to reduce weight and improve insulin resistance in animal models of metabolic syndrome. More recently resveratrol was evaluated in a randomized double blind trial in which obese individuals received placebo or resveratrol 150 mg per day for one month. At the end of the month the individuals receiving resveratrol showed mild but significant improvement in serum triglycerides, liver fat content, systolic blood pressure, and insulin resistance, all in association with improved mitochondrial function.[83] While the studies only showed a mild effect, resveratrol appears as a promising drug to help combat fat storage.

Lowering uric acid (*Approach 3*). Based on our experimental studies, lowering uric acid should also be a potential way to treat obesity. As we discussed, uric acid stimulates oxidative stress within the mitochondria, and this leads to changes in metabolism that favors the shunting of energy into fat. In animals, lowering serum and intracellular uric acid was found to block many of the effects of fructose to cause metabolic syndrome.[84-85]

This raises the clinical question of whether lowering uric acid might be another way to help combat obesity and metabolic syndrome. Serum uric acid varies greatly in humans, from levels of 2 mg/dl or lower to levels above 10 mg/dl. Serum uric acid levels greater than 5.2 or 5.5 mg/dl are also associated with increased risk for developing obesity, high blood pressure, insulin resistance, diabetes, chronic kidney disease and gout.[86-89] Hence, one might consider uric acid as a "new" cardiovascular risk factor and consider treatment for those individuals whose uric acid level is >5.2 mg/dl.

Pilot studies suggest that lowering uric acid might have beneficial effects on serum triglycerides, insulin resistance and blood pressure.[90-92] In a more recent trial, Dr. Dan Feig randomized obese adolescents to receive placebo, allopurinol, or probenecid for two months. During this period, the adolescents receiving placebo maintained serum uric acid levels of 5.9 mg/dl and gained 7.5 pounds. Allopurinol treatment lowered serum uric acid to 3.4 mg/dl and these individuals lost one pound. Probenecid reduced uric acid to an intermediate level and also had intermediate effects on weight. Both allopurinol and probenecid also reduced systolic and diastolic blood pressure significantly (Dan Feig, personal communication).

Nevertheless, it is still too early to recommend treatment to lower uric acid at this time. First, the evidence currently is based on pilot studies, and large definitive trials need to be performed. Allopurinol, which is one of the most powerful uric acid lowering drugs, is also contraindicated in pregnancy and may also be rarely associated with life-threatening toxic reactions.[93] While the risk for this toxic reaction can be substantially reduced by genetic screening (looking for the HLA-B58 genotype), this is not typically done in the clinical setting.[94] So, while I believe there will be a time when we are administering these drugs routinely to people with high uric acid levels, at this time it is not recommended.

In the meantime, restricting carbohydrates and umami-based foods high in purine content, will also have some benefit in lowering uric acid.[95-96] The effects are usually limited to 1 to 2 mg/dl, so while this is helpful, it is likely we may need to also include uric acid lowering therapies in the future.

Blocking Injury to the Mitochondria (*Approach 4*). While blocking AMPD, or lowering uric acid both have benefits on mitochondria, there are also other therapies that are being developed to block injury to the mitochondria. One therapy is relatively old, and consists of antioxidants—however, not all antioxidants get into the mitochondria. Two general antioxidants with significant promise are vitamin C and N-acetyl cysteine (NAC).[97-98] We have already discussed the benefits of vitamin C and I do recommend taking 500 mg daily—higher doses could theoretically be better, but may increase the risk for kidney stones, especially at doses of 2 grams or more.[99] Clinical experience with NAC in the treatment of obesity is lacking, although it appears to block obesity in sucrose-fed animals.[100]

There is also increasing interest in ubiquinol as it appears to be a specific mitochondrial antioxidant. Ubiquinol is a form of coenzyme Q-10, which is a component in mitochondria that is involved in ATP production. Ubiquinol is the reduced form of this enzyme, which means that it carries antioxidant properties. Since it is fat soluble, it can enter cells and mitochondria, where it may help protect against oxidative stress. Various groups are actively studying whether ubiquinol can help in the treatment of obesity or metabolic syndrome. At this point there are no published studies, but preliminary reports are encouraging.

Curing Obesity Requires Stimulating Mitochondria Repair and Growth

In this book we have presented evidence that weight is normally tightly regulated and stable. To change to a higher weight, animals must stimulate oxidative stress in their mitochondria, or energy factories, in which the energy that is ingested from food is preferentially shunted to fat as opposed to ATP. The low ATP state causes fatigue and further stimulates food intake. Leptin resistance also develops, leading to more food intake that helps to recover the ATP levels at the expense of increasing fat stores. The relative shunting of energy to fat leads to an accumulation of fat in the liver, blood and abdominal viscera, and insulin resistance develops.

In most animals, fat accumulation is transient, and there is a switch back to burning fat. This occurs with the migrating whale, the hibernating squirrel, the penguin incubating its egg, and the insect when it becomes a pupa. However, for humans there appears to be no end, and we keep engaging the pathway by eating foods rich in sugar and purines. With time the mitochondria become exhausted and start to decrease, locking one into an obese state. The body has reset its weight to a new level. Now, when weight loss is attempted, the body activates a hormonal response to regain the weight back to its new set point.[101]

I believe that the key to curing obesity is not simply blocking the switch, but also stimulating the repair and regrowth of mitochondria in our tissues. One way this can be monitored is by measuring mitochondrial DNA in peripheral white blood cells. Studies have shown that a low mitochondrial DNA is common in obese adolescents where it correlates with the presence of insulin resistance and elevated uric acid levels.[67] One of the best ways to stimulate mitochondria growth is by exercise, but resveratrol and AICAR also have promise. The best candidate, however, was discovered quite by accident.

The Kuna Indians and their Resistance to Diabetes and High Blood Pressure

Along the Atlantic coast of Panama is the San Blas Archipelago, a series of small islands that extend from Columbia to within 100 miles of the Canal Zone. Many of the islands are within a mile of the Panama coast, and passage to and from the mainland is easy. Approximately 500 years ago the Kuna Indians moved into these islands where they lived primarily on coconut milk, fried bananas, and fish. There was great benefit in moving to these islands, as they were windswept and dry, and free of mosquitoes present on the mainland that carry malaria, dengue and yellow fever. The islands are also separated from the ocean by a barrier reef that helped keep the Spanish Galleons away. The Kuna were a fortunate people, and as will be seen—more lucky than even they realized.

In the early 1940s, Colonel Robert Hardaway, who was Chief of the Medical Service at Gorgas Hospital in Ancón, a city within the Canal Zone, contacted Captain B. H. Kean, a physician in charge of the Laboratory, and told him he was struck by apparent differences in blood pressure between the West Indian (African Americans) and the Panamanians that were working in the Canal Zone. Kean became interested in this observation, and conducted a clinical study in which he measured blood pressure in the Panamanians and West Indians who worked in the Canal Zone, followed by a study of the Kuna Indians living in the San Blas Islands. His results were fascinating, as over 20 percent of West Indians working in Panama had high blood pressure with systolic blood pressures of 150 mm Hg or more, while only 6 percent of mainland Panamanians had similar blood pressure. However, the findings among the Kuna were the most striking of all, with a complete absence of high blood pressure among the 408 adults tested. In fact, many of the Kuna had low blood pressure, with systolic blood pressures less than 90 mm Hg.[102-103]

The reason the Kuna Indians were protected from hypertension was not discovered until a half century later. Dr. Norman Hollenberg, a physician scientist from Harvard, was interested in genes that might regulate blood pressure. Hollenberg had read Kean's paper about the Kuna, and he thought these people might carry a gene that protects against the development of hypertension. He first went to the San Blas Islands and repeated the original study, and confirmed that the Kuna living on these islands had an absence of hypertension, as well as a low frequency of diabetes and heart disease. Unfortunately, he found that the Kuna Indians who had moved to Panama City were not protected, and that as many as 45 percent of the Kuna living in Panama City who were over the age of 60 were hypertensive. The Kuna living in Panama City also had higher rates of diabetes and heart disease. These findings suggested that the Kuna were not carrying low blood pressure genes, but rather that there was something special about living in the San Blas Islands that was protective.[104-106]

One of the most important factors that regulate high blood pressure is salt intake. Many studies had shown that native populations that had low blood pressure typically had diets very low in salt content. However, the San Blas Kuna loved salt, and on average were eating more than 12 grams a day, which is more than in the United States. The San Blas Kuna also liked sugar, and actually ate more sugar (about 5 teaspoons equivalent daily) than the Kuna living in Panama City.[107] These observations made it all the more puzzling for why the Kuna had an absence of high blood pressure and diabetes. There was one major difference in the types of food that the Kuna were eating. The San Blas Kuna loved to make beverages with cocoa, which was a bitter drink since they added very little sugar. The average Kuna Indian would drink at least five cups a day, but they frequently abandoned this habit if they moved to Panama City.[107] As we will see below, a special compound in cocoa may hold promise for being one way to reverse the epidemic of obesity and diabetes.

Cocoa, a Cure for Obesity?

Chocolate originates from the plant, *Theobroma cacao*, and received its name from Karl Linnaeus, who named it the drink (*broma*) of the gods (*Theo*). Cocoa was harvested by the PreClassical Mayans as early as 600 B.C. where it was provided as a drink, often mixed with chilli, maize, or honey.[108] By the 16th century it was a revered drink of the Aztecs and was reserved for priests, officers and royalty, and also for the couriers that would travel long distances by foot. According to a written account by Bernal Díaz del Castillo, who was in the expedition with Hernando Cortéz that took the Aztec capital of Tenochtitlan, the king Montezuma would drink cocoa from a gold cup each night before he would visit his wives.[109] By the 1540s cocoa had been introduced to Spain, and it rapidly spread throughout Europe over the subsequent centuries. While the original cocoa did not have sugar added, this rapidly occurred once cocoa was introduced in Europe, and before long there were chocolate confectionaries and chocolate houses that have continued to this day. Chocolate became so loved that Stollwerck, a German company, constructed a 38-foot tall, 15-ton pavilion made completely of chocolate for the World's Columbian Exposition in Chicago in 1893.

The Love of Chocolate: The Columbia World Exposition of 1893

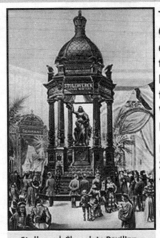

Stollwerck Chocolate Pavilion

The Columbian World Exposition of 1893 was held in Chicago to celebrate the 400th anniversary of the discovery of America by Columbus. It was famous for the first Ferris Wheel, the introduction of the hamburger and cracker jacks, and was one of the first fairs with electric lights. There was Buffalo Bill's Wild West Show, ragtime music by Scott Joplin, and Hawaiian hula and Egyptian belly dancing.

However, it was also a fair famous for chocolate, for Stollwerck, a German company, constructed a 38 foot tall, 15 ton pavilion made completely of chocolate. Milton Hershey, an entrepreneur, got his idea to make chocolate at this fair.

While the Spanish physician, Antonio Lavendan, wrote on the potential benefits of chocolate for angina and gout in the late 1700s, it was not until the last several decades that the cardiovascular benefits of chocolate have been appreciated.[110] The benefits of chocolate are due to the presence of flavanols and antioxidants present in the cocoa. Some of these compounds are destroyed during the processing of chocolate, but some is retained in dark chocolate. Studies comparing the effects of 100 grams of flavanol-rich dark chocolate with flavanol-poor white chocolate have shown that the former can improve blood pressure and insulin resistance, including in individuals with high blood pressure.[111] Effects on obesity are harder to show since most chocolate contains a fair amount of sugar and fat.

More recently, several compounds have been isolated from chocolate, of which the flavanol, epicatechin, may be the most important. We have collaborated with Francisco Villarreal from the University of California, San Diego, and have evidence that epicatechin can block many of the effects of fructose in rats. More importantly, epicatechin appears to be one of the most potent stimuli for mitochondrial biogenesis ever discovered. When it is given to aging mice, a marked increase in skeletal mitochondrial volume was observed in association with a 40 to 50 percent increase in exercise performance.[112] In humans the administration of epicatechin has been shown to improve mitochondrial function in patients with heart failure.

> *Chocolate contains one of the most potent compounds for stimulating mitochondrial growth and repair.*

Summary

The recognition that the energy factories of the cell are under attack in people with obesity have opened new doors for the future treatment of obesity. It is my belief that the prescription to cure obesity will still include restriction of carbohydrates, a daily exercise program, and counseling. However, there will be a day in which we also administer drugs that block the injury to the mitochondria (such as by blocking AMPD or fructokinase, or lowering serum uric acid) as well as drugs to stimulate mitochondrial growth and repair. Drugs such as resveratrol, AICAR and epicatechin hold great promise to regenerate our mitochondria and increase our energy and burn our fat. Other compounds have also been found that may increase mitochondria. For example, branched chain amino acids, such as leucine, isoleucine and valine have recently been shown to stimulate mitochondrial regeneration and increase life span in mice.[113] Leucine has also been shown to improve insulin resistance in mice.[114] So for those of you who wish to see the day when obesity can be cured, I believe it will not be long.

The story I have told, however, has some features that challenge current thinking. Before we end this book, let's briefly look at the arguments against the ideas we have presented.

SECTION 7

FUTURE CONSIDERATIONS

CHAPTER 24

SCIENTIFIC TRUTH, A MOVING FIELD

The concepts presented in this book challenge many current beliefs. What are the major arguments against the fat switch and the respective roles of fructose and uric acid?

This science-based decision by the nation's leading medical body reaffirms that no single food or ingredient is the sole cause of obesity. Rather, too many calories and too little exercise is a primary cause.

—Audrae Erickson, President, Corn Refiners Association, June 18, 2008, in response to the American Medical Association press release of June 17, 2008

The evidence that sucrose may have a role in coronary artery disease is "utter nonsense" and "would never pass an acceptable term paper in an undergraduate course in home economics."

—Keys and Keys, 1975[1] (quoted from Hujoel)[2]

The concepts proposed in this book will be challenging for many scientists and physicians. After all, we suggest that sugar (fructose) is causing obesity not only by its caloric content but by its metabolic effects. It suggests that uric acid, which has been ignored as a risk factor by the medical community for over 20 years, may have an underlying role in obesity, diabetes, and high blood pressure. However, as we have seen, the evidence supporting the hypothesis is strong. Nevertheless, it is important to discuss the countering viewpoint. While a variety of arguments have been made, we will concentrate only on the major criticisms.

How this Book Challenges Current Concepts

1. *Old.* Large proportions of food and little exercise driven by western culture is the cause of obesity.
   New. Large proportions of food and too little exercise driven by western culture is the response to the turning on of the fat switch.
2. *Old.* Metabolic Syndrome is an abnormal condition driven by insulin resistance.
   New. Metabolic Syndrome is the normal condition animals undertake to store fat.
3. *Old.* Uric acid is increased as a consequence of obesity and insulin resistance.
   New. Uric acid is increased by specific foods and causes obesity and insulin resistance.
4. *Old.* Fructose-containing sugars contribute to obesity due to their caloric content.
   New. Fructose-containing sugars cause obesity not by calories but by turning on the fat switch.
5. *Old.* Treatment of obesity requires caloric restriction, exercise, and behavioral modification.
   New. Effective treatment requires turning off the fat switch and improving the function of the mitochondria.

The Epidemiology Argument

Epidemiology is the study of populations and their health issues. One of their key roles is to look for associations with disease. For example, if there were an outbreak of salmonella infection and an epidemiology study showed that the infected individuals all went to a specific restaurant where they ate a particular type of food, then it might implicate that food as a potential source of the outbreak. Similar approaches have been used to look for factors that may predict the development of heart disease or diabetes. One of the most famous epidemiology groups to study this latter topic is the Framingham Heart Study Group, which was set up in 1948 to follow adults living in Framingham, Massachusetts, which was then a small town of only 28,000 people that were primarily of Irish and Italian descent. Since its original inception, the Framingham has recruited subsequent generations as well, allowing its studies to continue to the current day.

The Framingham Heart Study Group is responsible for identifying several major risk factors for heart disease, including smoking and elevated serum cholesterol. The Framingham also developed a scoring system that is commonly used today to assess the risk for an individual to develop heart disease. As such, the Framingham is perhaps the most respected group in the field of epidemiology, and the verdicts are often viewed as gospel in the field of medicine.

In 1999, the Framingham Heart Study Group published a study that concluded that uric acid is not a true cardiovascular risk factor and that it should not even be measured by the practicing physician.[3] In an accompanying editorial, Vaccarino and Krumholz viewed the study as definitive, and laid uric acid to rest, a requiem that has still been embraced by many professional societies.

The Framingham came to their conclusions by examining the relationship of uric acid with other known risk factors for heart disease, such as smoking, high blood pressure, obesity, and elevated cholesterol. They then determined if these risk factors were "independent" of each other in predicting heart disease. To do this, they performed special statistical tests and found that an elevated uric acid increased the risk for heart disease primarily when it was associated with high blood pressure, and that when one controlled for the presence of high blood pressure, the association of uric acid with heart disease disappeared. This was interpreted to mean that an elevated uric acid is not the cause of heart disease, but rather the association of uric acid with heart disease is due to the fact that people with high blood pressure who get heart disease happen to have high uric acid levels. This is similar to the argument that the reason coffee drinking is associated with heart disease is because many coffee drinkers smoke cigarettes, and it is the latter which is actually responsible.

The problem with this analysis is that causality has nothing to do with whether a factor is an independent risk factor or not. For example, let's say we performed a study of the general population and found that smoking, high blood pressure, high cholesterol, and wearing neck ties were all more common in individuals who had suffered a stroke. We then determine if these risk factors were independent of each other, and we find that smoking only increases the risk for stroke when it is associated with high blood pressure, and when one controls for the presence of high blood pressure, the association of smoking with stroke disappears. We then publish a paper and state that smoking is not a true risk factor for stroke, as its effects are removed when we control for high blood pressure. Of course you should object, as the reason smoking increases the risk for stroke is because it increases the risk for high blood pressure, and the latter is a well known cause of stroke.

Let's take another example of how one might be tricked by requiring a risk factor to be independent to have a causal role. Using such approach, I could argue that Osama Bin Laden was innocent in the terrorist attack on September 11, 2001 of the World Trade Center. After all, he didn't know how to fly, he wasn't on the list of passengers, and he was not present at the scene. While he may have been associated with the terrorists, he did not act independently of the terrorists who flew the airplanes as without these latter individuals, the buildings would not have been taken down. Based on epidemiological grounds, Bin Laden did not have a causal role in the terrorist attack, as he was not an independent risk factor.

The reason an elevated uric acid is not independent of high blood pressure and other cardiovascular risk factors in the Framingham Study is likely because uric acid has a causal role in high blood pressure, insulin resistance, and obesity and hence controlling for these risk factors may effectively remove how uric acid works, similar to why smoking was not independent of high blood pressure as a cause of stroke. For uric acid, the best argument for causality remains its relationship with blood pressure, in which all of Koch's postulates have been met.[4-5] An elevated uric acid increases blood pressure in laboratory animals. Serum uric acid both predicts and is associated with hypertension in humans. In pilot studies, lowering uric acid reduces blood pressure in people with hypertension.

No wonder uric acid was not independent of high blood pressure as a cause of heart disease in the Framingham study. Yet sadly this type of reasoning continues to persist among specialists, especially in the cardiology community.

The "Animal Models are Flawed" Argument

One of the favored arguments against the sugar and uric acid stories is that the large number of animal studies on which the hypotheses are based are all flawed because humans are not laboratory animals. I was even at a lecture given by a Harvard scientist who stated that while the studies in laboratory animals by Dr. Johnson's group and others were elegant, his father had told him never to trust animal studies when it comes to understanding human disease. This type of argument allows the proponent to rid hundreds of studies without having to comment on them, and embraces creationist thinking by implying we have nothing to learn from animal studies because humans are simply different. However, it should be evident from this book that a comparison of the biology with other animals can be enlightening and may provide key insights into disease. Remember, without studies in laboratory animals, we might still be asking what is the cause of tuberculosis (see Chapter 13).

A more targeted criticism of studies in laboratory animals is that the fructose is typically administered in large amounts to rats (such as 60 percent of their diet) when humans are ingesting only 10 to 15 percent of their diet as fructose.[6-7] Recall, however, that humans are much more sensitive to the effects of fructose because they have the uricase mutation. When we inhibited uricase in rats, they developed features of metabolic syndrome with even low doses of fructose.[8] Moreover, it is common in laboratory studies to give large doses of a factor in order to speed up the disease process. For example, insulin resistance occurs within two months in rats fed 60 percent fructose, but it takes 15 months if they are given a diet of 15 percent fructose.[9] Likewise, we were able to induce metabolic syndrome in 25 percent of adult men in just two weeks when we supplemented their diet with 200 g of fructose daily (equivalent to nine soft drinks a day).[10] This is much more than most people drink, but it is also true that metabolic syndrome normally takes years to develop and to see this occur in just two weeks was striking. Thankfully, these changes reversed when the study was over.

The Genetic Argument

Major advances in human genetics have occurred in the last decade, in part because of the mapping of all of the genes in human DNA. By using this new fund of knowledge, it is possible to screen the entire human genome for genes that might be involved in various diseases. Several groups looked at what genes might be involved in controlling uric acid levels, and they were able to identify one gene (the Glut 9 gene) that could account for 3 to 6 percent of the overall serum uric acid level.[11-12] The majority of the serum uric acid could not be predicted by genetics, and is consistent with the level of serum uric acid being driven primarily by diet. However, at least a small amount of serum uric acid can be predicted by whether you have a specific variant of the Glut 9 gene, which is a gene involved in the excretion of uric acid by the kidney.

The interesting finding was that the presence of this gene variant could predict gout, but not high blood pressure or diabetes.[12] Since an increase in uric acid is known to cause gout, the fact that this gene variant (which we call a polymorphism) did not predict high blood pressure suggested that the relationship of serum uric acid with high blood pressure did not reflect a causal relationship.

However, our work showed that the way uric acid causes diabetes and high blood pressure is by working on the mitochondria inside the cell. This contrasts with gout which results when uric acid precipitates into crystals in joints, which is outside of the cell. In this regard, this genetic variant of Glut 9 works by increasing the movement of uric acid out of cells,[13-14] and hence it would be expected to increase the risk for gout but have minimal if any effect on high blood pressure or insulin resistance.

The observation that it is the uric acid concentration inside the cell that is responsible for how it causes fat accumulation and insulin resistance can also explain why certain drugs, such as allopurinol, may be more effective than other uric acid lowering drugs such as probenecid in blocking these metabolic effects.[15] This is because allopurinol blocks the production of uric acid inside the cell whereas probenecid blocks the entry of uric acid into the cells but does not alter internal production.

The "Evidenced- Based Medicine" Argument

In recent years it has become fashionable to rate clinical practice based on "evidenced based medicine," in which conclusions are made from specific studies (usually interventions) and then used as a recommendation of proper practice. Another common approach is to perform a "meta-analysis" in which a group of studies, often with slightly different designs, are analyzed as a group and then conclusions provided to aid the clinician or scientist in decision making. While the principal of these approaches is fine, the problem is that that evidenced -based medicine is often being misused or misinterpreted because of a lack of understanding of the underlying physiology.

An easy example would be if I told you that I could prove that cigarettes do not cause lung cancer. For this study, I might randomize 100 people to not smoke, or to smoke five cigarettes per day. After two weeks I end the study, obtain chest X-rays, and show there is no lung cancer in either group. Of course, you would probably laugh at this experimental design, as you know that cancer does not develop in such a short time. This is because you understand the physiology, and you know that the tars present in cigarettes cause recurrent inflammation and toxicity to the lung that leads to the emergence of cancer only after years.

Similarly, a number of studies have concluded that fructose or sweeteners such as sucrose and HFCS are safe in humans and do not increase the risk for obesity or diabetes. These latter studies typically are by investigators funded by the beverage industry.[6,16-19] In most cases the studies are technically fine but suffer the same problem as the cigarette and cancer experiment.

For example, these investigators might argue that fructose does not cause weight gain, and then quote isocaloric studies in which calorie intake is kept equal between groups. Or they might argue that fructose does not raise blood pressure, and quote studies in which blood pressure is measured after an overnight fast (when the fructose effects are gone). Or they might quote studies in young healthy individuals in which administering fructose appears to have no effects at all.

The issue, of course, is understanding the physiology of how fructose (or sugar) causes disease. Fructose increases weight gain by causing leptin resistance, which then alters the appetite.[20] As such, changes in weight will not be seen if both control group and fructose group receive the same number of calories. It also takes time to cause leptin resistance, and even then it may be hard to show weight gain unless a high energy food source is available, such as diets high in fat.[20] The effects of fructose to increase blood pressure initially are only seen during the time fructose is administered, and is likely mediated by the release of uric acid.[21-23] After several weeks a diet high in fructose also increases fasting uric acid levels, likely because fructose also stimulates uric acid synthesis.[24] However, experimental studies show that persistent hypertension requires the development of subtle injury to the blood vessels in the kidney, which takes weeks to months in the animal.[25-26] Even then the development of high blood pressure may not manifest unless the subject is on a high salt diet.

The effects of fructose on metabolism also take time to develop. Young, healthy people are relatively resistant to the effects of fructose, in part because they absorb less, and also because they tend to have healthy blood vessels. However, over time, the repeated assault associated with high sugar intake increases the proteins involved in fructose absorption and metabolism, and the effects of excessive fructose intake become much more apparent in individuals who are obese or have insulin resistance.[27-29] So if your goal is to show that fructose is safe, then do a short term study in young healthy children or adults. In contrast, if you want to show that even short-term fructose can induce metabolic effects, then give the fructose to someone who is already fat and prediabetic.

Science, a Moving Field

Science is not an absolute truth but is a moving field and based on models, or hypotheses, that provide the best explanation to account for the observations of the time. Newtonian physics was perfect for its day, but required revision by Einstein and others as more refined techniques were developed that could measure features of the universe unknown to Newton. Today even Einstein's relativity theory is being modified based on new observations using more sophisticated equipment and technology. The revision, refinement, and occasionally paradigm shifts that occur with the advancement of science is what makes science exciting, and represents an evolution in knowledge towards the greater truth.

> *Science is not an absolute truth but moves forward based on models that both explain and predict observations.*

Fructose and uric acid are not alone in having been challenged as true cardiovascular risk factors. While high blood pressure was known to be associated with increased death by the early 1900s, controversy existed over whether treatment of high blood pressure would be good, as some investigators thought the high blood pressure was needed to aid blood flow through diseased vessels. John Hay, a Professor from Liverpool, once wrote, "There is some truth in saying that the greatest danger to man with high blood pressure lies in its discovery, because some fool is certain to try to reduce it."[30] Likewise, an elevated serum cholesterol was not always viewed as having a role in atherosclerosis, as noted in a 1948 textbook of chemistry by Peters and VanSlyke, where it is stated that "There is no satisfactory evidence that the incidence of atherosclerosis bears any relation to the concentration of cholesterol in the blood."[31]

One problem is that scientists often become so entrenched in prior theory that they can become blind, even when the data is in front of their eyes. A great example relates to the work of insect cytologist, Theophilus Painter, who in 1921 reported in the prestigious journal, Science, that humans have 48 chromosomes.[32] In his paper, he actually states that his counts varied from 45 to 48, and that the best preparations had 46 chromosomes. However, he concluded that humans have 48 chromosomes, and this conclusion was accepted by the medical community. For the next 30 years scientists would confirm that humans have 48 chromosomes using various methods.[33] It was not until 1956 that Joe Hin Tijo and Albert Levan reported that humans actually have 46 chromosomes.[34] This finding is all the more ironic as Levan had reported the presence of 48 chromosomes in humans only a few months before.[35] It is also a credit to Levan that he acknowledged his error and moved the field forward.

Just as there are those who religiously adhere to old theory, it is not uncommon for individuals who are presenting their new hypotheses to also become wed to theirs. Scientists can be in so love with their own hypotheses that they will keep finding explanations for data that challenges their hypothesis to levels that can reach absurdity. It is therefore healthy if the originator of the new hypothesis maintains a skeptical viewpoint. Richard Glassock, who is a leader in American medicine, has often said that a good scientist does not try to prove his hypothesis, but tries to disprove it. Likewise, I have always told the new scientists who join my laboratory that if their experiments confirm our hypothesis, it is great, but if the data challenges, or disproves, the hypothesis, that it is better. The goal is to get closer to the truth, and a hypothesis is only meant to be a means to this end.

The philosopher, Thomas Kuhn, once wrote that science proceeds as "a series of peaceful interludes punctuated by intellectually violent revolutions . . . One conceptual world view is replaced by another."[36] It is my hope that the concepts presented in this book will stimulate both basic and clinical investigation. If true, our work predicts that obesity and prediabetes will one day be curable, likely by both blocking the mechanisms by which sugar activates the switch, coupled with treatments that will allow recovery of the energy producing factories in the cell (mitochondria). Regardless, testing new ideas provides new knowledge that should help propel the field forward. This is all the more important given the gravity of the epidemic of obesity and diabetes, and our current inability to arrest its progression.

CHAPTER 25

AFTERTHOUGHTS: DIVINE MUTATIONS, HEROISM AND MIRACLES

> *In a way, the story of the struggles of humans to survive gives insight not only into the cause of obesity, but also into the world of heroism, miracles, and faith.*

Charles Darwin's masterpiece, *Origin of Species*, was published in 1859 and introduced evolution to both the public and the scientist.[37] The first edition sold out within hours of being released. The conceptual advances of this work provided the scientific framework to help us understand our own origins. As Darwin wrote, "It is not the strongest of the species that survives, nor the most intelligent that survives. It is the one that is the most adaptable to change."[37] As shown in this book, survival depends on having adequate fat stores to survive periods of food deprivation. "Survival of the fattest" thus spelled the fate for many species in history. Species that could improve their ability to store fat had the best chances to survive when times got tough. Humans were particularly successful at learning how to enhance their fat stores in response to foods. The uricase and vitamin C mutations enhanced the effects of fructose to increase fat stores. Unfortunately, these mutations have increased our susceptibility to becoming obese and diabetic today. James Neel was right. Our acquisition of thrifty genes, or more precisely, our loss of nonthrifty genes, is why many of us are fat today, coupled with the wide availability of foods that can activate the fat switch, such as sugar and beer.

As one reflects on this story, one realizes how fortunate we were to have acquired these mutations. Extinction is a common event. There have been at least five massive extinctions that each led to the demise of more than 50 percent of species living at that time.[38] Recall that during the Miocene there were 100 different ape species, for which only 5 survive today.[39] Consider the fact only *Homo sapiens* survive today, and related species in our genus, such as *Home erectus, Homo antecessor, Homo heidelbergensis* and Neanderthals (*Homo neanderthalensis*) no longer walk the earth. We are lucky to be alive.

But philosophically, can evolutionary mechanisms completely account for our survival? Evolution as described by Darwin was a slow process that occurred over thousands of years. More recently, Neil Eldredge and Stephen Jay Gould suggested that evolution can accelerate during periods of upheaval, for under conditions where an organism is disadvantaged; the potential for a spontaneous mutation to carry beneficial effects on survival is increased.[40] Nevertheless, mutations are rare, occurring in only one in 15 to 30 million nucleotides of DNA in each human.[41-43] This translates into approximately 100 to 200 mutations in the 20,000 genes present in each human.[41-43] In a population of millions of people, the potential for a survival mutation to surface might be expected. However, when the population is dwindling, the chances of a survival mutation become less and less. Recall that during the Mid-Miocene, falling temperatures caused a decrease in the availability of fruits, forcing our ancestral apes to retreat to isolated colonies where they went through repeated periods of starvation. Under these conditions in which the overall population was falling, the birth of an ape with the uricase mutation that could increase the ability to survive famine would have been an extremely fortuitous event.

Recently the discovery of epigenetics has provided a potential answer for how animals can survive when the chances for a survival mutation are low. Epigenetics refers to genetic changes that can be passed to the next generation which are not due to changes in the genes (DNA) themselves, but are rather caused by acquired changes in substances that regulate DNA (our genetic material).[44]   Epigenetics is especially important in pregnancy. For example, maternal malnutrition can trigger changes in the fetus that result in increased risk for obesity following birth.[45-46]   A study of women who became pregnant in World War II during a period of food rationing reported that the girls born to these mothers were more likely to be obese as adults.[47] Epigenetic changes can also be passed on for several generations. Thus, epigenetics could provide an alternative survival mechanism when a mutation fails to occur.

When All Else Fails

What happens to a population when both classical evolutionary mechanisms and epigenetics fail? Is extinction inevitable? I think not. A story that might be relevant to this question relates to the migration of modern humans (*Homo sapiens*) out of Africa. Our knowledge of early humans has been improved by our ability to track back thousands of generations by studying the DNA from the mitochondria. As is well known, every baby receives half of his or her DNA from the mother and the other half from the father—but this relates to our chromosomal DNA which resides in the nucleus of the cell. In contrast, mitochondria also carry DNA and this DNA is always passed from the mother to her children.[48]   This mitochondrial DNA will therefore remain the same in the maternal lineage for generations and generations unless a mutation occurs. When the latter happens, then that mutation will be spread to subsequent generations. By looking at the pattern of mutations, one can draw genealogy maps that date back thousands of years. Others have used the DNA present in the Y chromosome (which is only passed from male to male) to develop molecular genealogies in men. Studies in chromosomal DNA can also be used. Studies based on chromosomal DNA suggest that the first person with blue eyes lived approximately 6,000 to 10,000 years ago, likely in the agricultural settlements near the Black Sea.[49]   In essence, every individual with blue eyes is a descendent of this individual.

Using molecular genetics, coupled with the fossil record, it has been shown that the earliest modern humans (the "Mitochondrial Eve") lived in

Africa.[50-51] These peoples were hunters and gatherers and lived in the coastal plains near the border of Namibia and Angola approximately 200,000 years ago.[50] Some humans also lived in Eastern Africa; indeed, the earliest known fossil of a modern human is Kibish man, whose fossil bones were found between volcanic layers of rock near Kibish, Ethiopia, and have been dated to 195,000 years ago.[52] Today the hunter gatherer San people (Bushmen) of the Kalahari desert carry the greatest concentration of ancestral human genes, suggesting that they may be closest genetically to our ancestors.

For the next 100,000 years the early human population suffered through extensive droughts in Africa, and the population remained low.[53-54] Then, approximately 63,000 years ago, a massive volcanic eruption occurred on the island of Sumatra in Indonesia. The Toba supervolcano spewed ash into the atmosphere that led to the deposition of 6 inches of ash throughout southern Asia and a volcanic winter that lasted between 5 and 10 years. Rainfall became less and the droughts worsened. Temperatures fell worldwide to the lowest temperatures in the last 125,000 years, and persisted for up to 1800 years, possibly precipitating the last ice age in Europe.[55-56] Extinction of a number of species in southeast Asia has been documented. Around the same time, the human population plummeted by fivefold; it is estimated that the population fell to as few as 13,800 individuals.[57]

Whether this natural disaster was the reason or not for the fall in the population or in the subsequent migration remains debated, but it was during this period that some modern humans migrated out of Africa. The telltale sign is the presence of a mitochondrial DNA signature (the L3 clade) that was present in one of the women who made this trip and which is an ancestral marker for all European and Asian peoples. While there is some evidence that this group crossed by land, from Egypt through the Sinai and into Asia, some studies suggest the people followed a coastal route to the south.

If they followed a coastal route, this small band of individuals, who may have been as few as 150 individuals, crossed from Ethiopia to the Arabian peninsula by raft or boat at the place where the Red Sea is most narrow, a place known as the *Bab el Mandeb*, or "Gate of Tears." Today the strait separating the Horn of Africa from Arabia is approximately 10 to 20 miles of rough seas, but during this period of history the distance was likely less and may have only been a few miles.[58] While we do not know enough details of what really happened, I am struck with the likelihood that these humans took desperate chances to find a more hospitable place to live. Here the escape from famine was likely not driven by genetic or epigenetic changes, but rather by heroism and ingenuity.

Religion and Science

Our species has survived multiple times when extinction seemed imminent ("bottleneck" periods). We survived due to serendipitous genetic mutations that carried survival advantage (Darwinian evolution) and by epigenetic changes, with the latter primarily occurring during pregnancy. When this failed, humans survived by wit and courage. One can imagine how survival mutations, heroism, or "miracles" that helped promote survival could influence the development of religions. This raises an interesting question. Imagine that with each crisis, you flip a coin in which heads results in your survival and tails results in your extinction. If you think in "real time," then at each crisis you will flip the coin with a 50 percent chance of survival. Each time you advance, the odds for survival with the next crisis remains a laudable 50 percent. However, if you think retrospectively, then you realize that as a species we may have flipped heads for many times in a row, at a statistical chance that might seem impossible. Depending on which viewpoint you choose, you could make a case that evolutionary theory either supports or refutes religion and the existence of a higher being. But whether we read the story forwards or backwards, it is the same tale in the end. We are fortunate to be here, but it is critical as we move forward that we not only better understand our place in nature, but nature's place with us.

GLOSSARY

adipocyte: Specialized cells that make and store fat.

AMP: Adenosine monophosphate. A major breakdown product of DNA, RNA and ATP.

AMPD: AMP deaminase. An enzyme that utilizes AMP, generating downstream products such as uric acid. AMPD activation is associated with fat accumulation and an inhibition of AMPK.

AMPK: AMP kinase. An enzyme that utilizes AMP and has a major role in burning fat and protecting against diabetes.

ATP: Adenosine triphosphate. The primary source of energy for the cell.

diabetes, type 2:   A condition in which blood glucose increases in the blood. This is due to both a resistance of tissues to the effect of insulin (insulin resistance) as well as low grade damage to the islet cells in the pancreas resulting in inadequate insulin production for the level of blood glucose.

dopamine: A chemical secreted in the brain that is associated with a pleasure response.

epigenetic: Epigenetics refers to genetic changes that can be passed to the next generation which are not due to changes in the genes (DNA) themselves, but are rather caused by acquired changes in substances that regulate DNA (our genetic material).

estivation: A process similar to hibernation, but which occurs in hot temperatures.

foraging response: A late response in starvation in which the animal becomes agitated and starts searching for food.

fructokinase: The first enzyme in fructose metabolism, also known as ketohexokinase or KHK. Fructokinase metabolizes fructose to fructose-1-phosphate, and in the process causes transient depletion of ATP and activation of AMPD. This latter process is why fructose is so effective at causing features of metabolic syndrome.

fructose: A simple sugar, also known as fruit sugar or levulose. The primary sugar in fruits and honey. It is also present in sucrose and high fructose corn syrup.

ghrelin: A hormone that is secreted by the gut that has some opposite actions to leptin, suggesting it is a type of "hunger" hormone turned on by food deprivation.

glucose: A simple sugar that is the primary carbohydrate fuel in the body and which circulates in the blood. High levels of glucose (>125 mg/dl) in the fasting state is defined as diabetes.

glycogen: The primary storage form of carbohydrates in the animal, similar to starch in plants. Glycogen consists of multiple glucose molecules bound together.

high fructose corn syrup: A sweetener generated from corn in which corn syrup (made primarily of glucose) is converted by a series of enzymes into a mixture of glucose and fructose. The most common proportion is 55 percent fructose and 45 percent glucose (used in soft drinks) and 42 percent fructose and 58 percent glucose (used in pastries).

IMP: Inosine monophosphate. IMP is the product of AMPD and is a precursor of uric acid. IMP has also been found to amplify the umami taste.

impaired fasting glucose: Normally blood glucose levels are less than 100 mg/dl in the fasting state. Individuals with fasting blood glucose between 100 and 125 mg/dl are defined as having impaired fasting glucose. This is considered a prediabetic condition and is associated with insulin resistance and the metabolic syndrome.

insulin: A hormone released from the beta cells in the islets of the pancreas in response to a rise of glucose in the blood following a meal. Insulin stimulates the uptake and utilization of glucose into tissues.

insulin resistance: A prediabetic condition commonly observed in obese people in which the individual become resistant to the effect of insulin to reduce blood glucose levels. Blood glucose levels tend to be high (100-125 mg/dl in the fasting state) and insulin levels are also high.

ketoacids: Ketones and ketoacids are produced during the oxidation of fatty acids. In essence, ketoacids reflected the burning or utilization of fat.

leptin: Considered the principal satiety hormone. It is released from fat cells and is responsible for telling a person when they are full and should quit eating.

leptin resistance: A condition commonly observed in obese people in which the brain becomes resistant to the effects of leptin. Leptin resistance is associated with high levels of leptin in the blood.

metabolic syndrome: A cluster of signs associated with fat storage, including abdominal obesity, high serum triglycerides, low HDL cholesterol, impaired fasting glucose, and elevated blood pressure.

mitochondria: Small components within the cytoplasm of cells where the majority of ATP is produced. Equivalent to the energy factories of the cell.

polyol pathway: A series of enzymes that converts glucose to fructose. The first enzyme is aldose reductase, which converts glucose to sorbitol. The second enzyme is sorbitol dehydrogenase, which converts sorbitol to fructose.

purines: The building blocks for DNA, RNA, and ATP. Uric acid is also generated from diets high in purines. Umami foods typically have high purine content.

oxidative Stress: A condition in which there are high levels of oxidants that can damage tissues. Oxidative stress is increased in conditions associated with low grade inflammation, such as occurs in many individuals with metabolic syndrome and heart disease. Low grade oxidative stress to the mitochondria acts to increase fat accumulation and reduce ATP generation. High grade, or chronic, oxidative stress to mitochondria can cause their loss.

RNA World: Considered by many to represent a period of time in the past when life consisted solely of RNA with an absence of protein or DNA.

satiety: A sensation of fullness that leads to a cessation in eating.

starch: The primary storage form of carbohydrates in the plant, similar to glycogen in animals. Starch consists of multiple glucose molecules bound together.

sucrose: A disaccharide sugar consisting of fructose and glucose bound together. Also known as table sugar. It is primarily derived from the sugarcane and sugar beet. When ingested, it is degraded by an enzyme in the gut (sucrase) which releases the glucose and fructose that is then absorbed.

Thrifty gene: Refers to a hypothesis by James Neel that proposed that the reason so many people are obese and diabetic today is because we acquired genes in our past that protected us during periods of famine but that are counterproductive today, as they now increase our suscep-tibility to become fat and insulin resistant.

torpor: Refers to a hibernating animal in which body metabolism decreases markedly, with a fall in body temperature and a lowering of heart rate.

umami: One of five major tastes sensed by the taste buds (sweet, salt, bitter, sour, and umami). Umami is the savory taste, and is mediated by gluta-mate and IMP.

uric acid: A major breakdown product of DNA, RNA and ATP that circu-lates in the blood. High levels of uric acid can precipitate as crystals in joints causing the arthritic condition, gout. Uric acid levels are also commonly elevated in people with obesity, metabolic syndrome and heart disease.

uricase: An enzyme present in most mammals but which was lost in humans and great apes due to a mutation that occurred 15 million years ago. The enzyme acts to degrade uric acid. Animals that lack uricase have higher uric acid levels than other mammals.

xanthine oxidase: The enzyme that generates uric acid in the cell. It also produces oxidants in this process.

REFERENCES

PREFACE AND PROLOGUE

1.   Diamond J. The double puzzle of diabetes. Nature 2003;423:599-602.

2.   Neel JV. The study of natural selection in primitive and civilized human populations. Human biology; an international record of research 1958;30:43-72.

3.   Neel JV. Diabetes mellitus: a "thrifty" genotype rendered detrimental by "progress"? American journal of human genetics 1962;14:353-62.

4.   Barry JM. The site of origin of the 1918 influenza pandemic and its public health implications. J Transl Med 2004;2:3.

5.   Yach D, Stuckler D, Brownell KD. Epidemiologic and economic consequences of the global epidemics of obesity and diabetes. Nature medicine 2006;12:62-6.

6.   Hossain P, Kawar B, El Nahas M. Obesity and diabetes in the developing world--a growing challenge. The New England journal of medicine 2007;356:213-5.

7,   Ogden CL, Caroll MD, Curtin LR, McDowell MA, Tabak CJ, Flegal KM. Prevalence of overweight and obesity in the United States. 1999-2004. JAMA 2006;295:1549-55.

8.   Medico-Actuarial Mortality Investigation. Association of Life Insurance Medical Directors and the Actuarial Society of America 1912;1.

9,   Adams KF, Schatzkin A, Harris TB, et al. Overweight, obesity and mortality in a large prospective cohort of persons 50 to 71 years old. The New England journal of medicine 2006;355:763-78.

10.   Wellman NS, Friedberg B. Causes and consequences of adult obesity: health, social and economic impacts in the United States. Asia Pac J Clin Nutr 2002;11 Suppl 8:S705-9.

11.   Thompson D, Wolf AM. The medical-care cost burden of obesity. Obes Rev 2001;2:189-97.

12.   Devol R, Bedroussian A. An unhealthy America:The economic burden of chronic disease--Charting a new course to save lives and increase productiviety and economic growth: Milken Institute; 2007.

251

SECTION 1

1. Darwin C. On The Origin of Species by Means of Natural Selection, or The Preservation of Favoured Races in the Struggle for Life. First edition ed. London: John Murray; 1859.

2. Keesey RE, Powley TL. The regulation of body weight. Annu Rev Psychol 1986; 37:109-133.

3. Keesey RE, Powley TL. Body energy homeostasis. Appetite 2008;51:442-5.

4. Bairlein F. How to get fat: nutritional mechanisms of seasonal fat accumulation in migratory songbirds. Naturwissenschaften 2002;89:1-10.

5. Mrosovsky N, Sherry DF. Animal anorexias. Science (New York, NY 1980;207:837-42.

6. Martin SL. Mammalian hibernation: a naturally reversible model for insulin resistance in man? Diab Vasc Dis Res 2008;5:76-81.

7. Heldmaier G, Ruf T. Body temperature and metabolic rate during natural hypothermia in endotherms. J Comp physiol B 1992;162:696-706.

8. Lyman CP. Oxygen consumption, body temperature and heart rate of woodchucks entering hibernation. The American journal of physiology 1958;194:83-91.

9. Arrese EL, Soulages JL. Insect fat body: energy, metabolism, and regulation. Annu Rev Entomol 2010;55:207-25.

10. Hartman FA, Brownell KA. Liver lipids in hummingbirds. The Condor 1959;61:270-7.

11. Tryland M, Brun E. Serum chemistry of the minke whale from the northeastern Atlantic. J Wildl Dis 2001;37:332-41.

12. Van Beurden EK. Energy Metabolism of Dormant Australian Water-holding Frogs (Cyclorana platycephalus). Copeia 1980;4:787-99.

13. Pond CM. Morphological Aspects and the Ecological and Mechanical Consequences of Fat Deposition in Wild Vertebrates. Annual Rev Ecol Systematics 1978;9:519-70.

14. Shattock SG. On Normal Tumour-like Formations of Fat in Man and the Lower Animals. Proc R Soc Med 1909;2:207-70.

15. Jonsson N, Jonsson B, Hansen LP. Changes in Proximate Composition and Estimates of Energetic Costs During Upstream Migration and Spawning in Atlantic Salmon Salmo salar. J Animal Ecol 1997;66:425-36.

16. McVeigh BR, Healey MC, Wolfe F. Energy expenditures during spawning by chum salmon Oncorhynchus keta (Walbaum) in British Columbia. J Fish Biol 2007;71:1696-713.

17. Cranford JA. Hibernation in the western jumping mouse (Zapus princeps). J Mamm 1978;59:496-506.

18.   Dunbrack RL, Ramsay MA. The Allometry of Mammalian Adaptations to Seasonal Environments: A Critique of the Fasting Endurance Hypothesis. Oikos 1993;66:336-42.

19.   Bergmann C. Ü ber die Verh ä ltnisse der W ä rme ö konomie der Thiere zu ihrer Grösse Göttinger Studien 1847;3:595-708.

20.   Stillwell RC. Are latitudinal clines in body size adaptive? Oikos 2010;119 1387–90.

21.   Hays GC, Broderick AC, Glen F, Godley BJ. Change in body mass associated with long-term fasting in a marine reptile: the case of green turtles (Chelonia mydas) at Ascension Island. Can J Zool 2002;80:1299-302.

22.   Millar JS, Hickling GJ. Fasting Endurance and the Evolution of Mammalian Body Size Functional Ecology 1990;4:5-12.

23.   Nagy KA, Girard IA, Brown TK. Energetics of free-ranging mammals, reptiles, and birds. Annu Rev Nutr 1999;19:247-77.

24.   Peterson CC. Ecological energetics of the desert tortoise (Gopherus agassizii): effects of rainfall and drought. Ecology 1996;77:1831-44.

25.   Weis-Fogh T. Fat Combustion and Metabolic Rate of Flying Locusts (Schistocerca gregaria Forskal. Philosoph Transs Royal Soc London 1952;237:1--36.

26.   Alvarez LW, Alvarez W, Asaro F, Michel HV. Extraterrestrial cause for the cretaceous-tertiary extinction. Science (New York, NY 1980;208:1095-108.

27.   Pontzer H, Allen V, Hutchinson JR. Biomechanics of running indicates endothermy in bipedal dinosaurs. PLoS ONE 2009;4:e7783.

28.   Ortmann S, Heldmaier G. Regulation of body temperature andenergy requirements of hibernating alpine marmots (Marmota mamota). American journal of physiology 2000;278:R698-R704.

29.   Dausmann KH, Glos J, Ganzhorn JU, Heldmaier G. Physiology: hibernation in a tropical primate. Nature 2004;429:825-6.

30.   Hargrove JL. Adipose energy stores, physical work, and the metabolic syndrome: lessons from hummingbirds. Nutr J 2005;4:36.

31.   Lancereaux E. Le Diabete maigre et le Diabete gras, . L' Union Mid 1880.

32.   Third Report of the National Cholesterol Education Program (NCEP) Expert Panel on Detection, Evaluation, and Treatment of High Blood Cholesterol in Adults (Adult Treatment Panel III): National Heart, Lung, and Blood Institute, National Institutes of Health; 2001 May 2001. Report No.: NIH Publication No. 01-3670.

33.   Kylin E. [Studies of the hypertension-hyperglycemia-hyperuricemia syndrome] Studien uber das Hypertonie-Hyperglykamie-hyperurikamiesyndrome. Zentralblatt fur innere Medizin 1923;44:105-27.

34.   Haller H. [Epidermiology and associated risk factors of hyperlipoproteinemia]. Z Gesamte Inn Med 1977;32:124-8.

35.   Singer P. [Diagnosis of primary hyperlipoproteinemias]. Z Gesamte Inn Med 1977;32:129-33.

36.   Phillips GB. Sex hormones, risk factors and cardiovascular disease. Am J Med 1978;65:7-11.

37.   Reaven GM. Banting Lecture 1988. Role of insulin resistance in human disease. 1988. Nutrition 1997;13:65; discussion 4, 6.

38.   Ford ES, Giles WH, Mokdad AH. Increasing prevalence of the metabolic syndrome among u.s. Adults. Diabetes care 2004;27:2444-9.

39.   Florant GL, Lawrence AK, Williams K, Bauman WA. Seasonal changes in pancreatic B-cell function in euthermic yellow-bellied marmots. The American journal of physiology 1985;249:R159-65.

40.   Shafrir E, Ziv E, Kalman R. Nutritionally induced diabetes in desert rodents as models of type 2 diabetes: Acomys cahirinus (spiny mice) and Psammomys obesus (desert gerbil). ILAR J 2006;47:212-24.

41.   Conlon JM, Yano K, Chartrel N, Vaudry H, Storey KB. Freeze tolerance in the wood frog Rana sylvatica is associated with unusual structural features in insulin but not in glucagon. J Mol Endocrinol 1998;21:153-9.

42.   Fedorov VB, Goropashnaya AV, Toien O, et al. Elevated expression of protein biosynthesis genes in liver and muscle of hibernating black bears (Ursus americanus). Physiol Genomics 2009;37:108-18.

43.   Costa DP, F. T. Mass Changes and Metabolism during the Perinatal Fast: A Comparison between Antarctic (Arctocephalus gazella) and Galápagos Fur Seals (Arctocephalus galapagoensis). Physiological Zoology 1988;61:160-9.

44.   Frisch RE. Menarche and fatness: reexamination of the critical body composition hypothesis. Science (New York, NY 1978;200:1509-13.

45.   Frisch RE. Critical fatness hypothesis. The American journal of physiology 1997;273:E231-2.

46.   Frisch RE, McArthur JW. Menstrual cycles: fatness as a determinant of minimum weight for height necessary for their maintenance or onset. Science (New York, NY 1974;185:949-51.

47.   Frisch RE, Wyshak G, Vincent L. Delayed menarche and amenorrhea in ballet dancers. The New England journal of medicine 1980;303:17-9.

48.   Cahill GF, Jr. Fuel metabolim in starvation. Annu Rev Nutr 2006;26:1-22.

49.   Cahill GF, Jr., Veech RL. Ketoacids? Good medicine? Trans Am Clin Climatol Assoc 2003;114:149-61; discussion 62-3.

50.   Adolph EF, Heggeness FW. Age changes in body water and fat in fetal and infant mammals. Growth 1971;35:55-63.

51.   Keys A, Brozek J. Body fat in adult man. Physiol Rev 1953;33:245-325.

52.   Reynolds EL. The distribution of subcutaneous fat in childhood and adolescence. Monogr Soc Res Child Develop 1951;15:1-189.

53.   Christopoulou-Aletra H, Papavramidou N, Pozzilli P. Obesity in the Neolithic era: a Greek female figurine. Obes Surg 2006;16:1112-4.

54.   Bray GA. History of Obesity. In: Williams G, Frühbeck G, eds. Obesity: Science to Practice. London: John Wiley and Sons; 2009:604 pp.

55.   Wadd W. Cursory Remarks on Corpulence or Obesity Considered as a Disease with critical examination of ancient and modern opinions relative to the causes and cure. 3rd ed. London: Smith and Davy; 1816.

56.   Speke JH. Journal of Discovery of the Source of the Nile; 1864.

57.   Distant WL. Untitled. The Journal of the Anthropological Institute of Great Britain and Ireland 1896;25:277.

58.   Darwin C. The Descent of Man, and Selection in Relation to Sex. London: John Murray; 1871.

59.   Hollinshed R. Hollinshed's Chronicles of England, Scotland and Ireland; 1577.

60.   Kunkel D. Children and television advertising. In: Singer DG, Singer JL, eds. Handbook of Children and the media. Thousand Oaks: Sage; 2001:375-93.

61.   Gortmaker SL, Must A, Sobol AM, Peterson K, Colditz GA, Dietz WH. Television viewing as a cause of increasing obesity among children in the United States, 1986-1990. Arch Pediatr Adolesc Med 1996;150:356-62.

62.   Omram AR. The epidemiologic transition: a theory of the epidemiology of population change. Millbank Memorial Fund Q 1971;49:509-38.

63.   Ludwig DS. Childhood obesity-- The shape of things to come. The New England journal of medicine 2007;357:2325-7.

64.   Christakis NA, Fowler JH. The spread of obesity in a large social network over 32 years. The New England journal of medicine 2007;357:370-9.

65.   Mello MM, Studdert DM, Brennan TA. Obesity-- the new frontier of public health law. The New England journal of medicine 2006;354:2601-10.

66.   Zhang Y, Proenca R, Maffei M. Positional cloning of the mouse obese gene and its human homologue. Nature 1994;372:425-32.

67.   Rubaum-Keller I. Foodaholic-- the seven stages to permanent weight loss. Minneapolis: Mill City Press; 2011.

68.   Robinson TN. Reducing children's television viewing to prevent obesity: a randomized controlled trial. JAMA 1999;282:1561-7.

69.   Schultz Y, Flatt JP, Jequier E. Failure of dietary fat intake to promote fat oxidation: a factor favoring the development of obesity. The American journal of clinical nutrition 1989;50:307-14.

70.   Blaak EE. Basic disturbances in skeletal muscle fatty acid metabolism in obesity and   type 2 diabetes mellitus. The Proceedings of the Nutrition Society 2004;63:323-30.

71.   Westerterp KR. Dietary fat oxidation as a function of body fat. Current opinion in lipidology 2009;20:45-9.

72.   Raben A, Andersen HB, Christensen NJ, Madsen J, Holst JJ, Astrup A. Evidence   for an abnormal postprandial response to a high-fat mealin women predisposed to obesity. Am J Physiol Cell Physiol 1994;267:E549-59.

73.   Kim JY, Hickner RC, Cortright Rl, Dohm GL, Houmard JA. Lipid oxidation is reduced in obese human skeletal muscle. Am J Physiol Endocrinol Metab 2000;279:E1039-44.

74.   Kelley DE, He J, Menshikova EV, Ritov VB. Dysfunction of mitochondria in human skeletal muscle in type 2 diabetes. Diabetes 2002;51:2944-50.

75.   Gianotti TF, Sookoian S, Dieuzeide G, et al. A decreased mitochondrial DNA content is related to insulin resistance in adolescents. Obesity (Silver Spring) 2008;16:1591-5.

76.   Nair S, V PC, Arnold C, Diehl AM. Hepatic ATP reserve and efficiency of replenishing: comparison between obese and nonobese normal individuals. Am J Gastroenterol 2003;98:466-70.

77.   Hulens M, Vansant G, Lysens R, Claessens AL, Muls E. Exercise capacity in lean versus obese women. Scand J Med Sci Sports 2001;11:305-9.

78.   Lean ME. Pathophysiology of obesity. The Proceedings of the Nutrition Society 2000;59:331-6.

79.   Mattsson E, Larsson UE, Rossner S. Is walking for exercise too exhausting for obese women? Int J Obes Relat Metab Disord 1997;21:380-6.

80.   Okamoto M, Tan F, Suyama A, Okada H, Miyamoto T, Kishimoto T. The characteristics of fatigue symptoms and their association with the life style and the health status in school children. J Epidemiol 2000;10:241-8.

81.   Lennmarken C, Sandstedt S, von Schenck H, Larsson J. Skeletal muscle function and metabolism in obese women. JPEN J Parenter Enteral Nutr 1986;10:583-7.

82.   Ji H, Graczyk-Milbrandt G, Friedman MI. Metabolic inhibitors synergistically decrease hepatic energy status and increase food intake. American journal of physiology 2000;278:R1579-82.

83.   Friedman MI, Harris RB, Ji H, Ramirez I, Tordoff MG. Fatty acid oxidation affects food intake by altering hepatic energy status. The American journal of physiology 1999;276:R1046-53.

84.   Koch JE, Ji H, Osbakken MD, Friedman MI. Temporal relationships between eating behavior and liver adenine nucleotides in rats treated with 2,5-AM. The American journal of physiology 1998;274:R610-7.

85.   Astrup A, Buemann B, Christensen NJ, Toubro S. Failure to increase lipid oxidation in response to increasing dietary fat content in formerly obese women. Am J Physiol Cell Physiol 1994;266:E592-9.

86.   Jackman MR, Steig A, Higgins JA, et al. Weight regain after sustained weight reduction is accompanied by suppressed oxidation of dietary fat and adipocyte hyperplasia. American journal of physiology 2008;294:R1117-29.

SECTION 2

1.   Cahill GF, Jr. Fuel metabolism in starvation. Annu Rev Nutr 2006;26:1-22.

2.   Cahill GF, Jr. Starvation in man. The New England journal of medicine 1970;282:668-75.

3.   McGarry JD, Meier JM, Foster DW. The effects of starvation and refeeding on carbohydrate and lipid metabolism in vivo and in the perfused rat liver. The relationship between fatty acid oxidation and esterification in the regulation of ketogenesis. J Biol Chem 1973;248:270-8.

4.   Fisher NF, Lackey RW. The glycogen content of heart, liver and muscles of normal and diabetic dogs. The American journal of physiology 1925;72:43-9.

5.   Nilsson LH, Hultman E. Liver glycogen in man--the effect of total starvation or a carbohydrate-poor diet followed by carbohydrate refeeding. Scand J Clin Lab Invest 1973;32:325-30.

6.   Weis-Fogh T. Fat Combustion and Metabolic Rate of Flying Locusts (Schistocerca gregaria Forskal. Philosoph Transs Royal Soc London 1952;237:1--36.

7.   Youn JH, Youn MS, Bergman RN. Synergism of glucose and fructose in net glycogen synthesis in perfused rat livers. J Biol Chem 1986;261:15960-9.

8.   Muller C, Assimacopoulos-Jeannet F, Mosimann F, et al. Endogenous glucose production, gluconeogenesis and liver glycogen concentration in obese non-diabetic patients. Diabetologia 1997;40:463-8.

9.   Jinka TR, Carlson ZA, Moore JT, Drew KL. Altered thermoregulation via sensitization of A1 adenosine receptors in dietary-restricted rats. Psychopharmacology (Berl) 2010;209:217-24.

10.   Rigaud D, Hassid J, Meulemans A, Poupard AT, Boulier A. A paradoxical increase in resting energy expenditure in malnourished patients near death: the king penguin syndrome. The American journal of clinical nutrition 2000;72:355-60.

11.   Belkhou R, Cherel Y, Heitz A, Robin JP, Le Maho Y. Energy contribution of proteins and lipids during prolonged fasting in the rat. Nutr Res 1991;11:365-74.

12.   du Vigneaud V, Karr WG. Carbohydrate utilization I. Rate of disappearance of D-glucose from the blood. J Biol Chem 1925;66:281-300.

13.   Challet E, le Maho Y, Robin JP, Malan A, Cherel Y. Involvement of corticosterone in the fasting-induced rise in protein utilization and locomotor activity. Pharmacology, biochemistry, and behavior 1995;50:405-12.

14.   Cherel Y, Le Maho Y. Refeeding after the late increase in nitrogen excretion during prolonged fasting in the rat. Physiology & behavior 1991;50:345-9.

15. Mrosovsky N, Sherry DF. Animal anorexias. Science (New York, NY 1980;207:837-42.

16. Robin JP, Boucontet L, Chillet P, Groscolas R. Behavioral changes in fasting emperor penguins: evidence for a "refeeding signal" linked to a metabolic shift. The American journal of physiology 1998;274:R746-53.

17. Klaasen M. Metabolic constraints on longterm migration in birds. J Exp Biol 1996;199:57-64.

18. Landys MM, Piersma T, Guglielmo CG, Jukema J, Ramenofsky M, Wingfield JC. Metabolic profile of a long-distance migratory flight and stopover in a shorebird. Proc Royal Soc Biol 2005;272:295-302.

19. Jenni L, Jenni-Eiermann S, Spina F, Schwabl H. Regulation of protein breakdown and adrenocortical response to stress in birds during migratory flight. American journal of physiology 2000;278:R1182-9.

20. Dutton CJ, Taylor P. A comparison between pre- and posthibernation morphometry, hematology, and blood chemistry in viperid snakes. J Zoo Wildl Med 2003;34:53-8.

21. Rockall AG, Sohaib SA, Evans D, et al. Hepatic steatosis in Cushing's syndrome: a radiological assessment using computed tomography. European journal of endocrinology / European Federation of Endocrine Societies 2003;149:543-8.

22. Schaer M, Ginn PE. Iatrogenic Cushing's syndrome and steroid hepatopathy in a cat. J Am Anim Hosp Assoc 1999;35:48-51.

23. Kylin E. [Studies of the hypertension-hyperglycemia-hyperuricemia syndrome] Studien uber das Hypertonie-Hyperglykamie-hyperurikamiesyndrome. Zentralblatt fur innere Medizin 1923;44:105-27.

24. Grayson PC, Kim SY, Lavalley M, Choi HK. Hyperuricemia and incident hypertension: A systematic review and meta-analysis. Arthritis Care Res (Hoboken) 2010.

25. Kodama S, Saito K, Yachi Y, et al. Association between serum uric acid and development of type 2 diabetes. Diabetes care 2009;32:1737-42.

26. Masuo K, Kawaguchi H, Mikami H, Ogihara T, Tuck ML. Serum uric acid and plasma norepinephrine concentrations predict subsequent weight gain and blood pressure elevation. Hypertension 2003;42:474-80.

27. Lonardo A, Loria P, Leonardi F, et al. Fasting insulin and uric acid levels but not indices of iron metabolism are independent predictors of non-alcoholic fatty liver disease. A case-control study. Dig Liver Dis 2002;34:204-11.

28. Feig DI, Kang DH, Johnson RJ. Uric acid and cardiovascular risk. The New England journal of medicine 2008;359:1811-21.

29. Fischer AHL, Henrich T, Arendt D. The normal development of Platynereis dumerilii (Nereididae, Annelida). Frontiers in Zoology 2010;7:1-39.

30.   Zeeck E, Harder T, Beckmann M. Uric acid: The sperm-release pheromone of the marine polychaete: Platynereis dumerilii. J Chemical Ecology 1998;24:13-22.

31.   Gesteland RF, Cech TR, Atkins JF. The RNA World: the nature of modern RNA suggests a prebiotic RNA world. 3rd ed. New York City: Cold Spring Harbor Laboratory Press; 2006.

32.   Benner S. Life, the Universe, and the Scientific Method Gainesville: Ffame Press; 2010.

33.   Smith HW. From Fish to Philosopher. Boston: Little, Brown and Co; 1953.

34.   Keilin J. The biological significance of uric acid and guanine excretion. Biol Rev Cambridge Phil Soc 1959;34:265-96.

35.   Facchini F, Chen YD, Hollenbeck CB, Reaven GM. Relationship between resistance to insulin-mediated glucose uptake, urinary uric acid clearance, and plasma uric acid concentration. Jama 1991;266:3008-11.

36.   Lanaspa M, Sanchez-Lozada LG, Cicerchi C, et al. Uric acid-induced hepatic steatosis is mediated by generation of mitochondrial oxidative stress. (submitted)

37.   Ji H, Graczyk-Milbrandt G, Friedman MI. Metabolic inhibitors synergistically decrease hepatic energy status and increase food intake. American journal of physiology 2000;278:R1579-82.

38.   Friedman MI, Harris RB, Ji H, Ramirez I, Tordoff MG. Fatty acid oxidation affects food intake by altering hepatic energy status. The American journal of physiology 1999;276:R1046-53..

39.   Baldwin W, McRae S, Marek G, et al. Hyperuricemia as a mediator of the proinflammatory endocrine imbalance in the adipose tissue in a murine model of the metabolic syndrome. Diabetes 2011;60:1258-69.

40.   Nakagawa T, Hu H, Zharikov S, et al. A causal role for uric acid in fructose-induced metabolic syndrome. American journal of physiology 2006;290:F625-31.

41.   Reungjui S, Roncal CA, Mu W, et al. Thiazide diuretics exacerbate fructose-induced metabolic syndrome. J Am Soc Nephrol 2007;18:2724-31.

42.   Lanaspa M, Sautin Y, Ejaz A, et al. Uric acid and insulin resistance: What is the relationship? Curr Rheum Rev 2011;7:162-9.

43.   Ogino K, Kato M, Furuse Y, et al. Uric acid-lowering treatment with benzbromarone in patients with heart failure: a double-blind placebo-controlled crossover preliminary study. Circ Heart Fail 2010;3:73-81.

44.   Hoehn KL, Salmon AB, Hohnen-Behrens C, et al. Insulin resistance is a cellular antioxidant defense mechanism. Proceedings of the National Academy of Sciences of the United States of America 2009;106:17787-92.

45.   Block K, Gorin Y, Abboud HE. Subcellular localization of Nox4 and regulation in diabetes. Proceedings of the National Academy of Sciences of the United States of America 2009;106:14385-90.

46.   Mazzali M, Hughes J, Kim YG, et al. Elevated uric acid increases blood pressure in the rat by a novel crystal-independent mechanism. Hypertension 2001;38:1101-6.

47.   Sanchez-Lozada LG, Soto V, Tapia E, et al. Role of oxidative stress in the renal abnormalities induced by experimental hyperuricemia. American journal of physiology 2008;295:F1134-41.

48. Dikalova AE, Bikineyeva AT, Budzyn K, et al. Therapeutic targeting of mitochondrial superoxide in hypertension. Circulation research 2010;107:106-16.

49.   Watanabe S, Kang DH, Feng L, et al. Uric acid, hominoid evolution, and the pathogenesis of salt-sensitivity. Hypertension 2002;40:355-60.

50.   Kanellis J, Watanabe S, Li JH, et al. Uric acid stimulates monocyte chemoattractant protein-1 production in vascular smooth muscle cells via mitogen-activated protein kinase and cyclooxygenase-2. Hypertension 2003;41:1287-93.

51.   Kang DH, Park SK, Lee IK, Johnson RJ. Uric acid-induced C-reactive protein expression: implication on cell proliferation and nitric oxide production of human vascular cells. J Am Soc Nephrol 2005;16:3553-62.

52.   Roncal-Jimenez CA, Lanaspa MA, Rivard CJ, et al. Sucrose induces fatty liver and pancreatic inflammation in male breeder rats independent of excess energy intake. Metabolism: clinical and experimental 2011;60:1259-70.

53.   Shi Y, Evans JE, Rock KL. Molecular identification of a danger signal that alerts the immune system to dying cells. Nature 2003;425:516-21.

54.   Chen CJ, Kono H, Golenbock D, Reed G, Akira S, Rock KL. Identification of a key pathway required for the sterile inflammatory response triggered by dying cells. Nature medicine 2007;13:851-6.

55.   Kono H, Chen CJ, Ontiveros F, Rock KL. Uric acid promotes an acute inflammatory response to sterile cell death in mice. The Journal of clinical investigation 2010;120:1939-49.

56.   Zare F, Magnusson M, Bergstrom T, et al. Uric acid, a nucleic acid degradation product, down-regulates dsRNA-triggered arthritis. J Leukoc Biol 2006;79:482-8.

57.   Meotti FC, Jameson GN, Turner R, et al. Urate as a physiological substrate for myeloperoxidase: implications for hyperuricemia and inflammation. J Biol Chem 2011;286:12901-11.

58.   Shi Y, Galusha SA, Rock KL. Cutting edge: elimination of an endogenous adjuvant reduces the activation of CD8 T lymphocytes to transplanted cells and in an autoimmune diabetes model. J Immunol 2006;176:3905-8.

59.   Ma XJ, Tian DY, Xu D, et al. Uric acid enhances T cell immune responses to hepatitis B surface antigen-pulsed-dendritic cells in mice. World J Gastroenterol 2007;13:1060-6.

60.   Behrens MD, Wagner WM, Krco CJ, et al. The endogenous danger signal, crystalline uric acid, signals for enhanced antibody immunity. Blood 2008;111:1472-9.

61.   Orengo JM, Leliwa-Sytek A, Evans JE, et al. Uric acid is a mediator of the Plasmodium falciparum-induced inflammatory response. PLoS ONE 2009;4:e5194.

62.   Ames BN, Cathcart R, Schwiers E, Hochstein P. Uric acid provides an antioxidant defense in humans against oxidant- and radical-caused aging and cancer: a hypothesis. Proceedings of the National Academy of Sciences of the United States of America 1981;78:6858-62.

63.   Orowan E. The origin of man. Nature 1955;175:683-4.

64.   Barrera CM, Hunter RE, Dunlap WP. Hyperuricemia and locomotor activity in developing rats. Pharmacology, biochemistry, and behavior 1989;33:367-9.

65.   Hunter RE, Barrera CM, Dohanich GP, Dunlap WP. Effects of uric acid and caffeine on A1 adenosine receptor binding in developing rat brain. Pharmacology, biochemistry, and behavior 1990;35:791-5.

66.   Hellmann N, Jaenicke E, Decker H. Two types of urate binding sites on hemocyanin from the crayfish Astacus leptodactylus: an ITC study. Biophys Chem 2001;90:279-99.

67.   Terwilliger NB. Functional adaptations of oxygen-transport proteins. J Exp Biol 1998;201:1085-98.

68.   Perera IC, Lee YH, Wilkinson SP, Grove A. Mechanism for attenuation of DNA binding by MarR family transcriptional regulators by small molecule ligands. J Mol Biol 2009;390:1019-29.

69.   Wilkinson SP, Grove A. HucR, a novel uric acid-responsive member of the MarR family of transcriptional regulators from Deinococcus radiodurans. J Biol Chem 2004;279:51442-50.

70.   Wilkinson SP, Grove A. Negative cooperativity of uric acid binding to the transcriptional regulator HucR from Deinococcus radiodurans. J Mol Biol 2005;350:617-30.

71.   Barron AB, Sovik E, Cornish JL. The roles of dopamine and related compounds in reward-seeking behavior across animal phyla. Front Behav Neurosci 2010;4:163.

72.   Robertson HA, Carlson AD. Octopamine: presence in firefly lantern suggests a transmitter role. J Exp Zool 1976;195:159-64.

73.   Slamaa P, Reglier M. Xanthine oxidase-assisted catalysis by dopamine β-hydroxylase: Mechanistic considerations on the role of superoxide anion Comptes Rendus Chimie 2007;10:731-41.

74.   Fox IH, Palella TD, Kelley WN. Hyperuricemia: a marker for cell energy crisis. The New England journal of medicine 1987;317:111-2.

75. Martin SL. Mammalian hibernation: a naturally reversible model for insulin resistance in man? Diab Vasc Dis Res 2008;5:76-81.

76. Ortmann S, Heldmaier G. Regulation of body temperature andenergy requirements of hibernating alpine marmots (Marmota mamota). American journal of physiology 2000;278:R698-R704.

77. Russell RL, O'Neill PH, Epperson LE, Martin SL. Extensive use of torpor in 13-lined ground squirrels in the fall prior to cold exposure. J Comp physiol B 2010;180:1165-72.

78. Al-Badry KS, Taha HM. Hibernation-hypothermia and metabolism in hedgehogs. Changes in some organic components. Comp Biochem Physiol A Comp Physiol 1983;74:143-8.

79. Okamoto I, Kayano T, Hanaya T, Arai S, Ikeda M, Kurimoto M. Up-regulation of an extracellular superoxide dismutase-like activity in hibernating hamsters subjected to oxidative stress in mid- to late arousal from torpor. Comp Biochem Physiol C Toxicol Pharmacol 2006;144:47-56.

80. Toien O, Drew KL, Chao ML, Rice ME. Ascorbate dynamics and oxygen consumption during arousal from hibernation in Arctic ground squirrels. American journal of physiology 2001;281:R572-83.

81. Drew KL, Toien O, Rivera PM, Smith MA, Perry G, Rice ME. Role of the antioxidant ascorbate in hibernation and warming from hibernation. Comp Biochem Physiol C Toxicol Pharmacol 2002;133:483-92.

82. Nelson CJ, Otis JP, Martin SL, Carey HV. Analysis of the hibernation cycle using LC-MS-based metabolomics in ground squirrel liver. Physiol Genomics 2009;37:43-51.

83. Lanaspa MA, Garcia G, Cicerchi C et. al. Counteracting Roles of AMP Deaminase and AMP Kinase in the development of fatty liver PLoS One (*in revision*)

84. Lanaspa MA, Epperson E, Cicerchi C, et al Alterations in AMP handling during hibernation correlate with patterns of fat synthesis and fatty acid oxidation (submitted)

85. Buckner JS, Caldwell JM. Uric acid levels during last larval instar of Manduca Sexta, an abrupt transition from excretion to storage in fat body J Insect Physiol 1980;26:27-32.

86. Haunerland NH, Shirk PD. Regional and functional differentiation in the insect fat body Ann Rev Entomol 1995;40:121-45.

87. Ehresmann DD, Buckner JS, Graf G. Uric acid translocation from the fat body of Manduca Sexta during the pupal-adult transformation: Effects of 20-hydroxyecdysone J Insect Physiol 1990;36:173-80.

88. Ouyang J, Parakhia RA, Ochs RS. Metformin activates AMP kinase through inhibition of AMP deaminase. J Biol Chem 2011;286:1-11.

89.   Kubitzki K, Ziburski A. Seed Dispersal in Flood Plain Forests of Amazonia. Biotropica 1994;26:30-43.

90.   Junk WJ. Temporary fat storage,an adaptation of some fish species to the waterlevel fluctuations and related environmental changes of the Amazon river. Amazoniana 1985;9:315-51.

91.   Nagy S. Vitamin C contents of citrus fruit and their products: a review. Journal of agricultural and food chemistry 1980;28:8-18.

92.   Koike S, Kasai S, Yamazaki K, Furubayashi K. Fruit phenology of Prunus jamasakura and the feeding habit of the Asiatic black bear as a seed disperser. Ecol Res 2008;23:385-92.

93.   Auger J, Meyer SE, Black HL. Are American Black Bears (Ursus americanus) Legitimate Seed Dispersers for Fleshy-fruited Shrubs? Am Midl Naturalist 2002;147:352-67.

94.   McConkey K, Galleti M. Seed dispersal by the sun bear Helarctos malayanus in Central Borneo. J Trop Ecol 1999;15:237-41.

95.   Koike S, Morimoto H, Goto Y, Kozokai C, Yamazaki K. Frugivory of carnivores and seed dispersal of fleshy fruits in cool-temperate deciduous forests. J Forest Res 2008;13:215-22.

96.   Bairlein F. How to get fat: nutritional mechanisms of seasonal fat accumulation in migratory songbirds. Naturwissenschaften 2002;89:1-10.

97.   Knott CD. Changes in Orangutan Caloric Intake, Energy Balance, and Ketones in Response to Fluctuating Fruit Availability. Int J Primatol 1998;19:1061-79.

98.   Tappy L, Le KA. Metabolic effects of fructose and the worldwide increase in obesity. Physiol Rev 2010;90:23-46.

99.   Havel PJ. Dietary fructose: implications for dysregulation of energy homeostasis and lipid/carbohydrate metabolism. Nutrition reviews 2005;63:133-57.

100.   Johnson RJ, Segal MS, Sautin Y, et al. Potential role of sugar (fructose) in the epidemic of hypertension, obesity and the metabolic syndrome, diabetes, kidney disease, and cardiovascular disease. The American journal of clinical nutrition 2007;86:899-906.

101.   Gersch MS, Mu W, Cirillo P, et al. Fructose, but not dextrose, accelerates the progression of chronic kidney disease. American journal of physiology 2007;293:F1256-61.

102.   van den Berghe G, Bronfman M, Vanneste R, Hers HG. The mechanism of adenosine triphosphate depletion in the liver after a load of fructose. A kinetic study of liver adenylate deaminase. The Biochemical journal 1977;162:601-9.

103.   Avena NM, Rada P, Hoebel BG. Sugar bingeing in rats. Current protocols in neuroscience, Chapter 9:Unit9 23C.

104.   Teff KL, Elliott SS, Tschop M, et al. Dietary fructose reduces circulating insulin and leptin, attenuates postprandial suppression of ghrelin, and increases triglycerides in women. The Journal of clinical endocrinology and metabolism 2004;89:2963-72.

105.   Shapiro A, Mu W, Roncal C, Cheng KY, Johnson RJ, Scarpace PJ. Fructose-induced leptin resistance exacerbates weight gain in response to subsequent high-fat feeding. American journal of physiology 2008;295:R1370-5.

106.   Hargrove JL. Adipose energy stores, physical work, and the metabolic syndrome: lessons from hummingbirds. Nutr J 2005;4:36.

107.   Hartman FA, Brownell KA. Liver lipids in hummingbirds. The Condor 1959;61:270-7.

108.   Walker A, Teaford MF. The hunt for Proconsul. Scientific American 1989;260:76-82.

109.   Begun DR. Planet of the apes. Scientific American 2003;289:74-83.

110.   Skinner MF, Dupras TL, Moya-Sola S. Periodicity of linear enamel hypoplasia among Miocene Dryopithecus from Spain. J Paleopathol 1995:195-222.

111.   Kelley J, Andrews P, Alpagut B. A new hominoid species from the middle Miocene site of Pasalar, Turkey. Journal of human evolution 2008;54:455-79.

112.   Moya-Sola S, Kohler M. A Dryopithecus skeleton and the origins of great-ape locomotion. Nature 1996;379:156-9.

113.   Agusti J, Sanz de Siria A, Garces M. Explaining the end of the hominoid experiment in Europe. Journal of human evolution 2003;45:145-53.

114.   Stewart CB, Disotell TR. Primate evolution - in and out of Africa. Curr Biol 1998;8:R582-8.

115.   Andrews P, Kelley J. Middle Miocene dispersals of apes. Folia primatologica; international journal of primatology 2007;78:328-43.

116.   Begun DR. African and Eurasian Miocene hominoids and the origins of the Hominidae. In: Andrews P, Koufos G, DeBonis L, eds. Hominoid Evolution and Enviromental Change in the Neogene of Europe. Cambridge: Cambridge University Press; 2001:231-53.

117.   Neel JV. Diabetes mellitus: a "thrifty" genotype rendered detrimental by "progress"? American journal of human genetics 1962;14:353-62.

118.   Speakman JR. Thrifty genes for obesity, an attractive but flawed idea, and an alternative perspective: the 'drifty gene' hypothesis. Int J Obes (Lond) 2008;32:1611-7.

119.   Johnson RJ, Andrews P. Fructose, Uricase, and the Back-to-Africa Hypothesis. Evol Anthropol 2010;19 250-7.

120.   Stavric B, Johnson WJ, Clayman S, Gadd RE, Chartrand A. Effect of fructose administration on serum urate levels in the uricase inhibited rat. Experientia 1976;32:373-4.

121.   Stackhouse J, Presnell SR, McGeehan GM, Nambiar KP, Benner SA. The ribonuclease from an extinct bovid ruminant. FEBS Lett 1990;262:104-6.

122.   Whiteside JH, Olsen PE, Eglinton T, Brookfield ME, Sambrotto RN. Compound-specific carbon isotopes from earth's largest flood basalt eruptions directly linked to the end-Triassic mass extinction. Proceedings of the National Academy of Sciences of the United States of America 2010;107:6721-5.

123.   Moe OW. Uric acid nephrolithiasis: proton titration of an essential molecule? Curr Opin Nephrol Hypertens 2006;15:366-73.

124.   Nandi A, Mukhopadhyay CK, Ghosh MK, Chattopadhyay DJ, Chatterjee IB. Evolutionary significance of vitamin C biosynthesis in terrestrial vertebrates. Free radical biology & medicine 1997;22:1047-54.

125.   Graham JB, Dudley R, Aguilar NM, Gans C. Implications of the late Palaeozoic oxygen pulse for physiology and evolution. Nature 1995;375:117-20.

126.   King CG. The biological synthesis of ascorbic acid. World Rev Nutr Diet 1973;18:47-59.

127.   Pollock JI, Mullin RJ. Vitamin C biosynthesis in prosimians: evidence for the anthropoid affinity of Tarsius. American journal of physical anthropology 1987;73:65-70.

128.   Ohta Y, Nishikimi M. Random nucleotide substitutions in primate nonfunctional gene for L-gulono-gamma-lactone oxidase, the missing enzyme in L-ascorbic acid biosynthesis. Biochimica et biophysica acta 1999;1472:408-11.

129.   Alvarez LW, Alvarez W, Asaro F, Michel HV. Extraterrestrial cause for the cretaceous-tertiary extinction. Science (New York, NY 1980;208:1095-108.

130.   Johnson RJ, Gaucher EA, Sautin YY, Henderson GN, Angerhofer AJ, Benner SA. The planetary biology of ascorbate and uric acid and their relationship with the epidemic of obesity and cardiovascular disease. Medical hypotheses 2008;71:22-31.

131.   Vasdev S, Gill V, Parai S, Longerich L, Gadag V. Dietary vitamin E and C supplementation prevents fructose induced hypertension in rats. Mol Cell Biochem 2002;241:107-14.

132.   Mandl J, Szarka A, Banhegyi G. Vitamin C: update on physiology and pharmacology. Br J Pharmacol 2009;157:1097-110.

133.   Huang HY, Appel LJ, Choi MJ, et al. The effects of vitamin C supplementation on serum concentrations of uric acid: results of a randomized controlled trial. Arthritis and rheumatism 2005;52:1843-7.

134.   Banhegyi G, Braun L, Csala M, Puskas F, Mandl J. Ascorbate metabolism and its regulation in animals. Free radical biology & medicine 1997;23:793-803.

135.   Drew KL, Osborne PG, Frerichs KU, et al. Ascorbate and glutathione regulation in hibernating ground squirrels. Brain Res 1999;851:1-8.

136.   Perry GH, Dominy NJ, Claw KG, et al. Diet and the evolution of human amylase gene copy number variation. Nature genetics 2007;39:1256-60.

SECTION 3

1.   Wadd W. Cursory Remarks on Corpulence or Obesity Considered as a Disease with critical examination of ancient and modern opinions relative to the causes and cure. 3rd ed. London: Smith and Davy; 1816.

2.   Speke JH. Journal of Discovery of the Source of the Nile; 1864.

3.   Crane E. The World History of Beekeeping and Honey Hunting. New York: Routlege; 1999.

4.   Mazar A, Panitz-Cohen N. It Is the Land of Honey: Beekeeping at Tel Rehov. Near Eastern Archaeology 2007;70:202-19.

5.   Hajar R. Honey and Medicine. In: Selin H, ed. Encyclopaedia of the History of Science, Technology, and Medicine in Non-Western Cultures. New York: Springer-Verlag; 2008:1074-9.

6.   Breasted JH. Ancient Records of Egypt: The Eighteenth Dynasty. Chicago: University of Chicago Press; 1906.

7.   Sreebny LM. Sugar availability, sugar consumption and dental caries. Community Dent Oral Epiderniol 1982;10:1-7.

8.   Higuchi M, Iwani Y, Yamada T, Araya S. Levan synthesis and accumulation by human dental plaque. Arch Oral Biol 1970;15:563-7.

9.   Schwarz JC. La médecine dentaire dans l'Égypte pharaonique. In: Bulletin de la Société d'Égyptologie. Genève 2; 1979.

10.   Nriagu JO. Saturnine gout among Roman aristocrats. Did lead poisoning contribute to the fall of the Empire? The New England journal of medicine 1983;308:660-3.

11.   Allen FM, Stillman E, Fitz R. Total Dietary Regulation in the Treatment of Diabetes. Monographs of the Rockefeller Institute for Medical Research 1919;No. 11:1-646.

12.   Dwivedi G, Dwivedi S. Sushruta The clinician teacher par excellence. Indian J Chest Dis Allied Sci 2007;49:243-4.

13.   Frank LL. Diabetes mellitus in the texts of old Hindu medicine (Charaka, Susruta, Vagbhata). Am J Gastroenterol 1957;27:76-95.

14.   Bose RK. Discussion on diabetes in the tropics. II. Br Med J 1907;19:1053-4.

15.   Bhishagranta KKL. An English Translation of the Sushruta Samhita. Calcutta; 1907.

16.   Moseley B. A treatise on sugar. second ed. London: John Nichols; 1800.

17.   Sugar. In: Brougham L, ed. The Penny Cyclopaedia of the Society for the Diffusion of Useful Knowledge. London: Charles Knight and Co; 1842.

18.   Rosner F. The medical legacy of Moses Maimonides. Hoboken: KTAV Publishing House; 1998.

19.   Abdel-Halim RE. Obesity: 1000 years ago. Lancet 2005;366:204.

20.   Meyerhof M. Thirty-Three Clinical Observations by Rhazes (Circa 900 A.D.). Isis 1935;23:321-72.

21.   Papavramidou N, Christopoulou-Aletra H. Greco-Roman and Byzantine views on obesity. Obes Surg 2007;17:112-6.

22.   Rosner F. The Life of Moses Maimonides, a Prominent Medieval Physician. Einstein Quart J Biol Med 2002;19:125-8.

23.   Mintz S. Sweetness and Power. USA: Penguin Books; 1986.

24.   Galloway JH. The Sugar Cane Industry. Cambridge: Cambridge University Press; 1989.

25.   Smith WD. Complications of the commonplace: Tea, sugar and imperialism. J Interdisciplinary History 1992;23:259-78.

26.   Austen RA, Smith WD. Private tooth decay as public economic virtue: The slave:sugar triangle, consumerism, and European industrialization. In: Social Science History. Durham: Duke University Press; 1990:95-115.

27.   Venner T. Vita Recta ad Longum vitam (The right way to a long life). London: Abel Roper; 1660.

28.   Blankaart S. Borgerlyke Tafe: Om lang gesond sonder ziekten te leven. Amsterdam; 1683.

29.   Short T. A Discourse Concerning the Causes and Effects of Corpulency together with its method for prevention and cure. London: J Roberts; 1727.

30.   Flemyng M. A discourseon the nature, causes and cures of corpulency; 1760.

31.   Pennington NL, Baker CW. Sugar: A User's Guide to Sucrose. New York: Von Nostrand Reinhold; 1990.

32.   Deer N. The History of Sugar. London: Chapman and Hall; 1949-50.

33.   Warner F. A full and plan account of the gout. London: T Cadelll; 1768.

34.   Garrod AB. Observations on the blood and urine of gout, rheumatism and Bright's disease Medical Chirurgical Transaction 1848;31:83-.

35.   Ball GV. Two epidemics of gout. Bull Hist Med 1971;45:401-8.

36.   Bener A, Obineche E, Gillett M, Pasha MA, Bishawi B. Association between blood levels of lead, blood pressure and risk of diabetes and heart disease in workers. International archives of occupational and environmental health 2001;74:375-8.

37.   Ekong EB, Jaar BG, Weaver VM. Lead-related nephrotoxicity: a review of the epidemiologic evidence. Kidney international 2006;70:2074-84.

38.   Sanchez-Fructuoso AI, Torralbo A, Arroyo M, et al. Occult lead intoxication as a cause of hypertension and renal failure. Nephrol Dial Transplant 1996;11:1775-80.

39.   Marwood SF. Diabetes mellitus--some reflections. J R Coll Gen Pract 1973;23:38-45.

40. Fleming pr. Short History of Cardiology. Amsterdam: Editions Rodopi B.V.; 1997.

41. Rodnan GP, Beneder TG. Ancient therapeutic Arts in the Gout. Arthritis and rheumatism 1963;6:317-40.

42. Rush B. Observations upone the cause and cure of the gout. In: Medical Inquiries and Observations. Philadelphia: Johnson and Warner; 1809:245-322.

43. MacKinnon AU. The origin of the modern epidemic of coronary artery disease in England. J R Coll Gen Pract 1987;37:174-6.

44. Bright R. Tabular view of the morbid appearances in 100 cases connected with albuminous urine. Guy's Hosp Rep 1836;1:338-79.

45. Johnson G. On the Diseases of the Kidney. London: John W Parker and Son; 1852.

46. Mahomed FA. The etiology of Bright's disease and the prealbuminuric state. Med Chir Trans 1874;39:197-228.

47. Mahomed FA. On chronic bright's disease, and its essential symptoms. Lancet 1879;I:398-404.

48. Lancereaux E. Le Diabete maigre et le Diabete gras, . L' Union Mid 1880.

49. Duckworth D. A treatise on gout. London: C Griffin & Co; 1889.

50. Christie T. Notes on Diabetes mellitus, as it occurs in Ceylon. Edin Med Surg J 1811;7:285-99.

51. Watts W. On the symptoms varieties, and remote causes of diabetes. Lancet 1848;51:661-2.

52. Charles R. Discussion on diabetes in the tropics. I. Br Med J 1907;19:1051-3.

53. Bose CL. Discussion on diabetes in the tropics. III. Br Med J 1907;19:1054-6.

54. Cantle J. Discussion on diabetes in the tropics. Discussion. Br Med J 1907;19:1063.

55. Chakravarti S. Discussion on diabetes in the tropics. IV. Br Med J 1907;19:1056-7.

56. Charles R. Diabetes in the Tropics. Br Med J 1907;19:1051-64.

57. Fernando HM. Discussion on diabetes in the tropics. Discussion. Br Med J 1907;19:1060.

58. Mallick IM. Discussion on diabetes in the tropics. Discussion. Br Med J 1907;19:1061-2.

59. Sandwith PM. Discussion on diabetes in the tropics. VI. Br Med J 1907;19:1059-60.

60. Ziemann H. Discussion on diabetes in the tropics. Discussion. Br Med J 1907;19:1061.

61.   Helmchen LA, Henderson RM. Changes in the distribution of body mass index of white US men, 1890-2000. Annals of human biology 2004;31:174-81.

62.   Osler W. The Principles and Practice of Medicine. New York: D. Appleton and Co.; 1893.

63.   Emerson H, Larimore LD. Diabetes mellitus: A contribution to its epidemiology based chiefly on mortality statistics. Archives of internal medicine 1924;34:585-630.

64.   Banting F. The history of insulin. Edin Med J 1929;36:2-.

65.   Wright-St Clair RE. Early accounts of Maori diet and health. 1. The New Zealand medical journal 1969;70:327-31.

66.   Prior IA, Rose BS, Davidson F. Metabolic Maladies in New Zealand Maoris. Br Med J 1964;1:1065-9.

67.   Rose BS. Gout in Maoris. Seminars in arthritis and rheumatism 1975;5:121-45.

68.   Hrdlička A. Physiological and Medical observations among the Indians of Southwestern United States and Northern Mexico. Washington D.C.: U.S. Government Printing Office; 1908.

69.   Taubes G. Good calories, Bad Calories. New York: Alfred A Knopf; 2007.

70.   Campbell GD. Diabetes in Asians and Africans in and around Durban. South African medical journal = Suid-Afrikaanse tydskrif vir geneeskunde 1963;37:1195-208.

71.   Cohen AM. Effect of change in environment on he prevalence of diabetes among Yemenit and Kurdish communities. Israeli Med J 1960;19:137-42.

72.   Cohen AM, Bavly S, Poznanski R. Change of diet of Yemenite Jews in relation to diabetes and ischaemic heart-disease. Lancet 1961;2:1399-401.

73.   Concepcion I. Incidence of diabetes mellitus among Filipinos. J Phillipine Island MA 1922;2:57-.

74.   Albertsson MD. Diabetes in Iceland. Diabetes 1953;2:184-6.

75.   Joslin EP. The universality of diabetes: a survey of diabetic morbidity in Arizona. JAMA 1940;115:2033-8.

76.   Salsbury CG. Incidence of certain diseases among the Navajos. Arizona Med 1947;4:29-31.

77.   Stein JH, West KM, Robey JM, Tirador DF, McDonald GW. The high prevalence of abnormal glucose tolerance in the Cherokee Indians of North Carolina. Archives of internal medicine 1965;116:842-5.

78.   Hoy W, Kelly A, Jacups S, et al. Stemming the tide: reducing cardiovascular disease and renal failure in Australian Aborigines. Australian and New Zealand journal of medicine 1999;29:480-3.

79. Healey LA, Skeith MD, Decker JL, Bayani-Sioson PS. Hyperuricemia in Filipinos: interaction of heredity and environment. American journal of human genetics 1967;19:81-5.

80. Kagan A, Harris BR, Winkelstein W, Jr., et al. Epidemiologic studies of coronary heart disease and stroke in Japanese men living in Japan, Hawaii and California: demographic, physical, dietary and biochemical characteristics. Journal of chronic diseases 1974;27:345-64.

81. Donnison C. Blood Pressure in the African Native. Lancet 1929;i:6-7.

82. Williams A. The Blood Pressure of Africans. E African Med J 1941;18:109-17.

83. Joslin EP, Dublin LI, Marks HH. Studies in Diabetes mellitus. II. Its incidence and the factors underlying its variations. The American journal of the medical sciences 1934;187:433-57.

84. Saunders G, Bancroft H. Blood Pressure in African Americans. Nutrition reviews 1942;23:410-23.

85. Adams J. Some racial differences in blood pressure and morbidity in a group of white and colored workers. The American journal of the medical sciences 1930;184:342-50.

86. Johnson RJ, Segal MS, Sautin Y, et al. Potential role of sugar (fructose) in the epidemic of hypertension, obesity and the metabolic syndrome, diabetes, kidney disease, and cardiovascular disease. The American journal of clinical nutrition 2007;86:899-906.

87. Lee AJ, O'Dea K, Mathews JD. Apparent dietary intake in remote aboriginal communities. Aust J Public Health 1994;18:190-7.

88. Bell AC, Swinburn BA, Amosa H, Scragg R, Sharpe SJ. The impact of modernisation on the diets of adults aged 20-40 years from Samoan church communities in Auckland. Asia Pac J Public Health 1999;11:4-9.

89. Dresser C. Food consumption profiles of white and black persons aged 1-74 years: United States 1971-1974 Data from the National Health Survey, DHEW Publication No. (PHS) 79-1658. Hyattsville, MD: National Center for Health Statistics; 1979.

90. Kerr GR, Amante P, Decker M, Callen PW. Supermarket sales of high-sugar products in predominantly Black, Hispanic, and white census tracts of Houston, Texas. The American journal of clinical nutrition 1983;37:622-31.

91. Moynihan P, Petersen PE. Diet, nutrition and the prevention of dental diseases. Public Health Nutr 2004;7:201-26.

92. Hujoel P. Dietary carbohydrates and dental-systemic diseases. J Dent Res 2009;88:490-502.

93. Price WA. Nutrition and physical degeneration; a comparison of primitive and modern diets and their effects. New York: P.B. Hoeber; 1945.

94.   Sarnat H, Cohen S, Gat H. Changing patterns of dental caries in Ethiopian adolescents who immigrated to Israel. Community Dent Oral Epidemiol 1987;15:286-8.

95.   Cleave TL, Campbell GD. Diabetes, coronary thrombosis, and the saccharine disease. Bristol: John Wright and Sons; 1966.

96.   Griffin SO, Regnier E, Griffin PM, Huntley V. Effectiveness of fluoride in preventing caries in adults. J Dent Res 2007;86:410-5.

97.   Li Y. Fluoride: safety issues. J Indiana Dent Assoc. 1993;72:22-6.

98.   Bray GA, Nielsen SJ, Popkin BM. Consumption of high-fructose corn syrup in beverages may play a role in the epidemic of obesity. The American journal of clinical nutrition 2004;79:537-43.

99.   Platt R. Coronary disease and modern stress. Lancet 1951;1:51.

100.   Johnson RJ, Perez-Pozo SE, Sautin YY, et al. Hypothesis: could excessive fructose intake and uric acid cause type 2 diabetes? Endocr Rev 2009;30:96-116.

101.   Narayan KM, Boyle JP, Thompson TJ, Sorensen SW, Williamson DF. Lifetime risk for diabetes mellitus in the United States. JAMA 2003;290:1884-90.

102.   Joslin EP, Dublin LI, Marks HH. Studies in diabetes mellitus. III. Interpretation of the variations in diabetes incidence. The American journal of the medical sciences 1935;189:163-91.

103.   Mills CA. Diabetes mellitus: Sugar consumption in its etiology. Archives of internal medicine 1930;46:582-4.

104.   Keys A. Coronary heart disease--the global picture. Atherosclerosis 1975;22:149-92.

105.   Cleave TL, Campbell GD. The saccharine disease. American journal of proctology 1967;18:202-10.

106.   Yudkin J. Patterns and Trends in Carbohydrate Consumption and Their Relation to Disease. The Proceedings of the Nutrition Society 1964;23:149-62.

107.   Yudkin J. Evolutionary and historical changes in dietary carbohydrates. The American journal of clinical nutrition 1967;20:108-15.

108.   Yudkin J. Sugar and disease. Nature 1972;239:197-9.

109.   Murray JF. Mycobacterium tuberculosis and the cause of consumption: from discovery to fact. Am J Respir Crit Care Med 2004;169:1086-8.

110.   Malik VS, Popkin BM, Bray GA, Despres JP, Willett WC, Hu FB. Sugar-sweetened beverages and risk of metabolic syndrome and type 2 diabetes: a meta-analysis. Diabetes care 2010;33:2477-83.

111.   Ouyang X, Cirillo P, Sautin Y, et al. Fructose consumption as a risk factor for non-alcoholic fatty liver disease. J Hepatol 2008;48:993-9.

112.   Lanaspa M, Tapia E, Soto V, Sautin Y, Sanchez-Lozada LG. Uric acid and Fructose: Potential Biological Mechanisms. Sem Nephrol 2011; 31:426-32.

113.   Lanaspa M, Sanchez-Lozada LG, Cicerchi C, et al. Uric acid-induced hepatic steatosis is mediated generation of mitochondrial oxidative stress. (*submitted*)

114.   Shapiro A, Mu W, Roncal C, Cheng KY, Johnson RJ, Scarpace PJ. Fructose-induced leptin resistance exacerbates weight gain in response to subsequent high-fat feeding. American journal of physiology 2008;295:R1370-5.

115.   Stanhope KL, Schwarz JM, Keim NL, et al. Consuming fructose-sweetened, not glucose-sweetened, beverages increases visceral adiposity and lipids and decreases insulin sensitivity in overweight/obese humans. The Journal of clinical investigation 2009;119:1322-34.

116.   Perez-Pozo SE, Schold J, Nakagawa T, Sanchez-Lozada LG, Johnson RJ, Lillo JL. Excessive fructose intake induces the features of metabolic syndrome in healthy adult men: role of uric acid in the hypertensive response. Int J Obes (Lond) 2010;34:454-61.

117.   Roncal-Jimenez CA, Lanaspa MA, Rivard CJ, et al. Sucrose induces fatty liver and pancreatic inflammation in male breeder rats independent of excess energy intake. Metabolism: clinical and experimental 2011; 60:1259-70

118.   Nakagawa T, Hu H, Zharikov S, et al. A causal role for uric acid in fructose-induced metabolic syndrome. American journal of physiology 2006;290:F625-31.

119.   Shi L, van Meijgaard J. Substantial decline in sugar-sweetened beverage consumption among California's children and adolescents. Int J Gen Med 2010;3:221-4.

120.   Le KA, Tappy L. Metabolic effects of fructose. Curr Opin Clin Nutr Metab Care 2006;9:469-75.

121.   Ellwood KC, Michaelis OEt, Hallfrisch JG, O'Dorisio TM, Cataland S. Blood insulin, glucose, fructose and gastric inhibitory polypeptide levels in carbohydrate-sensitive and normal men given a sucrose or invert sugar tolerance test. The Journal of nutrition 1983;113:1732-6.

122.   Hallfrisch J, Ellwood K, Michaelis OEt, Reiser S, Prather ES. Plasma fructose, uric acid, and inorganic phosphorus responses of hyperinsulinemic men fed fructose. J Am Coll Nutr 1986;5:61-8.

123.   Hallfrisch J, Ellwood KC, Michaelis OEt, Reiser S, O'Dorisio TM, Prather ES. Effects of dietary fructose on plasma glucose and hormone responses in normal and hyperinsulinemic men. The Journal of nutrition 1983;113:1819-26.

124.   Hallfrisch J, Reiser S, Prather ES. Blood lipid distribution of hyperinsulinemic men consuming three levels of fructose. The American journal of clinical nutrition 1983;37:740-8.

125.   Reiser S, Bickard MC, Hallfrisch J, Michaelis OEt, Prather ES. Blood lipids and their distribution in lipoproteins in hyperinsulinemic subjects fed three different levels of sucrose. The Journal of nutrition 1981;111:1045-57.

126.   Van den Berghe G. Fructose: metabolism and short-term effects on carbohydrate and purine metabolic pathways. Progress in biochemical pharmacology 1986;21:1-32.

127.   Roncal-Jimenez CA, Lanaspa MA, Rivard CJ, et al. Sucrose induces fatty liver and pancreatic inflammation in male breeder rats independent of excess energy intake. Metabolism: clinical and experimental 2011;60:1259-70.

128.   Korieh A, Crouzoulon G. Dietary regulation of fructose metabolism in the intestine and in the liver of the rat. Duration of the effects of a high fructose diet after the return to the standard diet. Arch Int Physiol Biochim Biophys 1991;99:455-60.

129.   Weiser MM, Quill H, Isselbacher KJ. Effects of diet on rat intestinal soluble hexokinase and fructokinase activities. The American journal of physiology 1971;221:844-9.

130.   Knott CD. Changes in Orangutan Caloric Intake, Energy Balance, and Ketones in Response to Fluctuating Fruit Availability. Int J Primatol 1998;19:1061-79.

131.   Bazzano LA, Li TY, Joshipura KJ, Hu FB. Intake of fruit, vegetables, and fruit juices and risk of diabetes in women. Diabetes care 2008;31:1311-7.

132.   Madero M, Arriaga JC, Jalal D, et al. The effect of two energy-restricted diets, a low-fructose diet versus a moderate natural fructose diet, on weight loss and metabolic syndrome parameters: a randomized controlled trial. Metabolism: clinical and experimental 2011; 60:1551-9

133.   Dennison BA, Rockwell HL, Baker SL. Excess fruit juice consumption by preschool-aged children is associated with short stature and obesity. Pediatrics 1997;99:15-22.

134.   Palmer JR, Boggs DA, Krishnan S, Hu FB, Singer M, Rosenberg L. Sugar-sweetened beverages and incidence of type 2 diabetes mellitus in African American women. Archives of internal medicine 2008;168:1487-92.

135.   American Academy of Pediatrics: The use and misuse of fruit juice in pediatrics. Pediatrics 2001;107:1210-3.

136.   Le MT, Frye RF, Rivard C, et al. Effects of high fructose corn syrup and sucrose on the pharmacokinetics of fructose and acute metabolic and hemodynamic responses in healthy subjects. Metabolism: clinical and experimental 2011;in press.

137.   Ventura EE, Davis JN, Goran MI. Sugar content of popular sweetened beverages based on objective laboratory analysis: focus on fructose content. Obesity (Silver Spring) 2011;19:868-74.

138.   Sanchez-Lozada LG, Mu W, Roncal C, et al. Comparison of free fructose and glucose to sucrose in the ability to cause fatty liver. European journal of nutrition 2010;49:1-9.

139.   Bocarsly ME, Powell ES, Avena NM, Hoebel BG. High-fructose corn syrup causes characteristics of obesity in rats: increased body weight, body fat and triglyceride levels. Pharmacology, biochemistry, and behavior 2010;97:101-6.

140.   Masuo K, Kawaguchi H, Mikami H, Ogihara T, Tuck ML. Serum uric acid and plasma norepinephrine concentrations predict subsequent weight gain and blood pressure elevation. Hypertension 2003;42:474-80.

141.   Kodama S, Saito K, Yachi Y, et al. Association between serum uric acid and development of type 2 diabetes. Diabetes care 2009;32:1737-42.

142.   Baldwin W, McRae S, Marek G, et al. Hyperuricemia as a mediator of the proinflammatory endocrine imbalance in the adipose tissue in a murine model of the metabolic syndrome. Diabetes 2011;60:1258-69.

143.   Ogino K, Kato M, Furuse Y, et al. Uric acid-lowering treatment with benzbromarone in patients with heart failure: a double-blind placebo-controlled crossover preliminary study. Circ Heart Fail 2010;3:73-81.

SECTION 4

1.   Almond R, Pollard AJ. The Yeomanry of Robin Hood and Social Terminology in Fifteenth-Century England. Past Present 2001;170:52-77.

2.   Coss PR. Aspects of Cultural Diffusion in Medieval England: The Early Romances, Local Society and Robin Hood. Past Present 1985;108:35-79.

3.   Rogers J, Waldron T. DISH and the Monastic Way of Life. Int J Osteoarchaeol 2001;11:357-65.

4.   Harvey B. Living and Dying in England 1100 –1540. The Monastic Experience. . Oxford: Clarendon Press; 1993.

5.   Allen FM. Studies concerning glycosuria and diabetes. Cambridge, MA: Harvard University Press; 1913.

6.   Groen JJ, Tijong KB, Koster M, Willebrands AF, Verdonck G, Pierloot M. The influence of nutrition and ways of life on blood cholesterol and the prevalence of hypertension and coronary heart disease among Trapist and Benedictine monks. The American journal of clinical nutrition 1962;10:456-70.

7.   Ka T, Moriwaki Y, Takahashi S, et al. Effects of long-term beer ingestion on plasma concentrations and urinary excretion of purine bases. Hormone and metabolic research Hormon- und Stoffwechselforschung 2005;37:641-5.

8.   Choi HK, Atkinson K, Karlson EW, Willett W, Curhan G. Alcohol intake and risk of incident gout in men: a prospective study. Lancet 2004;363:1277-81.

9.   Choi HK, Curhan G. Beer, liquor, and wine consumption and serum uric acid level: the Third National Health and Nutrition Examination Survey. Arthritis and rheumatism 2004;51:1023-9.

10.   Yamamoto T, Moriwaki Y, Takahashi S, et al. Effect of beer on the plasma concentrations of uridine and purine bases. Metabolism: clinical and experimental 2002;51:1317-23.

11.   Lanaspa M, Sautin Y, Ejaz A, et al. Uric acid and insulin resistance: What is the relationship? Curr Rheum Rev 2011;7:162-9.

12.   Nishizawa T, Akaoka I, Nishida Y, Kawaguchi Y, Hayashi E, Yoshimura T. Some factors related to obesity in the Japanese sumo wrestler. The American journal of clinical nutrition 1976;29:1167-74.

13.   Khadiga A, Ati A, Mohammed S, Saad AM, Mohamed HE. Response of broiler chicks to dietary monosodium glutamate. Pakistan Vet J 2009;29:165-8.

14.   Feigelson M, Feigelson P. Relationships between hepatic enzyme induction, glutamate formation, and purine nucleotide biosynthesis in glucocorticoid action. J Biol Chem 1966;241:5819-26.

15.   Shigemura N, Shirosaki S, Sanematsu K, Yoshida R, Ninomiya Y. Genetic and molecular basis of individual differences in human umami taste perception. PLoS ONE 2009;4:e6717.

16.   Clifford AJ, Riumallo JA, Youn VR, Scrimshaw NS. Effect of Oral Purines on Serum and Urinary Uric Acid of Normal, Hyperuricemic and Gouty Humans. The Journal of nutrition 1976;106:428-50.

17.   He K, Du S, Xun P, et al. Consumption of monosodium glutamate in relation to incidence of overweight in Chinese adults: China Health and Nutrition Survey (CHNS). The American journal of clinical nutrition 2011;93:1328-36.

18.   Bunyan J, Murrell EA, Shah PP. The induction of obesity in rodents by means of monosodium glutamate. The British journal of nutrition 1976;35:25-39.

19.   Collison KS, Maqbool ZM, Inglis AL, et al. Effect of dietary monosodium glutamate on HFCS-induced hepatic steatosis: expression profiles in the liver and visceral fat. Obesity (Silver Spring) 2010;18:1122-34.

20.   Collison KS, Zaidi MZ, Saleh SM, et al. Effect of trans-fat, fructose and monosodium glutamate feeding on feline weight gain, adiposity, insulin sensitivity, adipokine and lipid profile. The British journal of nutrition 2011:1-10.

21.   Li X, Li W, Wang H, et al. Cats lack a sweet taste receptor. The Journal of nutrition 2006;136:1932S-4S.

22.   Quetin LB, Ross RM. Behavioral and Physiological Characteristics of the Antarctic Krill, Euphausia superba. American Zoologist 1991;31:49-63.

23.   Ikeda T. RNA content of the Antarctic Krill (Euphausa Superba Dana), an estimator of natural growth rate. Proc NIPR Symp Polar Bio 1989;2:26-33.

24.   Shin AC, Nicol S, King RA. Nucleic acid content as a potential growth rate estimator of Antarctic krill. Marine and Freshwater Behaviour and Physiology 2003;36:295 — 305.

REFERENCES

25. Tryland M, Brun E. Serum chemistry of the minke whale from the northeastern Atlantic. J Wildl Dis 2001;37:332-41.

26. Dubois JY, Jekel PA, Mulder PP, et al. Pancreatic-type ribonuclease 1 gene duplications in rat species. J Mol Evol 2002;55:522-33.

27. Beintema JJ, Scheffer AJ, van Dijk H, Welling GW, Zwiers H. Pancreatic ribonuclease distribution and comparisons in mammals. Nat New Biol 1973;241:76-8.

28. Wang XY, Li NZ, Yu L, Zhao H, Zhang YP. Duplication and functional diversification of pancreatic ribonuclease (RNASE1) gene. Chinese Science Bulletin 2010;55:2-6.

29. Peracaula R, Royle L, Tabares G, et al. Glycosylation of human pancreatic ribonuclease: differences between normal and tumor states. Glycobiology 2003;13:227-44.

30. McGregor IS, Gallate JE. Rats on the grog: novel pharmacotherapies for alcohol craving. Addict Behav 2004;29:1341-57.

31. Stefansson V. The Friendly Arctic. The story of five years in polar regions. . New York: MacMillan Co.; 1921.

32. Jenness D. The Eskimos of Northern Alaska: A Study in the Effect of Civilization. Geographical Review 1918;5:89-101.

33. Jenness D. The Copper Eskimos. Geographical Review 1917;4:81-91.

34. Lewis AJ, Peck EJ. The Life and Work of the Rev. E.J. Peck among the Eskimos. London: Hodder and Stoughton; 1905.

35. Heinbecker P. Studies on the metabolism of Eskimos. J Biol Chem 1928:461-75.

36. Ho KJ, Mikkelson B, Lewis LA, Feldman SA, Taylor CB. Alaskan Arctic Eskimo: responses to a customary high fat diet. The American journal of clinical nutrition 1972;25:737-45.

37. Donahoo W, Wyatt HR, Kriehn j, et al. Dietary fat increases energy intake across the range of typical consumption in the United States. Obesity (Silver Spring) 2008;16:64-9.

38. Weigle DS, Breen PA, Matthys CC, et al. A high-protein diet induces sustained reductions in appetite, ad libitum caloric intake, and body weight despite compensatory changes in diurnal plasma leptin and ghrelin concentrations. The American journal of clinical nutrition 2005;82:41-8.

39. Teff KL, Elliott SS, Tschop M, et al. Dietary fructose reduces circulating insulin and leptin, attenuates postprandial suppression of ghrelin, and increases triglycerides in women. The Journal of clinical endocrinology and metabolism 2004;89:2963-72.

276

40.   Austin GI, Ogden LG, Hill JO. Trends in Carbohydrate, Fat, and Protein Intake and Association with Energy Intake in Normal-Weight, Overweight, and Obese Individuals: 1971-2006. The American journal of clinical nutrition 2010.

41.Keys A. Coronary heart disease--the global picture. Atherosclerosis 1975;22:149-92.

42.   Keys A, Aravanis C, Blackburn HW, et al. Epidemiological studies related to coronary heart disease: characteristics of men aged 40-59 in seven countries. Acta Med Scand Suppl 1966;460:1-392.

43.   Sanchez-Lozada LG, Tapia E, Jimenez A, et al. Fructose-induced metabolic syndrome is associated with glomerular hypertension and renal microvascular damage in rats. American journal of physiology 2007;292:F423-9.

44.   Sanchez-Lozada LG, Tapia E, Santamaria J, et al. Mild hyperuricemia induces vasoconstriction and maintains glomerular hypertension in normal and remnant kidney rats. Kidney international 2005;67:237-47.

45.   Kanbay M, Sanchez-Lozada LG, Franco M, et al. Microvascular disease and its role in the brain and cardiovascular system: a potential role for uric acid as a cardiorenal toxin. Nephrol Dial Transplant 2011; 26:430-437.

46.   McClellan WS, Dubois EF. Clinical calorimetry. XLV. Prolonged meat diets with a study of kidney function and ketosis. J Biol Chem 1930;87:651-68.

47.   Howard BV, Van Horn L, Hsia J, et al. Low-fat dietary pattern and risk of cardiovascular disease: the Women's Health Initiative Randomized Controlled Dietary Modification Trial. Jama 2006;295:655-66.

48.   Harvey W. On corpulence in relation to disease. London: Henry Renshaw; 1872.

49.   Banting W. Letter on corpulence, Addressed to the Public. In. London: Harrison; 1869:10 pp.

50.   Geraci JR, Smith TG. Vitamin C in the Diet of Inuit Hunters From Holman, Northwest Territories. Arctic 1979;32:135-9.

51.   Risica PM, Ebbesson SO, Schraer CD, Nobmann ED, Caballero BH. Body fat distribution in Alaskan Eskimos of the Bering Straits region: the Alaskan Siberia Project. Int J Obes Relat Metab Disord 2000;24:171-9.

52.   Schaefer O. Are Eskimos more or less obese than other Canadians? A comparison of skinfold thickness and ponderal index of Canadian Eskimos. The American journal of clinical nutrition 1977;30:1623-8.

53.   van Marken Lichtenbelt WD, Vanhommerig JW, Smulders NM, et al. Cold-activated brown adipose tissue in healthy men. The New England journal of medicine 2009;360:1500-8.

54.   Mishmar D, Ruiz-Pesini E, Golik P, et al. Natural selection shaped regional mtDNA variation in humans. Proceedings of the National Academy of Sciences of the United States of America 2003;100:171-6.

REFERENCES

55.   Ruiz-Pesini E, Mishmar D, Brandon M, Procaccio V, Wallace DC. Effects of purifying and adaptive selection on regional variation in human mtDNA. Science (New York, NY 2004;303:223-6.

56.   Rasmussen K, Birket-Smith K, Mathiassen T, Freuchen P. The Danish Ethnographic and Geographic Expedition to Arctic America. Preliminary Reportof the Fifth Thule Expedition. Geographical Review 1925;15:521-62.

57.   Johnson RJ, with Gower T. The Sugar Fix. The high-fructose fallout that is making you fat and sick. 1st ed. New York: Rodale; 2008.

58.   Reungjui S, Roncal CA, Mu W, et al. Thiazide diuretics exacerbate fructose-induced metabolic syndrome. J Am Soc Nephrol 2007;18:2724-31.

59.   Gardner CD, Kiazand A, Alhassan S, et al. Comparison of the Atkins, Zone, Ornish, and LEARN diets for change in weight and related risk factors among overweight premenopausal women: the A TO Z Weight Loss Study: a randomized trial. JAMA 2007;297:969-77.

60.   Brenner BM, Meyer TW, Hostetter TH. Dietary protein intake and the progressive nature of kidney disease: the role of hemodynamically mediated glomerular injury in the pathogenesis of progressive glomerular sclerosis in aging, renal ablation, and intrinsic renal disease. The New England journal of medicine 1982;307:652-9.

61.   Atkins R. Dr. Atkins' New Diet Revolution. New York: Avon Books; 1998.

62.   Chen L, Caballero B, Mitchell DC, et al. Reducing consumption of sugar-sweetened beverages is associated with reduced blood pressure: a prospective study among United States adults. Circulation 2010;121:2398-406.

63.   Madero M, Arriaga JC, Jalal D, et al. The effect of two energy-restricted diets, a low-fructose diet versus a moderate natural fructose diet, on weight loss and metabolic syndrome parameters: a randomized controlled trial. Metabolism: clinical and experimental 2011; 60:1551-9

64.   Shi L, van Meijgaard J. Substantial decline in sugar-sweetened beverage consumption among California's children and adolescents. Int J Gen Med 2010;3:221-4.

65.   Kawasaki T, Akanuma H, Yamanouchi T. Increased fructose concentrations in blood and urine in patients with diabetes. Diabetes care 2002;25:353-7.

66.   Kawasaki T, Ogata N, Akanuma H. Plasma fructose significantly increased after the oral glucose loading in patients with type 2 diabetes. Diabetes 2003;52:A549.

67.   Taubes G. Good calories, Bad Calories. New York: Alfred A Knopf; 2007.

68.   Guglielmi FW, Boggio-Bertinet D, Federico A, et al. Total parenteral nutrition-related gastroenterological complications. Dig Liver Dis 2006;38:623-42.

69.   Nishimura M, Yamaguchi M, Naito S, Yamauchi A. Soybean oil fat emulsion to prevent TPN-induced liver damage: possible molecular mechanisms and clinical implications. Biol Pharm Bull 2006;29:855-62.

70.   Wang H, Khaoustov VI, Krishnan B, et al. Total parenteral nutrition induces liver steatosis and apoptosis in neonatal piglets. The Journal of nutrition 2006;136:2547-52.

71.   Nanri A, Mizoue T, Noda M, et al. Rice intake and type 2 diabetes in Japanese men and women: the Japan Public Health Center-based Prospective Study. The American journal of clinical nutrition 2010;92:1468-77.

72.   Mizoue T, Yamaji T, Tabata S, et al. Dietary patterns and glucose tolerance abnormalities in Japanese men. The Journal of nutrition 2006;136:1352-8.

73.   Longland AC, Byrd BM. Pasture nonstructural carbohydrates and equine laminitis. The Journal of nutrition 2006;136:2099S-102S.

74.   Brocklebank KJ, Hendry GAF. Characteristics of plant species which store different types of reserve carbohydratres. New Phytol 1989;112:255-60.

75.   Pilon-Smits E, Ebskamp M, Paul MJ, Jeuken M, Weisbeek PJ, Smeekens S. Improved Performance of Transgenic Fructan-Accumulating Tobacco under Drought Stress. Plant Physiol 1995;107:125-30.

76.   Hendry GAF. Evolutionary origins and natural functions of fructans-- a climatological, biogeographic and mechanistic appraisal. New Phytol 1993;123:3-14.

77.   Ali M, Rellos P, Cox TM. Hereditary fructose intolerance. J Med Genet 1998;35:353-65.

78.   Wexler DL, Penders JE, Bowen WH, Burne RA. Characteristics and cariogenicity of a fructanase-defective Streptococcus mutants strain. Infect Immun 1992;60:3673-81.

79.   Burne RA, Chen YY, Wexler DL, Kuramitsu H, Bowen WH. Cariogenicity of Streptococcus mutans strains with defects in fructan metabolism assessed in a program-fed specific-pathogen-free rat model. J Dent Res 1996;75:1572-7.

80.   Backhed F, Ding H, Wang T, et al. The gut microbiota as an environmental factor that regulates fat storage. Proceedings of the National Academy of Sciences of the United States of America 2004;101:15718-23.

81.   Ley RE, Backhed F, Turnbaugh P, Lozupone CA, Knight RD, Gordon JI. Obesity alters gut microbial ecology. Proceedings of the National Academy of Sciences of the United States of America 2005;102:11070-5.

82.   Ley RE, Turnbaugh PJ, Klein S, Gordon JI. Microbial ecology: human gut microbes associated with obesity. Nature 2006;444:1022-3.

83.   Turnbaugh PJ, Ley RE, Mahowald MA, Magrini V, Mardis ER, Gordon JI. An obesity-associated gut microbiome with increased capacity for energy harvest. Nature 2006;444:1027-31.

84.   Skinner MF, Dupras TL, Moya-Sola S. Periodicity of linear enamel hypoplasia among Miocene Dryopithecus from Spain. J Paleopathol 1995:195-222.

85.   Johnson RJ, Andrews P. Fructose, Uricase, and the Back-to-Africa Hypothesis. Evol Anthropol 2010;19 250-7.

86.   Andrews P. Palaeoecology of the Miocene fauna from Paşalar, Turkey. Journal of human evolution 1990;19:569-82.

87.   King T, Aiello L, Andrews P. Dental microwear of Griphopithecus alpani. Journal of human evolution 1999;36:3-31.

88.   Marshall AJ, Wrangham R. Evolutionary consequences of fallback foods. Int J Primatol 2007;28:1219-35.

89.   Johnson RJ, Rivard C, Lanaspa MA, et al Fructokinase, Fructans, Intestinal Permeability, and Metabolic Syndrome: An Equine Connection? J Equin Vet Sci 2012 (in press).

90.   van Eps AW, Pollitt CC. Equine laminitis induced with oligofructose. Equine Vet J 2006;38:203-8.

91.   Garner HE, Hutcheson DP, Coffman JR, Hahn AW, Salem C. Lactic acidosis: a factor associated with equine laminitis. J Anim Sci 1977;45:1037-41.

92.   Graham JP, Boland JJ, Silbergeld E. Growth promoting antibiotics in food animal production: an economic analysis. Public Health Rep 2007;122:79-87.

93.   Coates ME, Davies MK, Kon SK. The effect of antibiotics on the intestine of the chick. The British journal of nutrition 1955;9:110-9.

94.   Coates ME, Fuller R, Harrison GF, Lev M, Suffolk SF. A comparison of the growth of chicks in the Gustafsson germ-free apparatus and in a conventional environment, with and without dietary supplements of penicillin. The British journal of nutrition 1963;17:141-50.

95.   Onifade AA. Growth performance, carcass characteristics, organs measurement and haematology of broiler chickens fed a high fibre diet supplemented with antibiotics or dried yeast. Nahrung 1997;41:370-4.

96.   Wang Y, Lehane C, Ghebremeskel K, Crawford MA. Modern organic and broiler chickens sold for human consumption provide more energy from fat than protein. Public Health Nutr 2010;13:400-8.

97.   Nriagu JO. Saturnine gout among Roman aristocrats. Did lead poisoning contribute to the fall of the Empire? The New England journal of medicine 1983;308:660-3.

98.   Bener A, Obineche E, Gillett M, Pasha MA, Bishawi B. Association between blood levels of lead, blood pressure and risk of diabetes and heart disease in workers. International archives of occupational and environmental health 2001;74:375-8.

99.   Wedeen RP. Irregular gout: humoral fantasy or saturnine malady. Bull N Y Acad Med 1984;60:969-79.

100.   Lancereaux E. Lancereaux, E.: Note relative a un cas de paralysie saturnine avec alteration des cordons nerveux et des muscles paralyses. . Gaz Med Paris 1862;17:709-13.

101.   Ball GV. Two epidemics of gout. Bull Hist Med 1971;45:401-8.

102.   Lin JL, Ho HH, Yu CC. Chelation therapy for patients with elevated body lead burden and progressive renal insufficiency. A randomized, controlled trial. Annals of internal medicine 1999;130:7-13.

103.   Ekong EB, Jaar BG, Weaver VM. Lead-related nephrotoxicity: a review of the epidemiologic evidence. Kidney international 2006;70:2074-84.

104.   Emerson H, Larimore LD. Diabetes mellitus: A contribution to its epidemiology based chiefly on mortality statistics. Archives of internal medicine 1924;34:585-630.

SECTION 5

1.   Cameron JS, Hicks J. Frederick Akbar Mahomed and his role in the description of hypertension at Guy's Hospital. Kidney international 1996;49:1488-506.

2.   Mahomed FA. The etiology of Bright's disease and the prealbuminuric state. Med Chir Trans 1874;39:197-228.

3.   Medico-Actuarial Mortality Investigation. Association of Life Insurance Medical Directors and the Actuarial Society of America 1912;1.

4.   Johnson RJ, Titte S, Cade JR, Rideout BA, Oliver WJ. Uric acid, evolution and primitive cultures. Semin Nephrol 2005;25:3-8.

5.   Kearney PM, Whelton M, Reynolds K, Muntner P, Whelton PK, He J. Global burden of hypertension: analysis of worldwide data. Lancet 2005;365:217-23.

6.   Allen FM, Sherrill JW. The treatment of arterial hypertension. J Metabol Research 1922;2:429-545.

7.   Dahl LK. Possible role of salt intake in the development of essential hypertension. In: Cottier P, Bock K, editors. Essential Hypertension - an International Symposium 1960; Berlin: Springer; 1960. p. 53-65.

8.   MacGregor GA. Sodium is more important than calcium in essential hypertension. Hypertension 1985;7:628-40.

9.   Guyton AC, Coleman TG, Cowley AV, Jr., Scheel KW, Manning RD, Jr., Norman RA, Jr. Arterial pressure regulation. Overriding dominance of the kidneys in long-term regulation and in hypertension. The American journal of medicine 1972;52:584-94.

10.   Major outcomes in high-risk hypertensive patients randomized to angiotensin-converting enzyme inhibitor or calcium channel blocker vs diuretic: The Antihypertensive and Lipid-Lowering Treatment to Prevent Heart Attack Trial (ALLHAT). Jama 2002;288:2981-97.

11.   Carmelli D, Cardon LR, Fabsitz R. Clustering of hypertension, diabetes, and obesity in adult male twins: same genes or same environments? American journal of human genetics 1994;55:566-73.

12.   Barker DJ, Osmond C, Golding J, Kuh D, Wadsworth ME. Growth in utero, blood pressure in childhood and adult life, and mortality from cardiovascular disease. BMJ (Clinical research ed 1989;298:564-7.

13.   Brenner BM, Garcia DL, Anderson S. Glomeruli and blood pressure. Less of one, more the other? Am J Hypertens 1988;1:335-47.

14.   Hughson MD, Douglas-Denton R, Bertram JF, Hoy WE. Hypertension, glomerular number, and birth weight in African Americans and white subjects in the southeastern United States. Kidney international 2006;69:671-8.

15.   Moritz A, Oldt M. Arteriolar sclerosis in hypertensive and nonhypertensive individuals. Am J Pathol 1937;13:679-728.

16.   Johnson RJ, Herrera-Acosta J, Schreiner GF, Rodriguez-Iturbe B. Subtle acquired renal injury as a mechanism of salt-sensitive hypertension. The New England journal of medicine 2002;346:913-23.

17.   Rodriguez-Iturbe B. Renal infiltration of immunocompetent cells: cause and effect of sodium-sensitive hypertension. Clin Exp Nephrol 2010;14:105-11.

18.   Mahomed FA. On chronic bright's disease, and its essential symptoms. Lancet 1879;I:398-404.

19.   Davis NC. The cardiovascular and renal relations and manifestations of gout. JAMA 1897;29:261-2.

20.   Huchard H. Arteriolosclerosis: Including its cardiac form. JAMA 1909;53:1129.

21.   Haig A. Uric acid as a Factor in the Causation of Disease. A contribution to the pathology of high arterial tension, headache, epilepsy, mental depression, gout, rheumatism, diabetes, Bright's disease, and other disorders. First ed. London: J & A Churchill; 1892.

22.   Mazzali M, Hughes J, Kim YG, et al. Elevated uric acid increases blood pressure in the rat by a novel crystal-independent mechanism. Hypertension 2001;38:1101-6.

23.   Watanabe S, Kang DH, Feng L, et al. Uric acid, hominoid evolution, and the pathogenesis of salt-sensitivity. Hypertension 2002;40:355-60.

24.   Grayson PC, Kim SY, Lavalley M, Choi HK. Hyperuricemia and incident hypertension: A systematic review and meta-analysis. Arthritis Care Res (Hoboken) 2010.

25.   Feig DI, Kang DH, Johnson RJ. Uric acid and cardiovascular risk. The New England journal of medicine 2008;359:1811-21.

26.   Feig DI, Johnson RJ. The role of uric acid in pediatric hypertension. J Ren Nutr 2007;17:79-83.

27.   Feig DI, Soletsky B, Johnson RJ. Effect of Allopurinol on the Blood Pressure of Adolescents with Newly Diagnosed Essential Hypertension. JAMA 2008;300:922-30.

28.   Kanbay M, Huddam B, Azak A, et al. Allopurinol improves endothelial dysfunction and eGFR in asymptomatic hyperuricemic subjects with normal renal function: A prospective, randomized study CJASN 2011; 6:1887-94.

29.   Choi HK, Liu S, Curhan G. Intake of purine-rich foods, protein, and dairy products and relationship to serum levels of uric acid: the Third National Health and Nutrition Examination Survey. Arthritis and rheumatism 2005;52:283-9.

30.   Oliver WJ, Cohen EL, Neel JV. Blood pressure, sodium intake, and sodium related hormones in the Yanomamö Indians, a "no-salt" culture. Circulation 1975;52:146-51.

31.   Johnson RJ, Sautin YY, Oliver WJ, et al. Lessons from comparative physiology: could uric acid represent a physiologic alarm signal gone awry in western society? Journal of comparative physiology 2009;179:67-76.

32.   Emmerson BT. Effect of oral fructose on urate production. Annals of the rheumatic diseases 1974;33:276-80.

33.   Perheentupa J, Raivio K. Fructose-induced hyperuricaemia. Lancet 1967;2:528-31.

34.   Le MT, Frye RF, Rivard CJ, et al. Effects of high-fructose corn syrup and sucrose on the pharmacokinetics of fructose and acute metabolic and hemodynamic responses in healthy subjects. Metabolism: clinical and experimental 2012; 61:641-651.

35.   Choi JW, Ford ES, Gao X, Choi HK. Sugar-sweetened soft drinks, diet soft drinks, and serum uric acid level: The third national health and nutrition examination survey. Arthritis and rheumatism 2007;59:109-16.

36.   Nguyen S, Choi HK, Lustig RH, Hsu CY. Sugar-sweetened beverages, serum uric acid, and blood pressure in adolescents. The Journal of pediatrics 2009;154:807-13.

37.   Jalal DI, Smits G, Johnson RJ, Chonchol M. Increased fructose associates with elevated blood pressure. J Am Soc Nephrol 2010;21:1543-9.

38.   Sanchez-Lozada LG, Tapia E, Bautista-Garcia P, et al. Effects of febuxostat on metabolic and renal alterations in rats with fructose-induced metabolic syndrome. American journal of physiology 2008;294:F710-8.

39.   Brown CM, Dulloo AG, Yepuri G, Montani JP. Fructose ingestion acutely elevates blood pressure in healthy young humans. American journal of physiology 2008;294:R730-7.

40.   Perez-Pozo SE, Schold J, Nakagawa T, Sanchez-Lozada LG, Johnson RJ, Lillo JL. Excessive fructose intake induces the features of metabolic syndrome in healthy adult men: role of uric acid in the hypertensive response. Int J Obes (Lond) 2010;34:454-61.

41.   Chen L, Caballero B, Mitchell DC, et al. Reducing Consumption of Sugar-Sweetened Beverages Is Associated With Reduced Blood Pressure. A Prospective Study Among United States Adults. Circulation 2010;in press.

42.   Chen L, Caballero B, Mitchell DC, et al. Reducing consumption of sugar-sweetened beverages is associated with reduced blood pressure: a prospective study among United States adults. Circulation 2010;121:2398-406.

43.   He FJ, Marrero NM, MacGregor GA. Salt intake is related to soft drink consumption in children and adolescents: a link to obesity? Hypertension 2008;51:629-34.

44.   Singh AK, Amlal H, Haas PJ, et al. Fructose-induced hypertension: essential role of chloride and fructose absorbing transporters PAT1 and Glut5. Kidney international 2008;74:438-47.

45.   Heo SH, Lee SH. High levels of serum uric acid are associated with silent brain infarction. J Neurol Sci 2010;297:6-10.

46.   Kim SY, Guevara JP, Kim KM, Choi HK, Heitjan DF, Albert DA. Hyperuricemia and risk of stroke: A systematic review and meta-analysis. Arthritis and rheumatism 2009;61:885-92.

47.   Kanbay M, Sanchez-Lozada LG, Franco M, et al. Microvascular disease and its role in the brain and cardiovascular system: a potential role for uric acid as a cardiorenal toxin. Nephrol Dial Transplant 2011; 26:430-437.

48.   Chamorro A, Obach V, Cervera A, Revilla M, Deulofeu R, Aponte JH. Prognostic significance of uric acid serum concentration in patients with acute ischemic stroke. Stroke; a journal of cerebral circulation 2002;33:1048-52.

49.   Muir SW, Harrow C, Dawson J, et al. Allopurinol use yields potentially beneficial effects on inflammatory indices in those with recent ischemic stroke: a randomized, double-blind, placebo-controlled trial. Stroke; a journal of cerebral circulation 2008;39:3303-7.

50.   Khan F, George J, Wong K, McSwiggan S, Struthers AD, Belch JJ. Allopurinol treatment reduces arterial wave reflection in stroke survivors. Cardiovasc Ther 2008;26:247-52.

51.   Desai RV, Ahmed MI, Fonarow GC, et al. Effect of serum insulin on the association between hyperuricemia and incident heart failure. The American journal of cardiology 2010;106:1134-8.

52. Ekundayo OJ, Dell'Italia LJ, Sanders PW, et al. Association between hyperuricemia and incident heart failure among older adults: a propensity-matched study. Int J Cardiol 2010;142:279-87.

53. Hare JM, Mangal B, Brown J, et al. Impact of oxypurinol in patients with symptomatic heart failure. Results of the OPT-CHF study. Journal of the American College of Cardiology 2008;51:2301-9.

54. Langlois M, De Bacquer D, Duprez D, De Buyzere M, Delanghe J, Blaton V. Serum uric acid in hypertensive patients with and without peripheral arterial disease. Atherosclerosis 2003;168:163-8.

55. Montalcini T, Gorgone G, Gazzaruso C, Sesti G, Perticone F, Pujia A. Relation between serum uric acid and carotid intima-media thickness in healthy postmenopausal women. Intern Emerg Med 2007;2:19-23.

56. Patetsios P, Rodino W, Wisselink W, Bryan D, Kirwin JD, Panetta TF. Identification of uric acid in aortic aneurysms and atherosclerotic artery. Ann N Y Acad Sci 1996;800:243-5.

57. Suarna C, Dean RT, May J, Stocker R. Human atherosclerotic plaque contains both oxidized lipids and relatively large amounts of alpha-tocopherol and ascorbate. Arteriosclerosis, thrombosis, and vascular biology 1995;15:1616-24.

58. Johnson RJ, Kang DH, Feig D, et al. Is there a pathogenetic role for uric acid in hypertension and cardiovascular and renal disease? Hypertension 2003;41:1183-90.

59. Noman A, Ang DS, Ogston S, Lang CC, Struthers AD. Effect of high-dose allopurinol on exercise in patients with chronic stable angina: a randomised, placebo controlled crossover trial. Lancet 2010;375:2161-7.

60. Goicoechea M, de Vinuesa SG, Verdalles U, et al. Effect of allopurinol in chronic kidney disease progression and cardiovascular risk. Clin J Am Soc Nephrol 2010;5:1388-93.

61. Abrams B. Gout as an early warning of concomitant sleep apnea. J Clin Rheumatol 2010;16:305.

62. Drager LF, Lopes HF, Maki-Nunes C, et al. The impact of obstructive sleep apnea on metabolic and inflammatory markers in consecutive patients with metabolic syndrome. PLoS ONE 2010;5:e12065.

63. Zharikov SI, Swenson ER, Lanaspa M, Block ER, Patel JM, Johnson RJ. Could uric acid be a modifiable risk factor in subjects with pulmonary hypertension? Medical hypotheses 2010;74:1069-74.

64. Maynard SE, Min JY, Merchan J, et al. Excess placental soluble fms-like tyrosine kinase 1 (sFlt1) may contribute to endothelial dysfunction, hypertension, and proteinuria in preeclampsia. The Journal of clinical investigation 2003;111:649-58.

285

65.   Redman CW, Beilin LJ, Bonnar J, Wilkinson RH. Plasma-urate measurements in predicting fetal death in hypertensive pregnancy. Lancet 1976;1:1370-3.

66.   Laughon SK, Catov J, Powers RW, Roberts JM, Gandley RE. First trimester uric acid and adverse pregnancy outcomes. Am J Hypertens 2011;24:489-95.

67.   Wolak T, Sergienko R, Wiznitzer A, Paran E, Sheiner E. High Uric Acid Level During the First 20 Weeks of Pregnancy is Associated with Higher Risk for Gestational Diabetes Mellitus and Mild Preeclampsia. Hypertens Pregnancy 2010.

68.   Laughon SK, Catov J, Provins T, Roberts JM, Gandley RE. Elevated first-trimester uric acid concentrations are associated with the development of gestational diabetes. Am J Obstet Gynecol 2009;201:402 e1-5.

69.   Laughon SK, Catov J, Roberts JM. Uric acid concentrations are associated with insulin resistance and birthweight in normotensive pregnant women. Am J Obstet Gynecol 2009;201:582 e1-6.

70.   Kang DH, Finch J, Nakagawa T, et al. Uric acid, endothelial dysfunction and pre-eclampsia: searching for a pathogenetic link. Journal of hypertension 2004;22:229-35.

71.   Bainbridge SA, Roberts JM. Uric Acid as a Pathogenic Factor in Preeclampsia. Placenta 2008;29S:67-72.

72.   Clausen T, Slott M, Solvoll K, Drevon CA, Vollset SE, Henriksen T. High intake of energy, sucrose, and polyunsaturated fatty acids is associated with increased risk of preeclampsia. Am J Obstet Gynecol 2001;185:451-8.

73.   Maller O, Turner RE. Taste in acceptance of sugars by human infants. J Comp Physiol Psychol 1973;84:496-501.

74.   Blumenthal DM, Gold MS. Neurobiology of food addiction. Curr Opin Clin Nutr Metab Care 2010;13:359-65.

75.   Avena NM, Rada P, Hoebel BG. Evidence for sugar addiction: behavioral and neurochemical effects of intermittent, excessive sugar intake. Neuroscience and biobehavioral reviews 2008;32:20-39.

76.   Rubaum-Keller I. Foodaholic-- the seven stages to permanent weight loss. Minneapolis: Mill City Press; 2011.

77.   Avena NM, Rada P, Hoebel BG. Sugar bingeing in rats. Current protocols in neuroscience / editorial board, Jacqueline N Crawley [et al 2006;Chapter 9:Unit9 23C.

78.   Pecina S, Cagniard B, Berridge KC, Aldridge JW, Zhuang X. Hyperdopaminergic mutant mice have higher "wanting" but not "liking" for sweet rewards. J Neurosci 2003;23:9395-402.

79.   Spangler R, Wittkowski KM, Goddard NL, Avena NM, Hoebel BG, Leibowitz SF. Opiate-like effects of sugar on gene expression in reward areas of the rat brain. Brain Res Mol Brain Res 2004;124:134-42.

80. Rada P, Avena NM, Hoebel BG. Daily bingeing on sugar repeatedly releases dopamine in the accumbens shell. Neuroscience 2005;134:737-44.

81. Colantuoni C, Rada P, McCarthy J, et al. Evidence that intermittent, excessive sugar intake causes endogenous opioid dependence. Obes Res 2002;10:478-88.

82. Johnson PM, Kenny PJ. Dopamine D2 receptors in addiction-like reward dysfunction and compulsive eating in obese rats. Nat Neurosci 2010;13:635-41.

83. Stice E, Yokum S, Blum K, Bohon C. Weight gain is associated with reduced striatal response to palatable food. J Neurosci 2010;30:13105-9.

84. Volkow ND, Wang GJ, Telang F, et al. Low dopamine striatal D2 receptors are associated with prefrontal metabolism in obese subjects: possible contributing factors. Neuroimage 2008;42:1537-43.

85. Wang GJ, Volkow ND, Logan J, et al. Brain dopamine and obesity. Lancet 2001;357:354-7.

86. Klein TA, Neumann J, Reuter M, Hennig J, von Cramon DY, Ullsperger M. Genetically determined differences in learning from errors. Science (New York, NY 2007;318:1642-5.

87. Stice E, Spoor S, Bohon C, Small DM. Relation between obesity and blunted striatal response to food is moderated by TaqIA A1 allele. Science (New York, NY 2008;322:449-52.

88. de Araujo IE, Oliveira-Maia AJ, Sotnikova TD, et al. Food reward in the absence of taste receptor signaling. Neuron 2008;57:930-41.

89. Bernal SY, Dostova I, Kest A, et al. Role of dopamine D1 and D2 receptors in the nucleus accumbens shell on the acquisition and expression of fructose-conditioned flavor-flavor preferences in rats. Behavioural brain research 2008;190:59-66.

90. Purnell JQ, Klopfenstein BA, Stevens AA, et al. Brain functional magnetic resonance imaging response to glucose and fructose infusions in humans. Diabetes Obes Metab 2011;13:229-34.

91. Cha SH, Wolfgang M, Tokutake Y, Chohnan S, Lane MD. Differential effects of central fructose and glucose on hypothalamic malonyl-CoA and food intake. Proceedings of the National Academy of Sciences of the United States of America 2008;105:16871-5.

92. Colantuoni C, Schwenker J, McCarthy J, et al. Excessive sugar intake alters binding to dopamine and mu-opioid receptors in the brain. Neuroreport 2001;12:3549-52.

93. Goldman LS, Genel M, Bezman RJ, Slanetz PJ. Diagnosis and treatment of attention-deficit/hyperactivity disorder in children and adolescents. Council on Scientific Affairs, American Medical Association. JAMA 1998;279:1100-7.

94. Increasing prevalence of parent-reported attention-deficit/hyperactivity disorder among children --- United States, 2003 and 2007. MMWR Morb Mortal Wkly Rep 2010;59:1439-43.

95. White JW, Wolraich M. Effect of sugar on behavior and mental performance. The American journal of clinical nutrition 1995;62:242S-7S; discussion 7S-9S.

96. Prinz RJ, Roberts WA, Hantman E. Dietary correlates of hyperactive behavior in children. J Consult Clin Psychol 1980;48:760-9.

97. Wolraich ML, Lindgren SD, Stumbo PJ, Stegink LD, Appelbaum MI, Kiritsy MC. Effects of diets high in sucrose or aspartame on the behavior and cognitive performance of children. The New England journal of medicine 1994;330:301-7.

98. Wolraich M, Milich R, Stumbo P, Schultz F. Effects of sucrose ingestion on the behavior of hyperactive boys. The Journal of pediatrics 1985;106:675-82.

99. Johnson RJ, Gold MS, Johnson DR, et al. Attention-deficit/hyperactivity disorder: is it time to reappraise the role of sugar consumption? Postgrad Med 2011;123:39-49.

100. Volkow ND, Wang GJ, Kollins SH, et al. Evaluating dopamine reward pathway in ADHD: clinical implications. JAMA 2009;302:1084-91.

101. Zametkin AJ, Nordahl TE, Gross M, et al. Cerebral glucose metabolism in adults with hyperactivity of childhood onset. The New England journal of medicine 1990;323:1361-6.

102. Pagoto SL, Curtin C, Lemon SC, et al. Association between adult attention deficit/hyperactivity disorder and obesity in the US population. Obesity (Silver Spring) 2009;17:539-44.

103. Agranat-Meged AN, Deitcher C, Goldzweig G, Leibenson L, Stein M, Galili-Weisstub E. Childhood obesity and attention deficit/hyperactivity disorder: a newly described comorbidity in obese hospitalized children. Int J Eat Disord 2005;37:357-9.

104. Altfas JR. Prevalence of attention deficit/hyperactivity disorder among adults in obesity treatment. BMC Psychiatry 2002;2:9.

105. Barrera CM, Ruiz ZR, Dunlap WP. Uric acid: a participating factor in the symptoms of hyperactivity. Biological psychiatry 1988;24:344-7.

106. David O, Clark J, Voeller K. Lead and hyperactivity. Lancet 1972;2:900-3.

107. Church WH, Rappolt G. Nigrostriatal catecholamine metabolism in guinea pigs is altered by purine enzyme inhibition. Experimental brain research Experimentelle Hirnforschung 1999;127:147-50.

108. Barrera CM, Hunter RE, Dunlap WP. Hyperuricemia and locomotor activity in developing rats. Pharmacology, biochemistry, and behavior 1989;33:367-9.

109. Hudson JI, Pope HG, Jr. Affective spectrum disorder: does antidepressant response identify a family of disorders with a common pathophysiology? Am J Psychiatry 1990;147:552-64.

110. Moore SC, Carter LM, van Goozen S. Confectionery consumption in childhood and adult violence. Br J Psychiatry 2009;195:366-7.

111. Ellis H. A study of British genius. London: Hurst and Blackett; 1903.

112. Orowan E. The origin of man. Nature 1955;175:683-4.

113. Stetten D, Jr., Hearon JZ. Intellectual level measured by army classification battery and serum uric acid concentration. Science (New York, NY 1959;129:1737.

114. Bloch S, Brackenridge CJ. Psychological, performance and biochemical factors in medical students under examination stress. Journal of psychosomatic research 1972;16:25-33.

115. Cervini C, Zamopa AM. Uric acid and intelligence. Annals of the rheumatic diseases 1982;41:435.

116. Kasl SV, Brooks GW, Rodgers WL. Serum uric acid and cholesterol in achievement behavior and motivation. II. The relationship to college attendance, extracurricular and social activities, and vocational aspirations. JAMA 1970;213:1291-9.

117. Kasl SV, Brooks GW, Rodgers WL. Serum uric acid and cholesterol in achievement behavior and motivation. I. The relationship to ability, grades, test performance, and motivation. JAMA 1970;213:1158-64.

118. Brooks GW, Mueller E. Serum urate concentrations among university professors; relation to drive, achievement, and leadership. Jama 1966;195:415-8.

119. Montoye HJ, Mikkelsen WM. Serum uric acid and achievement in high school. Arthritis and rheumatism 1973;16:359-62.

120. Stephan BC, Wells JC, Brayne C, Albanese E, Siervo M. Increased fructose intake as a risk factor for dementia. J Gerontol A Biol Sci Med Sci 2010;65:809-14.

121. Schretlen DJ, Inscore AB, Jinnah HA, Rao V, Gordon B, Pearlson GD. Serum uric acid and cognitive function in community-dwelling older adults. Neuropsychology 2007;21:136-40.

122. Ruggiero C, Cherubini A, Lauretani F, et al. Uric acid and dementia in community-dwelling older persons. Dement Geriatr Cogn Disord 2009;27:382-9.

123. Schretlen DJ, Inscore AB, Vannorsdall TD, et al. Serum uric acid and brain ischemia in normal elderly adults. Neurology 2007;69:1418-23.

124. Afsar B, Elsurer R, Covic A, Johnson RJ, Kanbay M. Relationship between Uric Acid and Subtle Cognitive Dysfunction in Chronic Kidney Disease. American journal of nephrology 2011;34:49-54.

125. Craft S. The role of metabolic disorders in Alzheimer disease and vascular dementia: two roads converged. Arch Neurol 2009;66:300-5.

126. Cao D, Lu H, Lewis TL, Li L. Intake of sucrose-sweetened water induces insulin resistance and exacerbates memory deficits and amyloidosis in a transgenic mouse model of Alzheimer disease. J Biol Chem 2007;282:36275-82.

127.   Farris W, Mansourian S, Chang Y, et al. Insulin-degrading enzyme regulates the levels of insulin, amyloid beta-protein, and the beta-amyloid precursor protein intracellular domain in vivo. Proceedings of the National Academy of Sciences of the United States of America 2003;100:4162-7.

128.   Watson GS, Baker LD, Cholerton BA, et al. Effects of insulin and octreotide on memory and growth hormone in Alzheimer's disease. J Alzheimers Dis 2009;18:595-602.

129.   Mielke JG, Taghibiglou C, Liu L, et al. A biochemical and functional characterization of diet-induced brain insulin resistance. Journal of neurochemistry 2005;93:1568-78.

130.   Ross AP, Bartness TJ, Mielke JG, Parent MB. A high fructose diet impairs spatial memory in male rats. Neurobiol Learn Mem 2009;92:410-6.

131.   Stranahan AM, Norman ED, Lee K, et al. Diet-induced insulin resistance impairs hippocampal synaptic plasticity and cognition in middle-aged rats. Hippocampus 2008;18:1085-8.

132.   Jurdak N, Lichtenstein AH, Kanarek RB. Diet-induced obesity and spatial cognition in young male rats. Nutr Neurosci 2008;11:48-54.

133.   Torres C, Aragon A, Gonzalez M, et al. Decreased kidney function of unknown cause in Nicaragua: a community-based survey. Am J Kidney Dis 2010;55:485-96.

134.   Nanayakkara S, Komiya T, Ratnatunga N, et al. Tubulointerstitial damage as the major pathological lesion in endemic chronic kidney disease among farmers in North Central Province of Sri Lanka. Environ Health Prev Med 2011.

135.   Roncal-Jimenez CA, Lanaspa MA, Rivard CJ, et al. Sucrose induces fatty liver and pancreatic inflammation in male breeder rats independent of excess energy intake. Metabolism: clinical and experimental 2011; 60:1259-70

136.   Lionetti E, Catassi C. New clues in celiac disease epidemiology, pathogenesis, clinical manifestations, and treatment. Int Rev Immunol 2011;30:219-31.

137.   Garcia-Manzanares A, Lucendo AJ. Nutritional and dietary aspects of celiac disease. Nutr Clin Pract 2011;26:163-73.

138.   Smecuol E, Bai JC, Vazquez H, et al. Gastrointestinal permeability in celiac disease. Gastroenterology 1997;112:1129-36.

139.   Riordan AM, Ruxton CH, Hunter JO. A review of associations between Crohn's disease and consumption of sugars. European journal of clinical nutrition 1998;52:229-38.

140.   Vogelsang H. Do changes in intestinal permeability predict disease relapse in Crohn's disease? Inflamm Bowel Dis 2008;14 Suppl 2:S162-3.

141.   Shen L, Su L, Turner JR. Mechanisms and functional implications of intestinal barrier defects. Dig Dis 2009;27:443-9.

142.   Strader AD. Ileal transposition provides insight into the effectiveness of gastric bypass surgery. Physiology & behavior 2006;88:277-82.

143.   Rubino F, Marescaux J. Effect of duodenal-jejunal exclusion in a non-obese animal model of type 2 diabetes: a new perspective for an old disease. Ann Surg 2004;239:1-11.

144.   Andreelli F, Amouyal C, Magnan C, Mithieux G. What can bariatric surgery teach us about the pathophysiology of type 2 diabetes? Diabetes Metab 2009;35:499-507.

145.   Duez H, Lamarche B, Uffelman KD, Valero R, Cohn JS, Lewis GF. Hyperinsulinemia is associated with increased production rate of intestinal apolipoprotein B-48-containing lipoproteins in humans. Arteriosclerosis, thrombosis, and vascular biology 2006;26:1357-63.

146.   Cirillo P, Gersch MS, Mu W, et al. Ketohexokinase-dependent metabolism of fructose induces proinflammatory mediators in proximal tubular cells. J Am Soc Nephrol 2009;20:545-53.

147.   Nakayama T, Kosugi T, Gersch M, et al. Dietary fructose causes tubulointerstitial injury in the normal rat kidney. American journal of physiology 2010;298:F712-20.

148.   Shoham DA, Durazo-Arvizu R, Kramer H, et al. Sugary soda consumption and albuminuria: results from the National Health and Nutrition Examination Survey, 1999-2004. PLoS ONE 2008;3:e3431.

149.   Gersch MS, Mu W, Cirillo P, et al. Fructose, but not dextrose, accelerates the progression of chronic kidney disease. American journal of physiology 2007;293:F1256-61.

SECTION 6

1.   Hill JO, Peters JC, Wyatt HR. Using the energy gap to address obesity: A commentary. Journal of the American Dietetic Association 2009;109:1848-53.

2.   Hill JO, Peters JC, Catenacci VA, Wyatt HR. International strategies to address obesity. Obes Rev 2008;9 Suppl 1:41-7.

3.   Keesey RE, Hirvonen MD. Body weight set-points: determination and adjustment. The Journal of nutrition 1997;127:1875S-83S.

4.   Bairlein F. How to get fat: nutritional mechanisms of seasonal fat accumulation in migratory songbirds. Naturwissenschaften 2002;89:1-10.

5.   MacLean PS, Higgins JA, Wyatt HR, et al. Regular exercise attenuates the metabolic drive to regain weight after long-term weight loss. American journal of physiology 2009;297:R793-802.

REFERENCES

6.   Van Horn L, Johnson RK, Flickinger BD, Vafiadis DK, Yin-Piazza S. Translation and implementation of added sugars consumption recommendations: a conference report from the American Heart Association Added Sugars Conference 2010. Circulation 2010;122:2470-90.

7.   Johnson RK, Appel LJ, Brands M, et al. Dietary sugars intake and cardiovascular health: a scientific statement from the American Heart Association. Circulation 2009;120:1011-20.

8.   Jacob RA, Spinozzi GM, Simon VA, et al. Consumption of cherries lowers plasma urate in healthy women. The Journal of nutrition 2003;133:1826-9.

9.   Madero M, Arriaga JC, Jalal D, et al. The effect of two energy-restricted diets, a low-fructose diet versus a moderate natural fructose diet, on weight loss and metabolic syndrome parameters: a randomized controlled trial. Metabolism: clinical and experimental 2011; 60:1551-9

10.   American Academy of Pediatrics: The use and misuse of fruit juice in pediatrics. Pediatrics 2001;107:1210-3.

11.   Mercola J, Pearsal KD. Sweet Deception. Nashville: Nelson Books; 2006.

12.   de Araujo IE, Oliveira-Maia AJ, Sotnikova TD, et al. Food reward in the absence of taste receptor signaling. Neuron 2008;57:930-41.

13.   Adcock LH, Gray CH. The metabolism of sorbitol in the human subject. The Biochemical journal 1957;65:554-60.

14.   Barngrover DA, Dills WL, Jr. The involvement of liver fructokinase in the metabolism of D-xylulose and xylitol in isolated rat hepatocytes. The Journal of nutrition 1983;113:522-30.

15.   Burt BA. The use of sorbitol- and xylitol-sweetened chewing gum in caries control. J Am Dent Assoc 2006;137:190-6.

16.   Hamalainen MM, Makinen KK. Metabolism of glucose, fructose and xylitol in normal and streptozotocin-diabetic rats. The Journal of nutrition 1982;112:1369-78.

17.   Forster H, Heller L, Hellmund U, Boecker S. [Parenteral feeding. Biochemical and clinical findings during continuous long-term infusion of glucose, fructose, sorbitol and xylitol. 2. Clinical aspects, discussion and results]. Fortschr Med 1975;93:1257-61.

18.   Liu S, Choi HK, Ford E, et al. A prospective study of dairy intake and the risk of type 2 diabetes in women. Diabetes care 2006;29:1579-84.

19.   Choi HK, Atkinson K, Karlson EW, Willett W, Curhan G. Purine-rich foods, dairy and protein intake, and the risk of gout in men. The New England journal of medicine 2004;350:1093-103.

20.   Choi HK, Liu S, Curhan G. Intake of purine-rich foods, protein, and dairy products and relationship to serum levels of uric acid: the Third National Health and Nutrition Examination Survey. Arthritis and rheumatism 2005;52:283-9.

21.   Hino A, Adachi H, Enomoto M, et al. Habitual coffee but not green tea consumption is inversely associated with metabolic syndrome: an epidemiological study in a general Japanese population. Diabetes research and clinical practice 2007;76:383-9.

22.   Tan DS. Coffee consumption and risk of type 2 diabetes mellitus. Lancet 2003;361:702; author reply 3.

23.   Campos H, Baylin A. Coffee consumption and risk of type 2 diabetes and heart disease. Nutrition reviews 2007;65:173-9.

24.   Kiyohara C, Kono S, Honjo S, et al. Inverse association between coffee drinking and serum uric acid concentrations in middle-aged Japanese males. The British journal of nutrition 1999;82:125-30.

25.   Choi HK, Curhan G. Coffee, tea, and caffeine consumption and serum uric acid level: the third national health and nutrition examination survey. Arthritis and rheumatism 2007;57:816-21.

26.   Choi HK, Willett W, Curhan G. Coffee consumption and risk of incident gout in men: a prospective study. Arthritis and rheumatism 2007;56:2049-55.

27.   Kela U, Vijayvargiya R, Trivedi CP. Inhibitory effects of methylxanthines on the activity of xanthine oxidase. Life sciences 1980;27:2109-19.

28.   Gao X, Curhan G, Forman JP, Ascherio A, Choi HK. Vitamin C Intake and Serum Uric Acid Concentration in Men. The Journal of rheumatology 2008.

29.   Gomez-Cabrera MC, Domenech E, Romagnoli M, et al. Oral administration of vitamin C decreases muscle mitochondrial biogenesis and hampers training-induced adaptations in endurance performance. The American journal of clinical nutrition 2008;87:142-9.

30.   Bruyere O, Malaise O, Neuprez A, Collette J, Reginster JY. Prevalence of vitamin D inadequacy in European postmenopausal women. Curr Med Res Opin 2007;23:1939-44.

31.   Pinelli NR, Jaber LA, Brown MB, Herman WH. Serum 25-hydroxy vitamin d and insulin resistance, metabolic syndrome, and glucose intolerance among Arab Americans. Diabetes care 2010;33:1373-5.

32.   Harel Z, Flanagan P, Forcier M, Harel D. Low vitamin D status among obese adolescents: prevalence and response to treatment. J Adolesc Health 2011;48:448-52.

33.   Barchetta I, Angelico F, Del Ben M, et al. Strong association between non alcoholic fatty liver disease (NAFLD) and low 25(OH) vitamin D levels in an adult population with normal serum liver enzymes. BMC Med 2011;9:85.

34.   Douard V, Suzuki T, Sabbagh Y, et al. Dietary fructose inhibits lactation-induced adaptations in rat 1,25-(OH)2D3 synthesis and calcium transport. FASEB J 2011.

35.   Chen W, Roncal Jimenez CA, Lanaspa M, et al. Uric acid suppresses 1-alpha hydroxylase Vitamin D in vitro and in vivo. Kidney international 2012 in press.

36.   Marriott BP, Cole N, Lee E. National estimates of dietary fructose intake increased from 1977 to 2004 in the United States. The Journal of nutrition 2009;139:1228S-35S.

37.   Flegal KM, Carroll MD, Ogden CL, Curtin LR. Prevalence and trends in obesity among US adults, 1999-2008. JAMA 2010;303:235-41.

38.   Brownell KD, Frieden TR. Ounces of prevention--the public policy case for taxes on sugared beverages. The New England journal of medicine 2009;360:1805-8.

39.   Malik VS, Popkin BM, Bray GA, Despres JP, Willett WC, Hu FB. Sugar-sweetened beverages and risk of metabolic syndrome and type 2 diabetes: a meta-analysis. Diabetes care 2010;33:2477-83.

40.   Shi L, van Meijgaard J. Substantial decline in sugar-sweetened beverage consumption among California's children and adolescents. Int J Gen Med 2010;3:221-4.

41.   Avena NM, Long KA, Hoebel BG. Sugar-dependent rats show enhanced responding for sugar after abstinence: evidence of a sugar deprivation effect. Physiology & behavior 2005;84:359-62.

42.   Avena NM, Rada P, Hoebel BG. Sugar bingeing in rats. Current protocols in neuroscience / editorial board, Jacqueline N Crawley [et al 2006;Chapter 9:Unit9 23C.

43.   Johnson RJ, Segal MS, Sautin Y, et al. Potential role of sugar (fructose) in the epidemic of hypertension, obesity and the metabolic syndrome, diabetes, kidney disease, and cardiovascular disease. The American journal of clinical nutrition 2007;86:899-906.

44.   Brownell KD, Farley T, Willett WC, et al. The public health and economic benefits of taxing sugar-sweetened beverages. The New England journal of medicine 2009;361:1599-605.

45.   Ludwig DS, Peterson KE, Gortmaker SL. Relation between consumption of sugar-sweetened drinks and childhood obesity: a prospective, observational analysis. Lancet 2001;357:505-8.

46.   Johnson RJ, Murray R. Fructose, exercise, and health. Curr Sports Med Rep 2010;9:253-8.

47.   Murray R. The effects of consuming carbohydrate-electrolyte beverages on gastric emptying and fluid absorption during and following exercise. Sports Med 1987;4:322-51.

48.   Murray R, Paul GL, Seifert JG, Eddy DE, Halaby GA. The effects of glucose, fructose, and sucrose ingestion during exercise. Med Sci Sports Exerc 1989;21:275-82.

49.   Muller C, Assimacopoulos-Jeannet F, Mosimann F, et al. Endogenous glucose production, gluconeogenesis and liver glycogen concentration in obese non-diabetic patients. Diabetologia 1997;40:463-8.

50.   Helge JW, Richter EA, Kiens B. Interaction of training and diet on metabolism and endurance during exercise in man. The Journal of physiology 1996;492 (Pt 1):293-306.

51.   Melanson EL, Gozansky WS, Barry DW, Maclean PS, Grunwald GK, Hill JO. When energy balance is maintained, exercise does not induce negative fat balance in lean sedentary, obese sedentary, or lean endurance-trained individuals. J Appl Physiol 2009;107:1847-56.

52.   Youn JH, Youn MS, Bergman RN. Synergism of glucose and fructose in net glycogen synthesis in perfused rat livers. J Biol Chem 1986;261:15960-9.

53.   Bruynseels K, Bergans N, Gillis N, et al. On the inhibition of hepatic glycogenolysis by fructose. A 31P-NMR study in perfused rat liver using the fructose analogue 2,5-anhydro-D-mannitol. NMR Biomed 1999;12:145-56.

54.   Ercan-Fang NG, Nuttall FQ, Gannon MC. Uric acid inhibits liver phosphorylase a activity under simulated in vivo conditions. Am J Physiol Endocrinol Metab 2001;280:E248-53.

55.   Banting W. Letter on corpulence, Addressed to the Public. In. London: Harrison; 1869:10 pp.

56.   Atkins R. Dr. Atkins' New Diet Revolution. New York: Avon Books; 1998.

57.   Foster GD, Wyatt HR, Hill JO, et al. A randomized trial of a low-carbohydrate diet for obesity. The New England journal of medicine 2003;348:2082-90.

58.   Gardner CD, Kiazand A, Alhassan S, et al. Comparison of the Atkins, Zone, Ornish, and LEARN diets for change in weight and related risk factors among overweight premenopausal women: the A TO Z Weight Loss Study: a randomized trial. JAMA 2007;297:969-77.

59.   Volek JS, Phinney SD. The Art and Science of Low Carbohydrate Living: Beyond Obesity, LLC; 2011.

60.   Boulter PR, Hoffman RS, Arky RA. Pattern of sodium excretion accompanying starvation. Metabolism: clinical and experimental 1973;22:675-83.

61.   Cahill GF, Jr. Starvation in man. The New England journal of medicine 1970;282:668-75.

62.   Shafiee MA, Charest AF, Cheema-Dhadli S, et al. Defining conditions that lead to the retention of water: the importance of the arterial sodium concentration. Kidney international 2005;67:613-21.

63.   Haskell WL, Blair SN, Hill JO. Physical activity: health outcomes and importance for public health policy. Prev Med 2009;49:280-2.

64.   Holloszy JO, Coyle EF. Adaptations of skeletal muscle to endurance exercise and their metabolic consequences. J Appl Physiol 1984;56:831-8.

65.   Kim JY, Hickner RC, Cortright Rl, Dohm GL, Houmard JA. Lipid oxidation is reduced in obese human skeletal muscle. Am J Physiol Endocrinol Metab 2000;279:E1039-44.

66.   Kelley DE, He J, Menshikova EV, Ritov VB. Dysfunction of mitochondria in human skeletal muscle in type 2 diabetes. Diabetes 2002;51:2944-50.

67.   Gianotti TF, Sookoian S, Dieuzeide G, et al. A decreased mitochondrial DNA content is related to insulin resistance in adolescents. Obesity (Silver Spring) 2008;16:1591-5.

68.   Lennmarken C, Sandstedt S, von Schenck H, Larsson J. Skeletal muscle function and metabolism in obese women. JPEN J Parenter Enteral Nutr 1986;10:583-7.

69.   Ji H, Graczyk-Milbrandt G, Friedman MI. Metabolic inhibitors synergistically decrease hepatic energy status and increase food intake. American journal of physiology 2000;278:R1579-82.

70.   Friedman MI, Harris RB, Ji H, Ramirez I, Tordoff MG. Fatty acid oxidation affects food intake by altering hepatic energy status. The American journal of physiology 1999;276:R1046-53.

71.   Koch JE, Ji H, Osbakken MD, Friedman MI. Temporal relationships between eating behavior and liver adenine nucleotides in rats treated with 2,5-AM. The American journal of physiology 1998;274:R610-7.

72.   Phinney SD, Bistrian BR, Wolfe RR, Blackburn GL. The human metabolic response to chronic ketosis without caloric restriction: physical and biochemical adaptation. Metabolism: clinical and experimental 1983;32:757-68.

73.   Appel LJ, Clark JM, Yeh HC, et al. Comparative effectiveness of weight-loss interventions in clinical practice. The New England journal of medicine 2011;365:1959-68.

74.   Steinmann B, Gitzelmann R, Van den Berghe G. Disorders of Fructose Metabolism. In: Scriver C, Beaudet A, Sly W, Valle D, eds. The Metabolic and Molecular Basis of Inherited Disease. New York: McGraw-Hill; 2001:1489-520.

75.   Ouyang J, Parakhia RA, Ochs RS. Metformin activates AMP kinase through inhibition of AMP deaminase. J Biol Chem 2011;286:1-11.

76.   Knowler WC, Barrett-Connor E, Fowler SE, et al. Reduction in the incidence of type 2 diabetes with lifestyle intervention or metformin. The New England journal of medicine 2002;346:393-403.

77.   Knowler WC, Fowler SE, Hamman RF, et al. 10-year follow-up of diabetes incidence and weight loss in the Diabetes Prevention Program Outcomes Study. Lancet 2009;374:1677-86.

78.   Baggott JE, Vaughn WH, Hudson BB. Inhibition of 5-aminoimidazole-4-carboxamide ribotide transformylase, adenosine deaminase and 5'-adenylate deaminase by polyglutamates of methotrexate and oxidized folates and by 5-aminoimidazole-4-carboxamide riboside and ribotide. The Biochemical journal 1986;236:193-200.

79.   Bergeron R, Previs SF, Cline GW, et al. Effect of 5-aminoimidazole-4-carboxamide-1-beta-D-ribofuranoside infusion on in vivo glucose and lipid metabolism in lean and obese Zucker rats. Diabetes 2001;50:1076-82.

80.   Pold R, Jensen LS, Jessen N, et al. Long-term AICAR administration and exercise prevents diabetes in ZDF rats. Diabetes 2005;54:928-34.

81.   Giri S, Rattan R, Haq E, et al. AICAR inhibits adipocyte differentiation in 3T3L1 and restores metabolic alterations in diet-induced obesity mice model. Nutr Metab (Lond) 2006;3:31.

82.   Narkar VA, Downes M, Yu RT, et al. AMPK and PPARdelta agonists are exercise mimetics. Cell 2008;134:405-15.

83.   Timmers S, Konings E, Bilet L, et al. Calorie restriction-like effects of 30 days of resveratrol supplementation on energy metabolism and metabolic profile in obese humans. Cell metabolism 2011;14:612-22.

84.   Baldwin W, McRae S, Marek G, et al. Hyperuricemia as a mediator of the proinflammatory endocrine imbalance in the adipose tissue in a murine model of the metabolic syndrome. Diabetes 2011;60:1258-69.

85.   Nakagawa T, Hu H, Zharikov S, et al. A causal role for uric acid in fructose-induced metabolic syndrome. American journal of physiology 2006;290:F625-31.

86.   Kodama S, Saito K, Yachi Y, et al. Association between serum uric acid and development of type 2 diabetes. Diabetes care 2009;32:1737-42.

87.   Masuo K, Kawaguchi H, Mikami H, Ogihara T, Tuck ML. Serum uric acid and plasma norepinephrine concentrations predict subsequent weight gain and blood pressure elevation. Hypertension 2003;42:474-80.

88.   Grayson PC, Kim SY, Lavalley M, Choi HK. Hyperuricemia and incident hypertension: A systematic review and meta-analysis. Arthritis Care Res (Hoboken) 2010.

89.   Feig DI, Kang DH, Johnson RJ. Uric acid and cardiovascular risk. The New England journal of medicine 2008;359:1811-21.

90.   Feig DI, Soletsky B, Johnson RJ. Effect of Allopurinol on the Blood Pressure of Adolescents with Newly Diagnosed Essential Hypertension. JAMA 2008;300:922-30.

91.   Ogino K, Kato M, Furuse Y, et al. Uric acid-lowering treatment with benzbromarone in patients with heart failure: a double-blind placebo-controlled crossover preliminary study. Circ Heart Fail 2010;3:73-81.

92.   Bluestone R, Lewis B, Mervart I. Hyperlipoproteinaemia in gout. Annals of the rheumatic diseases 1971;30:134-7.

93.   Anderson BE, Adams DR. Allopurinol hypersensitivity syndrome. J Drugs Dermatol 2002;1:60-2.

94.   Jung J-W, Kim Y-S, Joo K-W, et al. HLA-B58 can help the clinical decision on starting allopurinol in patients with chronic renal insufficiency. Nephrol Dial Transplant 2011; in press.

95.   Fam AG. Gout, diet, and the insulin resistance syndrome. The Journal of rheumatology 2002;29:1350-5.

96.   Dessein PH, Shipton EA, Stanwix AE, Joffe BI, Ramokgadi J. Beneficial effects of weight loss associated with moderate calorie/carbohydrate restriction, and increased proportional intake of protein and unsaturated fat on serum urate and lipoprotein levels in gout: a pilot study. Annals of the rheumatic diseases 2000;59:539-43.

97.   Dai DF, Chen T, Szeto H, et al. Mitochondrial Targeted Antioxidant Peptide Ameliorates Hypertensive Cardiomyopathy. Journal of the American College of Cardiology 2011.

98.   Dikalova AE, Bikineyeva AT, Budzyn K, et al. Therapeutic targeting of mitochondrial superoxide in hypertension. Circulation research 2010;107:106-16.

99.   Massey LK, Liebman M, Kynast-Gales SA. Ascorbate increases human oxaluria and kidney stone risk. The Journal of nutrition 2005;135:1673-7.

100.   Souza GA, Ebaid GX, Seiva FR, et al. N-Acetylcysteine an Allium plant compound improves high-sucrose diet-induced obesity and related effects. Evid Based Complement Alternat Med 2008.

101.   Sumithran P, Prendergast LA, Delbridge E, et al. Long-term persistence of hormonal adaptations to weight loss. The New England journal of medicine 2011;365:1597-604.

102.   Kean BH. Blood pressure studies on West Indians and Panamanians living on the isthmus of Panama. Arch Int Med 1941;68:466-75.

103.   Kean BH. The blood pressure of the Cuna Indians. Am J Trop Med Hyg 1944;24:341-3.

104.   Hollenberg NK, Martinez G, McCullough M, et al. Aging, acculturation, salt intake, and hypertension in the Kuna of Panama. Hypertension 1997;29:171-6.

105.   Hollenberg NK. Vascular action of cocoa flavanols in humans: the roots of the story. Journal of cardiovascular pharmacology 2006;47 Suppl 2:S99-102; discussion S19-21.

106.   Bayard V, Chamorro F, Motta J, Hollenberg NK. Does flavanol intake influence mortality from nitric oxide-dependent processes? Ischemic heart disease, stroke, diabetes mellitus, and cancer in Panama. International journal of medical sciences 2007;4:53-8.

107.   McCullough ML, Chevaux K, Jackson L, et al. Hypertension, the Kuna, and the epidemiology of flavanols. Journal of cardiovascular pharmacology 2006;47 Suppl 2:S103-9; discussion 19-21.

108.   Hurst WJ, Tarka SM, Jr., Powis TG, Valdez F, Jr., Hester TR. Cacao usage by the earliest Maya civilization. Nature 2002;418:289-90.

109.   Dillinger TL, Barriga P, Escarcega S, Jimenez M, Salazar Lowe D, Grivetti LE. Food of the gods: cure for humanity? A cultural history of the medicinal and ritual use of chocolate. The Journal of nutrition 2000;130:2057S-72S.

110.   Corti R, Flammer AJ, Hollenberg NK, Luscher TF. Cocoa and cardiovascular health. Circulation 2009;119:1433-41.

111.   Grassi D, Necozione S, Lippi C, et al. Cocoa reduces blood pressure and insulin resistance and improves endothelium-dependent vasodilation in hypertensives. Hypertension 2005;46:398-405.

112.   Nogueira L, Ramirez-Sanchez I, Perkins GA, et al. (-)-Epicatechin enhances fatigue resistance and oxidative capacity in mouse muscle. The Journal of physiology 2011;589:4615-31.

113.   D'Antona G, Ragni M, Cardile A, et al. Branched-chain amino acid supplementation promotes survival and supports cardiac and skeletal muscle mitochondrial biogenesis in middle-aged mice. Cell metabolism 2010;12:362-72.

114.   Macotela Y, Emanuelli B, Bang AM, et al. Dietary leucine--an environmental modifier of insulin resistance acting on multiple levels of metabolism. PLoS ONE 2011;6:e21187.

SECTION 7

1.   Keys AB, Keys M. How to eat well and stay well the Mediterranean way. 1st ed. Garden City, NY: Doubleday; 1975 page 58.

2.   Hujoel P. Dietary carbohydrates and dental-systemic diseases. J Dent Res 2009;88:490-502.

3.   Culleton BF, Larson MG, Kannel WB, Levy D. Serum uric acid and risk for cardiovascular disease and death: the Framingham Heart Study. Annals of internal medicine 1999;131:7-13.

4.   Feig DI, Kang DH, Johnson RJ. Uric acid and cardiovascular risk. The New England journal of medicine 2008;359:1811-21.

5.   Feig DI, Soletsky B, Johnson RJ. Effect of Allopurinol on the Blood Pressure of Adolescents with Newly Diagnosed Essential Hypertension. JAMA 2008;300:922-30.

6.   Livesey G. Fructose ingestion: dose-dependent responses in health research. The Journal of nutrition 2009;139:1246S-52S.

7.   White JS. Fructose as cause of metabolic syndrome is poorly supported. Int J Obes (Lond) 2010.

8.   Lanaspa M, Tapia E, Soto V, Sautin Y, Sanchez-Lozada LG. Uric acid and Fructose: Potential Biological Mechanisms. Sem Nephrol 2011; 31:426-32.

9.   Blakely SR, Hallfrisch J, Reiser S, Prather ES. Long-term effects of moderate fructose feeding on glucose tolerance parameters in rats. The Journal of nutrition 1981;111:307-14.

10.   Perez-Pozo SE, Schold J, Nakagawa T, Sanchez-Lozada LG, Johnson RJ, Lillo JL. Excessive fructose intake induces the features of metabolic syndrome in healthy adult men: role of uric acid in the hypertensive response. Int J Obes (Lond) 2010;34:454-61.

11.   Dehghan A, Kottgen A, Yang Q, et al. Association of three genetic loci with uric acid concentration and risk of gout: a genome-wide association study. Lancet 2008;372:1953-61.

12.   Yang Q, Kottgen A, Dehghan A, et al. Multiple genetic loci influence serum urate levels and their relationship with gout and cardiovascular disease risk factors. Circ Cardiovasc Genet 2010;3:523-30.

13.   Bibert S, Hess SK, Firsov D, et al. Mouse GLUT9: evidences for a urate uniporter. American journal of physiology 2009;297:F612-9.

14.   Anzai N, Ichida K, Jutabha P, et al. Plasma urate level is directly regulated by a voltage-driven urate efflux transporter URATv1 (SLC2A9) in humans. J Biol Chem 2008;283:26834-8.

15.   George J, Carr E, Davies J, Belch JJ, Struthers A. High-dose allopurinol improves endothelial function by profoundly reducing vascular oxidative stress and not by lowering uric acid. Circulation 2006;114:2508-16.

16.   Forshee RA, Storey ML, Allison DB, et al. A critical examination of the evidence relating high fructose corn syrup and weight gain. Crit Rev Food Sci Nutr 2007;47:561-82.

17.   White JS. Straight talk about high-fructose corn syrup: what it is and what it ain't. The American journal of clinical nutrition 2008;88:1716S-21S.

18.   Sievenpiper JL, de Souza RJ, Mirrahimi A, et al. Effect of Fructose on Body Weight in Controlled Feeding Trials. A Systematic Review and Meta-analysis Ann Intern Med 2012; 156:291-304

19.   Sievenpiper JL, de Souza RJ, Kendall CW, Jenkins DJ. Is fructose a story of mice but not men? Journal of the American Dietetic Association 2011;111:219-20; author reply 20-2.

20.   Shapiro A, Mu W, Roncal C, Cheng KY, Johnson RJ, Scarpace PJ. Fructose-induced leptin resistance exacerbates weight gain in response to subsequent high-fat feeding. American journal of physiology 2008;295:R1370-5.

21. Nakagawa T, Hu H, Zharikov S, et al. A causal role for uric acid in fructose-induced metabolic syndrome. American journal of physiology 2006;290:F625-31.

22. Le MT, Frye RF, Rivard C, et al. Effects of high fructose corn syrup and sucrose on the pharmacokinetics of fructose and acute metabolic and hemodynamic responses in healthy subjects. Metabolism: clinical and experimental 2012; 61:641-651.

23. Brown CM, Dulloo AG, Yepuri G, Montani JP. Fructose ingestion acutely elevates blood pressure in healthy young humans. American journal of physiology 2008;294:R730-7.

24. Emmerson BT. Effect of oral fructose on urate production. Annals of the rheumatic diseases 1974;33:276-80.

25. Watanabe S, Kang DH, Feng L, et al. Uric acid, hominoid evolution, and the pathogenesis of salt-sensitivity. Hypertension 2002;40:355-60.

26. Johnson RJ, Herrera-Acosta J, Schreiner GF, Rodriguez-Iturbe B. Subtle acquired renal injury as a mechanism of salt-sensitive hypertension. The New England journal of medicine 2002;346:913-23.

27. Hallfrisch J, Ellwood K, Michaelis OEt, Reiser S, Prather ES. Plasma fructose, uric acid, and inorganic phosphorus responses of hyperinsulinemic men fed fructose. J Am Coll Nutr 1986;5:61-8.

28. Hallfrisch J, Ellwood KC, Michaelis OEt, Reiser S, O'Dorisio TM, Prather ES. Effects of dietary fructose on plasma glucose and hormone responses in normal and hyperinsulinemic men. The Journal of nutrition 1983;113:1819-26.

29. Hallfrisch J, Reiser S, Prather ES. Blood lipid distribution of hyperinsulinemic men consuming three levels of fructose. The American journal of clinical nutrition 1983;37:740-8.

30. Hay J. The significance of a raised blood pressure. Br Med J 1931;2:43-7.

31. Peters JP, VanSlyke DD. Quantitative Clinical Chemistry. Baltimore: Williams and Wilkins; 1948.

32. Painter TS. The Y-chromosome in mammals. Science (New York, NY 1921;53:503-4.

33. Gartler SM. The chromosome number in humans: a brief history. Nature genetics 2006;7:655-60.

34. Tijo JH, Levan A. The chromosome number of man. Hereditas 1956;42:1-6.

35. Levan A. Chromosome studies on some human tumors and tissues of normal origin, grown in vivo and in vitro at the Sloan–Kettering Institute. Cancer 1956;9:648-63.

36. Kuhn TS. The Structure of Scientific Revolutions. First edition ed. Chicago: University of Chicago Press; 1962.

37.   Darwin C. On The Origin of Species by Means of Natural Selection, or The Preservation of Favoured Races in the Struggle for Life. First edition ed. London: John Murray; 1859.

38.   Raup DM, Sepkoski JJ, Jr. Mass extinctions in the marine fossil record. Science (New York, NY 1982;215:1501-3.

39.   Begun DR. Planet of the apes. Sci Am 2003;289:74-83.

40.   Eldredge N, Gould SJ. Punctuated equilibriua: an alternative to phyletic gradualism. In: Schopf TJM, ed. Models in Paleobiology. San Francisco: Cooper and Co.; 1972:82-115.

41.   Roach JC, Glusman G, Smit AF, et al. Analysis of genetic inheritance in a family quartet by whole-genome sequencing. Science (New York, NY 2010;328:636-9.

42.   Xue Y, Wang Q, Long Q, et al. Human Y chromosome base-substitution mutation rate measured by direct sequencing in a deep-rooting pedigree. Curr Biol 2009;19:1453-7.

43.   Nachman MW, Crowell SL. Estimate of the mutation rate per nucleotide in humans. Genetics 2000;156:297-304.

44.   Heerwagen MJ, Miller MR, Barbour LA, Friedman JE. Maternal Obesity and Fetal Metabolic Programming: A Fertile Epigenetic Soil. American journal of physiology 2010.

45.   Barker DJ, Osmond C, Golding J, Kuh D, Wadsworth ME. Growth in utero, blood pressure in childhood and adult life, and mortality from cardiovascular disease. BMJ (Clinical research ed 1989;298:564-7.

46.   Breier BH, Vickers MH, Ikenasio BA, Chan KY, Wong WP. Fetal programming of appetite and obesity. Mol Cell Endocrinol 2001;185:73-9.

47.   Ravelli AC, van Der Meulen JH, Osmond C, Barker DJ, Bleker OP. Obesity at the age of 50 y in men and women exposed to famine prenatally. The American journal of clinical nutrition 1999;70:811-6.

48.   Giles RE, Blanc H, Cann HM, Wallace DC. Maternal inheritance of human mitochondrial DNA. Proceedings of the National Academy of Sciences of the United States of America 1980;77:6715-9.

49.   Eiberg H, Troelsen J, Nielsen M, et al. Blue eye color in humans may be caused by a perfectly associated founder mutation in a regulatory element located within the HERC2 gene inhibiting OCA2 expression. Hum Genet 2008;123:177-87.

50.   Stringer CB, Andrews P. Genetic and fossil evidence for the origin of modern humans. Science (New York, NY 1988;239:1263-8.

51.   Cann RL, Stoneking M, Wilson AC. Mitochondrial DNA and human evolution. Nature 1987;325:31-6.

52.   McDougall I, Brown FH, Fleagle JG. Stratigraphic placement and age of modern humans from Kibish, Ethiopia. Nature 2005;433:733-6.

53.   Scholz CA, Johnson TC, Cohen AS, et al. East African megadroughts between 135 and 75 thousand years ago and bearing on early-modern human origins. Proceedings of the National Academy of Sciences of the United States of America 2007;104:16416-21.

54.   Cohen AS, Stone JR, Beuning KR, et al. Ecological consequences of early Late Pleistocene megadroughts in tropical Africa. Proceedings of the National Academy of Sciences of the United States of America 2007;104:16422-7.

55.   Williams MAJ, Ambrose S, van Der Kaars S, et al. Environmental impact of the 73 ka Toba super-eruption in South Asia. Palaeogeog Palaeoclimat Palaeoecol 2009;284:295-314.

56.   Ambrose SH. Late Pleistocene human population bottlenecks, volcanic winter, and differentiation of modern humans. Journal of human evolution 1998;34:623-51.

57.   Laval G, Patin E, Barreiro LB, Quintana-Murci L. Formulating a historical and demographic model of recent human evolution based on resequencing data from noncoding regions. PLoS ONE 2010;5:e10284.

58.   Bailey GN, Reynolds SC, King GC. Landscapes of human evolution: models and methods of tectonic geomorphology and the reconstruction of hominin landscapes. Journal of human evolution 2010.

ACKNOWLEDGMENTS

The approach I used in this book reflects a "planetary biology" approach to obesity, a concept developed by Dr. Steven Benner that involves a multidisciplinary approach to solving disease, including the use of biology, chemistry, evolutionary science, and history and as such I dedicate this book to Dr. Benner. I also thank the many collaborators and friends that formed the scientific basis for this book, especially Miguel A. Lanaspa-Garcia and Laura Gabriela Sánchez-Lozada, both who had instrumental roles in identifying the central mechanisms involved in triggering the fat switch in the mitochondria. I especially thank those whose work and ideas opened new doors that effectively altered the course of science upon which I was headed, especially Bernardo Rodriguez-Iturbe and the late Jaime Herrera-Acosta, George Schreiner, and Marilda Mazzali, Duk-Hee Kang, John Kanellis, Takahiko Nakagawa, Yuri Sautin, Takuji Ishimoto, and Daniel Feig. I also thank other scientists and physicians who worked in my laboratory and whose work was critical to the concepts presented in this book, including Katherine Gordon, Wei Mu, Carlos Roncal, Christopher Rivard, Olena Glushakova, David Long, Karen Price, Sirirat Reungjui, Marcelo Heinig, Pietro Cirillo, Wei Chen, Myphuong Le, Waichi Sato, Michael and Chris Gersch, Takahiro Nakayama, Tomoki Kosugi, and Uday Khosla. I also thank my collaborators Jim Hill, Magdalena Madero, Enrique Perez-Pozo, Julian Lopez Lillo, Jacek Manitius, Manal Abdelmalak, Anna Mae Diehl, Mehmet Kanbay, Reem Asad, Ebaa Ku, Philip Scarpace, George Henderson, Alexander Angerhofer, Witcha Imaram, Paul MaClean, Holly Wyatt, Martha Franco, Diana Jalal, Hui Yao Lan, Xueqing Yu, Jillian Sullivan, Shikha Sundaram, Elaine Epperson, Sandy Martin, Michel Chonchol, Bruce Rideout, the late Bill Oliver, Salah Kivlighn, Titte R Srinivas, Mark Segal, Eric Gaucher, Stephen Dreskin, Tanja Hess, Steven Benner, Eric Gaucher, Peter Andrews, Nancy Zahniser and Nicole Avena. Thanks to John Lewis, Elaine Armantrout, Joe Doolin, Francisco Tejeda and Bernardo Rodriguez-Iturbe for providing excellent critiques of the manuscript. Special thanks to Fred Lisaius and Nick Jurich for artwork in the book, and to Nathan Greenlee for setting up the websites (http:/fatswitchbook.com/ and http://fructosedoctor.com/). To my mentors, Bill Couser and Seymour Klebanoff, who got me excited about science, to Stewart Cameron whose early work on uric acid was an inspiration, to Timothy Van Dyke, Rick Silva, Laura Simon and Paul Tabor who helped guide me through the roads of inventorship, to Dr. Mercola for inviting me to publish my book via his website, and to my wife Olga and my children, Tracy and Ricky, I also provide thanks.

INDEX

Notes

Notes

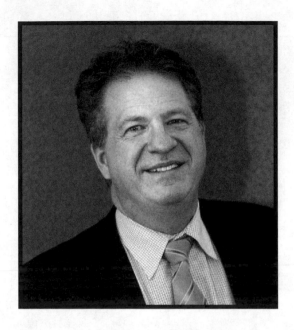

Richard J. Johnson, M.D., has been a practicing physician and clinical scientist for over 25 years. His research has been funded by the National Institute of Health since the late 1980s. He is a member of the American Society for Clinical Investigation and has published over 500 papers and lectured in over 40 countries. He has a special interest in the role of fructose in obesity and authored *The Sugar Fix* with Timothy Gower in 2008 (Rodale). He is currently a Professor of Medicine at the University of Colorado in Denver. He lives in Aurora, Colorado with his wife, Olga, and children, Ricky and Tracy.